INTEGRATED DIAGNOSTIC IMAGING
Digital PACS in Medicine

To Andrée, Tom and Charlotte

INTEGRATED DIAGNOSTIC IMAGING

Digital PACS in Medicine

Editor

J.P.J. de Valk

ELSEVIER
AMSTERDAM · LONDON · NEW YORK · TOKYO 1992

ELSEVIER SCIENCE PUBLISHERS B.V.
P.O. Box 211
1000 AE Amsterdam
The Netherlands

Library of Congress Cataloging in Publication Data

```
Integrated diagnostic imaging : digital PACS in medicine / editor,
  J.P.J. de Valk.
      p.   cm.
    Includes bibliographical references and index.
    ISBN (invalid) 0-444-81426-2 (alk. paper)
    1. Picrutc archiving and communication systems in medicine.
  I. Valk, Johannes Petrus Joseph de, 1954-   .
    [DNLM: 1. Diagnostic Imaging.  2. Image Processing, Computer
  -Assisted.  3. Radiology Information Systems.   WN 200 I5851]
  R857.P52I58   1992
  616.07'54--dc20
  DNLM/DLC
  for Library of Congress                                    92-49513
                                                                CIP
```

ISBN 0-444-81426-4

Printed on acid-free paper

Printed in the Netherlands

Preface

Much work, although often fragmentary, has been published by professionals, with sometimes very different backgrounds, on PACS (picture archiving and communication system) related issues up till today. The aim of this book is to provide in particular medical professionals, having a clear technical interest in medical imaging for daily use in a hospital environment, with a state of the art overview. This includes case studies done so far all around the world. The combination of both the historical perspective and the opinions as described by the authors of the individual chapters provides the reader with a realistic view on PACS in many aspects.

The collection of the individual chapters of this book took about two years, including sometimes major revisions (many things change in two years!). The selection of the invited authors has been based on various criteria. They are involved in a clinical environment and renowned in the professional PACS world, particularly in the world region where they are located. The majority of the invited 28 potential authors, selected accordingly, reacted positively, resulting in the final 19 chapters presented here.

The purpose was to produce a book by professionals in the medical environment for medical professionals. As can be seen in the list of contributors, all of them are based in a medical environment, with many of them having PACS project experience. Nearly half of the first authors have an MD degree, including radiologists.

All authors were asked to write a chapter according to the same guidelines, without interaction, to maximize independency of one another. This approach has resulted in a clear display of each individual perception and historical interpretation of the past, present, and future status of systems worldwide, without too much disturbing overlap. Where applicable, the authors have described their own practical case experience. Most of these case studies are very specialized into one subtopic of the medical imaging area, which altogether gives good insight into the complexity and problems of the total field, indicating practical guidelines at the same time.

The resulting book gives an outline of the history, status and future of (digital) medical image handling in the hospital environment during the final two decades of this century, as perceived and experienced by the professionals working in this field of medicine.

It is interesting to see how differently a period of 20 years can be assessed from the perspectives of professionals in the medical and technological science.

Although two decades seem very short from a common human perspective, it is rather long from the point of view of modern (medical) technology.

Just consider that the introduction of computerized medical equipment such as the CT-scanner has taken less than 10 years before it became generally accepted and affordable. Product cycles of personal computer types are sometimes even quoted less than three months currently!

From the early eighties several 'acronyms' have made their way into the professional world of medical image handling, focusing on storage and communication primarily.

Without doubt the first, and mostly used and acknowledged one, is 'PACS', also used in the previous part of this introduction. Most readers will know the word and what it stands for already. This acronym expresses pretty well the main need that professionals had and still have regarding their medical images. Above all, image archiving and communication has to be addressed properly before any sophisticated image processing can even start, let alone be an integrated and successful part of medical routine.

The second acronym that has much been heard starting from the middle of the eighties is 'IMAC(S)' (image management and communication (system)). The main reason to coin a second acronym, although maybe a bit confusing, was probably to put more emphasis on the need for a true and reliable management of the tremendous amount of digital image data that has to be handled in a hospital environment. It has become obvious that apart from technological issues, which can be handled better if time passes on, organizational issues will have to be addressed first.

The third, and last acronym in this summary, should be 'IDS' (integrated diagnostic system). This expression stresses the importance of the end-user aspects of the system looked at. After al, the medical profession is only interested in the use of any system to reach the true goal of medical imaging, being the support of diagnosis, needed for patient care. Integration with all other patient data is crucial to reach this goal, and of course, the resulting system should be user-transparant. The definition of IDS encompasses more than PACS or even IMAC(S); it includes all management and integration aspects and is exactly tailored according to the clinical end-user's needs, instead of a mere engineer's dream or an interesting scientific experiment.

There is no intent whatsoever in this introduction or book to make a choice between launched acronyms or professional opinions. Actually, over time, it has been clearly shown that there are a couple of project approaches to realize a system in practice, although actually total hospital systems are still not in full clinical operation (early 1992). An early categorization and overview of these approaches can be found in the article by de Valk et al. (1987), and the several approaches are illustrated by the separate practical pilots as described in most of the chapters of this book. The main difference is between bottom-up, more departmentally oriented smaller systems and top-down, more integrated, larger and sometimes even hospital-wide systems. The possibility of integration with other (existing) departmental or hospital information systems is one of the key features of any system: leading to the so-called 'open systems approach', which is nowadays widely advocated.

As indicated above, the acronym PACS is still the best known and accepted one in the professional world, and is therefore maintained throughout the book (also in this introduction in many cases where IMAC(S) or, even more appropriate, IDS could have been used).

There has been no intention, however, to write (another) handbook or report on PACS in a systematic way. The preservation of the individual opinions and perspectives of the many professionals contributing is considered to be the major strength of this book.

Since 1980 many conferences and events have been partially or fully dedicated to PACS. A few examples to be mentioned here are the SPIE PACS/Medical Imaging Conferences in the U.S.A., the IMAC conferences that were held in the U.S.A. and Japan, and several mainly radiology-oriented conferences, of which the annual RSNA in Chicago is the most famous and renowned one. Several groups with a noticeable record in PACS have been organising workshops and demonstrations, and especially for Europe the EuroPACS organisation (Bakker and de Valk, 1988), which was founded in 1984 during the first NATO Advanced Study Institute focusing on medical imaging, has acted as an − even more or less worldwide − umbrella for such events. The EuroPACS Newsletter has been a successful communication vehicle from the early beginning, also functioning as a historical logbook.

The three parts of the world that have been most active in the PACS field are the U.S.A., Western Europe and Japan. This is clearly reflected in the contributions to this book. For an assessment of the PACS developments status in the past, as started early in the U.S.A. and Japan, see de Valk et al. (1987, 1988).

It is interesting to compare the viewpoints from the different parts of the world on the developments thusfar worldwide, which was amongst the tasks that some authors tried to accomplish in their chapter. In the U.S.A., the whole PACS area has been strongly influenced by academia, whereas in Japan the degree of involvement of the industry has been much higher from the beginning. In Europe there is some kind of mixture of these two driving forces, which has also been expressed during the past EuroPACS events.

Although there are still no really hospital-wide functioning integrated PAC systems for diagnostic imaging, it seemed best to select authors based on their experience within hospitals with the set-up of PACS projecs that are (still) going on currently, as described in this book.

There are many different opinions on the legal aspects and the cost – benefit analysis of PACS. One should realise that there is a clear difference between show-projects (also called 'pilot projects', which often originate from prestige objectives) and future systems with a positive cost – benefit analysis that everybody would like to have here and now. But since nobody can wait forever, many small bottom-up systems are currently implemented which are used for aims that could not be reached before, such as the fast communication of digital images between a central imaging department (radiology) and, e.g., intensive care units.

Predictions on costs – benefits of non-existing systems are prone to irrealistic guesses, which cannot be verified. Only a thorough evaluation of current system implementations with the full involvement of all contributing parties can lead to reliable results, and then only if all these parties are willing to be fully exposed and provide the true data on the trials. One should realise that some of these data tend to be very sensitive and hence highly confidential, however, and therefore not openly communicated by the industry.

Talking about involvement of parties, it is appropriate to stress the importance of standardization in the field of digital medical imaging. The ongoing work of the American College of Radiology with the National Electrical Manufacturers Association in the ACR/NEMA Committee on Digital Communication (DICOM) of medical images has to be mentioned here before all other activities. Recently worldwide standardisation efforts have been started, but is is clear that until now the ACR/NEMA work is still the standard reference point and as such has been acknowledged by all (potential) PACS end-users all over the world.

Integration has been one of the keywords in PACS for many years now. This can be related to integration of patient data, but also to the integration of hospital departments and their functions and existing systems, even if non-digital (yet). Clearly the organisational consequences of a PACS implementation have been underestimated in the past. It is obvious that technology alone, although becoming more suitable and affordable, is not the critical issue (any more).

On one hand the chapters of this book can be perfectly read on a stand-alone basis, on the other hand, the interested and active reader can make comparisons between them and draw his own conclusions from the noticed similarities and dissimilarities. It has been tried to guarantee a maximum level of objectivity by inviting authors that have no clear relationship to hardware or software industry or similar organisations. Most authors have provided some graphical information, sometimes pictures showing their local case status, which can give an impression of reality. As stated before, the set-up of this book is meant to be unique if compared with the existing work in the field, and can be seen as complementary to that. The listed references at the ends of the individual chapters give a good stronghold to a comprehensive bibliography of useful reading material.

Finally, on the sequence of the 19 chapters the following explication can be given. The U.S.A. chapters preceed the European chapters, followed by the Japanese chapters. The chapters within a particular region of the world are ordered alphabetically, first by country, next by author. There has been a tendency for authors with a more technical background to write more in a reviewing style, whereas the authors with a medical background have focused more on their case and specific medical issues within that case. It seemed appropriate to maintain that individual approach, as the goal was to create a comprehensive overview of the field rather than a structured and more rigid sort of handbook.

As always, the predictions of the future (let us say until 2000) are the most difficult to make, and all attempts by authors who exposed themselves by doing so should be highly appreciated. Let us wait and see how a book like this would look in the year 2000!

Woerden, July 1992   Jan Peter J. DE VALK

Bakker, A.R., and J.P.J. de Valk (1988) EuroPACS, a catalyst for PACS in Europe, *Med. Inform.* 13, 279 – 280.

de Valk, J.P.J., A.R. Bakker, K. Bijl, W. Heijser, D.E. Boekee and G.L. Reijns (1987) PACS reviewed: possible and coming soon? *J. Med. Imaging* 1, 77 – 84.

de Valk, J.P.J., A.R. Bakker, K. Bijl, B.M. ter Haar Romeny, F. Linnebank and G.L. Reijns (1988) Photograph avoiding complex systems: PACS in Japan, *J. Med. Imaging* 2, 50 – 55.

Contributors

M. AKISADA
Tama Health Management Center
Tachikawa-shi
Tokyo
Japan

W.H. ANDERSON
Department of Diagnostic
  Radiology
University of Kansas Medical
  Center
Kansas City, KS
U.S.A.

F.H. BARNEVELD
  BINKHUYSEN
Department of Radiology
Academic Medical Center
University of Amsterdam
Amsterdam
the Netherlands

G. BATTAGLIA
Department of Radiology
University of Brescia
Brescia
Italy

Y. BIZAIS
Imagerie Médicale Multimodalité
Faculté de Médecine de Nantes
Nantes
France

A. CHIESA
Department of Radiology
University of Brescia
Brescia
Italy

P. CHIRON
Imagerie Médicale Multimodalité
Faculté de Médecine de Nantes
Nantes
France

L. DALLA PALMA
Department of Radiology
University of Trieste
Trieste
Italy

J.P.J. DE VALK
De Vlist 2
Woerden
the Netherlands

S.J. DWYER III
Department of Radiological
  Sciences
UCLA School of Medicine
University of California
Los Angeles, CA
U.S.A.

D.A. ECKARD
Department of Diagnostic
  Radiology
University of Kansas Medical
  Center
Kansas City, KS
U.S.A.

G. FORBES
Department of Diagnostic
  Radiology
Mayo Clinic
Rochester, MN
U.S.A.

Y. GANDON
Départment d'Imagerie Médicale
Hôpital de Pontchaillou
Rennes
France

G. GELL
Institut für Medizinische
  Informatik, Statistik und
  Dokumentation
Universität Graz
Graz
Austria

B. GIBAUD
INSERM U335
Service de Neurochirurgie
Hôpital de Pontchaillou
Rennes
France

P. GIRIBONA
U.S.L. n. 1 Triestina - C.E.V.A.B.
Research Area of Trieste
Trieste
Italy

W. GUIJT
Department of Diagnostic
  Radiology
St. Radboud University Hospital
Nijmegen
the Netherlands

L.A. HARRISON
Department of Diagnostic
  Radiology
University of Kansas Medical
  Center
Kansas City, KS
U.S.A.

K.S. HENSLEY
Department of Diagnostic
  Radiology
University of Kansas Medical
  Center
Kansas City, KS
U.S.A.

J.C. HONEYMAN
Department of Radiology
University of Florida Medical
  Center
Gainesville, FL
U.S.A.

H.K. HUANG
Medical Imaging Division
Department of Radiological
  Sciences
UCLA School of Medicine
University of California
Los Angeles, CA
U.S.A.

I. KIMURA
Department of Radiology and
  Nuclear Medicine
Kyoto University Hospital
Sakyo-ku
Kyoto
Japan

M. KIMURA
Institute of Clinical Medicine
University of Tsukuba
Tsukuba-shi
Japan

Y. KITAZOE
Medical Information Center
Kochi Medical School
Okoh-cho
Nanko-ku
Kochi
Japan

M. KOMORI
Department of Biomedical
    Informatics
Kyoto University Hospital
Sakyo-ku
Kyoto
Japan

J. KONISHI
Department of Radiology and
    Nuclear Medicine
Kyoto University Hospital
Sakyo-ku
Kyoto
Japan

S. KUSANO
Department of Radiology
National Defense Medical College
Tokorozawa-shi
Saitama
Japan

T. MAEDA
Department of Radiology
Kochi Medical School
Okoh-cho Kohasu
Nanko-ku
Kochi
Japan

R. MAROLDI
Department of Radiology
University of Brescia
Brescia
Italy

R. MATTHEUS
Radiology Department
Free University Hospital (VUB)
Brussel
Belgium

M.A. McFADDEN
Department of Diagnostic
    Radiology
University of Kansas Medical
    Center
Kansas City, KS
U.S.A.

K. MINATO
Department of Biomedical
    Informatics
Kyoto University Hospital
Sakyo-ku
Kyoto
Japan

G.L. MOSCATELLI
Department of Radiology
University of Brescia
Brescia
Italy

S.K. MUN
Department of Radiology
Georgetown University Hospital
Washington, D.C.
U.S.A.

M.D. MURPHEY
Department of Diagnostic
  Radiology
University of Kansas Medical
  Center
Kansas City, KS
U.S.A.

Y. NAKANO
Department of Radiology and
  Nuclear Medicine
Kyoto University Hospital
Sakyo-ku
Kyoto
Japan

H. NISHIMOTO
Department of Radiology
Kochi Medical School
Okoh-cho
Nanko-ku
Kochi
Japan

M. NISHIOKA
Department of Radiology
Kochi Medical School
Okoh-cho
Nanko-ku
Kochi
Japan

S. OHARA
Department of Radiology
Kochi Medical School
Okoh-cho
Nanko-ku
Kochi
Japan

Y. OKADA
Department of Radiology
Kitasato University East Hospital
Sagamihara-shi
Kanagawa
Japan

K. OKAJIMA
Department of Radiology and
  Nuclear Medicine
Kyoto University Hospital
Sakyo-ku
Kyoto
Japan

P.E. PETERS
Institut für Klinische Radiologie
Universität Münster
Münster
Germany

O. RATIB
Digital Imaging Unit
University Hospital of Geneva
Geneva
Switzerland

A.H. ROWBERG
Center for Imaging Systems
  Optimization
Department of Radiology
University of Washington Medical
  Center
Seattle, WA
U.S.A.

S.H.J. RUIJS
Department of Diagnostic
  Radiology
St. Radboud University Hospital
Nijmegen
the Netherlands

Y. SAIDA
Institute of Clinical Medicine
University of Tsukuba
Tsukuba-shi
Japan

K. SATOH
Research and Development Center
Hitachi Medical Corporation
Kashiwa
Chiba
Japan

J.-M. SCARABIN
INSERM U335
Service de Neurochirurgie
Hôpital de Pontchaillou
Rennes
France

F. STACUL
Department of Radiology
University of Trieste
Trieste
Italy

B.K. STEWART
Department of Radiological
    Sciences
UCLA School of Medicine
Los Angeles, CA
U.S.A.

A.W. TEMPLETON
Department of Diagnostic
    Radiology
University of Kansas Medical
    Center
Kansas City, KS
U.S.A.

B.M. TER HAAR ROMENY
Department of Radiology
University Hospital of Utrecht
Computer Vision Research Group
Utrecht
the Netherlands

Y. TOHYAMA
Department of Radiology
Kochi Medical School
Okoh-cho
Nanko-ku
Kochi
Japan

W. UKOVICH
D.E.E.I.
University of Trieste
Trieste
Italy

L.J.Th.O. VAN ERNING
Department of Diagnostic
    Radiology
St. Radboud University Hospital
Nijmegen
the Netherlands

P. VASSALLO
Institute of Clinical Radiology
University of Münster
Münster
Germany

W. WIESMANN
Department of Radiological
    Diagnostic
St. Marien-Hospital
Ham
Germany

M. WILTGEN
Institut für Medizinische
  Informatik, Statistik und
  Dokumentation
Universität Graz
Graz
Austria

M. YACHIDA
Department of Radiology
Kochi Medical School
Okoh-cho
Nanko-ku
Kochi
Japan

G.L. ZICK
Center for Imaging Systems
  Optimization
Department of Electrical
  Engineering
University of Washington
Seattle, WA
U.S.A.

Contents

PACS in Japan

PACS in the U.S.A.

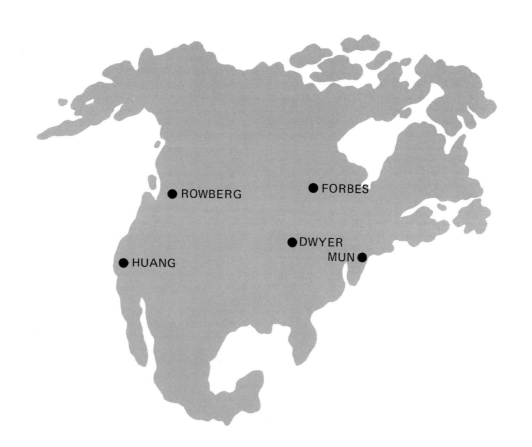

Integrated Diagnostic Imaging
Editor: J.P.J. De Valk
© *Elsevier Science Publishers B.V., 1992*

Chapter 1

Radiology image management networks

Samuel J. Dwyer III, Arch W. Templeton, Mark D. Murphey,
Linda A. Harrison, Donald A. Eckard, William H. Anderson,
Janice C. Honeyman, Brent K. Stewart, Kenneth S. Hensley
and Michael A. McFadden

1. Introduction

The goal of image management networks is to enhance patient care by improving communication between diagnostic radiologists and their referring physicians. Specific tasks are required of any image management network. The image data must be efficiently acquired from all interfaced imaging modalities. The data must be rapidly transmitted among the designated nodes on the network. Gray scale image workstations are used to display and manipulate the transmitted data. The acquired, transmitted, displayed and manipulated image data needs to be electronically archieved. Present or new radiology department's and hospital's information management systems should be connected with the network. Integrating all of these tasks has proven difficult.

Implementing and using an image management network has numerous potential advantages. Multiple sites throughout the department and hospital can share acquired image data. Geographically separated patient care areas and doctor's office areas can simultaneously retrieve, transmit, display, and manipulate patient image data. Multiple imaging examinations can be organized into an integrated consultation. Images and their consultation reports are rapidly shared with referring physician(s). These advantages were recognized in the early 1980s and have been the driving force for the extensive research and testing that have characterized a decade of image management networking projects (Duerinckx, 1982).

Radiology image management networks ideally perform multiple functions (Templeton et al., 1984, 1985, 1988; Cox et al., 1986, 1988; Huang, 1987) (fig. 1). Completed examinations are acquired from any imaging technology employing digital interfaces. The digital image data is formatted to the network protocol by the acquisition node. Each node on the network maintains an up-

RADIOLOGY IMAGE MANAGEMENT NETWORK

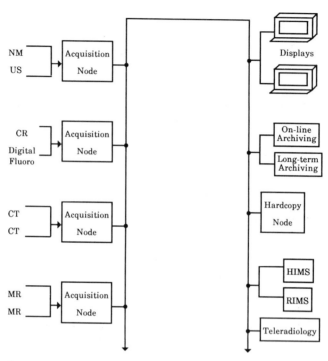

Fig. 1. A radiology image management network illustrating connection of the digital imaging modalities of nuclear medicine (NM), ultrasound (US), computed radiography (CR), digital fluorography (DF), computed tomography (CT), and magnetic resonance (MR). The image data is transmitted to the display workstations, on-line and long-term archiving and hard copy nodes. The hospital information management system (HIMS) and the radiology information management system (RIMS) are connected to the network. Teleradiology image data is also connected to the network.

dated database directory. A message is broadcast throughout the network stating that a new examination is available. This examination is transmitted to a designated interactive gray scale workstation. Examinations are reviewed at the display workstation and a consultation report is generated and entered into the patient's image file. While generated the consultation report, the radiologist selects images for the referring physician and identifies desired images for hard copy. Hard copy recordings are generated on the network hard copy nodes. All images or an appropriate subset of manipulated images are transmitted to the on-line archiving node. If there is no activity in a patient's file for 30 days, the image file is deleted from the on-line archiving node. This period of 30 days provides for the high demand, on-line access required for seriously ill patients in the hospital. Prior to its deletion, all stored image data is transmitted to the long-term archiving node at full contrast and spatial resolution. Image data is archived for five to seven years. This period of archiving is typical of that used in departmental libraries.

The difficulties in operating a radiology image management network are many and significant. Interfaces connecting imaging equipment to a network are still not commonly available. A huge amount of digital image data has to be acquired, transmitted, displayed and manipulated, and archived. Interactive display workstations are not totally acceptable to radiologists. The low brightness levels of gray scale monitors is one difficulty encountered in all diagnostic work. Another problem is the need for rapid display of multiple images on a single screen. Electronic archiving of terabytes of image data is still a significant technological challenge.

2. Acquiring imaging data

The successful acquisition of digital image data into a radiology image management network requires several steps. The completion of these steps involves a knowledge of all digital radiology technologies, the amount and format of image data being generated, and their interfaces. When the patient examination is completed, the image data is transferred into the acquisition node. Next, the formatted image is entered into the distributed database operational on the network. An updated patient image directory is broadcast periodically throughout the network. The acquired image data is transmitted to a designated gray scale display workstation and to an on-line archiving node.

2.1. Digital radiology systems

Digital image data equipment used extensively in all departments of radiology include nuclear medicine (NM), ultrasonography (US), computed tomography (CT), magnetic resonance (MR), and digitized fluorography (DF). In the average radiology department, 22 – 26% of the daily workload uses these imaging modalities (Oestmann et al., 1990). Screen – film imaging examinations still account for about 75% of a department's workload. Digital radiology systems are replacing conventional screen – film examinations. Computed radiography (CR) phosphor plate systems are capable of performing chest examinations, an examination which accounts for one-third of all examinations performed. The declining costs and increasing capabilities of digital hardware insures that digital radiology systems will be phased into departments, hospitals, and clinics. Digital radiography and fluorography systems provide a strong emphasis for the implementation of image management networks.

One of the first digital systems was a digital scan projection radiography chest imaging system, (Barnes et al., 1985). Collimated X-rays passing through the patient were detected by an electronic detector array. Scatter radiation was reduced by the use of moving slits. The image matrix was 1024 × 1024 × 8 bits, with a pixel size of 0.5 mm. Resolution was measured at 1 cycle/mm with a scan time of 4.9 s and a skin exposure of 25 mR.

Scanning equalization radiography (SER) was developed to accommodate the large contrast ranges contained in a chest examination (Wandtke and Plewes, 1989). The X-ray source is pulsed by a modified grid pulse system. X-rays passing through the patient are detected by a screen and a photomultiplier tube. The signal from the detector determines the appropriate length of time for each X-ray exposure, and thus provides an adaptive contrast control for specific regions of the chest. The X-ray beam scans across the patient in five seconds.

A digitized fluorography system (fig. 2) uses an image intensifier, a 1023 line television chain, and a video digitizer that produces a 1 K × 1 K × 8 bit digital array (Cox et al., 1990). Field sizes include 34, 40, and 47 cm. Spatial resolution is 1.8 cycles/mm with a pixel size of 0.4 mm. Frame rates vary from 1 to 15 images/s. Skin exposure is 20 mR for a chest examination using the 47 cm field of view. These 1 K × 1 K × 8 bit images have proven very adequate for a number of examinations.

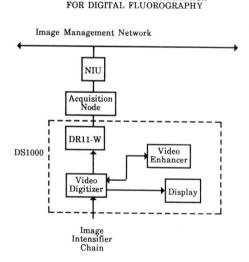

Fig. 2. A digital interface for a digital fluorography system.

Computed radiology (CR) systems provide diagnostic results equivalent to screen – film examinations (Sonoda et al., 1983). These systems are based upon scanning laser-stimulated luminescence. A storage phosphor plate consisting of europium-activated barium fluorohalide receptors replaces the screen – film in conventional cassettes. The latent image is read out by a laser beam scanner. The resultant digital image is enhanced and printed by a laser film recorder and/or displayed on a gray scale workstation. The resultant digital image is 2 K × 2 K × 10 bits with a pixel size of 0.2 mm/pixel. The storage phosphor plate is reusable. Exposure techniques are the same or less than those used for screen – film examinations. Patients radiation exposure is reduced.

Laser film digitizers are employed to convert analog radiographic films into digital arrays of 2 K × 2 K × 12 bits or 4 K × 4 K × 12 bits. These digitizers linearly map the optical densities of the radiographic film into pixels with 12 bit digital numbers.

2.2. Interfaces and amounts of image data generated

Each digital imaging modality requires a method for accessing and transferring the image data into the acquisition node. The electronic devices for accomplishing this function are called interfaces. The hardware and software for these digital interfaces remains limited. The amount of digital image data generated by most imaging modalities is large requiring interface throughput rates of up to 8 Mbytes/s. The current ACR-NEMA interface standard calls for a 50 pin

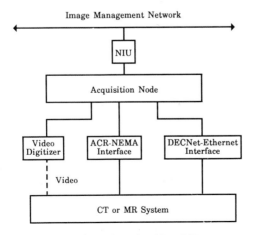

Fig. 3. Three interfaces for CT or MR systems.

Table 1
The amount of digital data generated by KU Department.

Examination	Patients per day	Images per patient	Mbytes per day
Body CT	21	20 – 40	441
Head CT	16	16 – 20	168
NM, static	26	4 – 8	14
NM, dynamic	9	15	2.3
Ultrasound	34	30 – 42	376
DSA	8	12 – 16	67
CR	14	4	59
MR head	6	50	40
MR body	5	70	46

Total generated per day: 1.2 Gbytes.

connector and data transfer rates of 8 Mbytes/s. The ACR-NEMA standard was developed by a joint committee of the American College of Radiology (ACR) and the National Electronics Manufacturers Association (NEMA). An improved ACR-NEMA interface standard is in the process of being voted upon. A variety of digital interfaces have been tried. Figure 3 illustrates an implemented digital interface for a digital fluorography system. This interface is a direct memory access unit (DR11-W) developed by Digital Equipment Corporation. Figure 3 illustrates several other interfaces that have been used with CT and MR systems. Interfaces for computed radiography systems are specifically designed for the manufacturers equipment and are not available.

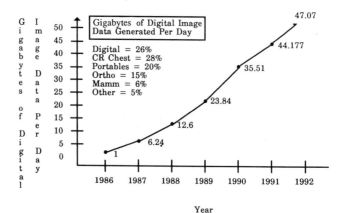

Fig. 4. An estimate of the number of Gbytes of digital image data generated per day. The 1.21 Gbytes estimated in table 1 is for the period 1986 – 1987.

The amount of digital image data now generated by our department is large and rapidly growing. Table 1 is a conservative estimate of 1 Gbyte each working day. Figure 4 is an estimate of the growth of digital imaging data in our department.

2.3. Problems of the acquisition nodes

Patient examinations and the resultant image data generation occur in peaks. No method exists yet for designing intelligent interfaces which could sample the stream of generated image data and automatically establish a protocol for transmitting the data into the acquisition node. Acquisition nodes require digital interfaces to each imaging modality connected to the image management network. The hardware and software required are usually not available. Additionally, most imaging equipment uses medium performance computers so as to reduce costs. Thus, certain interfaces will actually lower the performance of the imaging system.

3. Networks

The network portion of a digital image management system distributes the image data. Computer resources are shared via the network. User interface to the network provides for access to the image data. There are two types of networks, local-area networks (LAN) and wide-area networks (WAN).

3.1. Local-area networks

A local-area network (LAN) is a technology which allows privately owned computers and computer-related devices to communicate with each other. The maximum length of LANs is no more than several kilometers and serves a limited geographic area, at maximum a metropolitan area. They can interconnect large computers with high-speed computer peripherals. They can also connect minicomputers, microcomputers, terminals, workstations and business equipment in the same office building or between buildings. Since LANs are independent, stand-alone networks with short cable lengths high transmission rates are thus possible. They are not constrained to follow public communication protocols. The declining costs of microcomputer systems, computer devices, and LANs offer radiology departments a cost-effective method for managing image data and patient consultations.

The transmission media selected for a LAN depends upon signaling rates. Twisted-pair cables can signal between 1 and 10 Mbits/s. Coaxial cables can signal between 10 and 50 Mbits/s while fiber optic cables can signal at

10 Mbits/s to 4 Gbits/s. Throughput rates are generally one-fifth to one-eighth
the signaling rates, due to the large system overheads.

An important consideration of a LAN is its topology. Topology refers to the
specific arrangement of computers and computer-devices and the interconnections between them. A star topology contains a centralized hub through which
all data passes. They are easy to implement, the links are independent of each
other and the cost is reasonable. However, star topology is vulnerable to hub
failure. A bus topology uses a single communication circuit which is shared by
every node (multiple access) and connected by network interface units (NIUs).
It is easy to attach new devices to the bus. Data throughput is good. However,
messages can interfere with each other and the most active nodes tend to 'hog'
the bus. A tree topology is a series of buses connected together by a high-speed
backbone. This type of topology provides for variable signaling rates depending
upon user demand.

A ring topology has all nodes connected together in a ring configuration.
Each node is connected to two other nodes by repeaters. Rings provide high
transmission rates. Transmission capacity is shared fairly. Implementation is
low in cost. However, cable installation is difficult. Monitoring devices are
needed to remove stray packets of data.

LANs use baseband signaling. With baseband signaling, the signal is not
modulated – demodulated, thereby providing for high-speed transmission. The
digital data is encoded into electrical signals using a self-clocking Manchester
code. Two common methods of accessing the network are the broadcast-bus access method and the ring access method. In the broadcast-bus access method

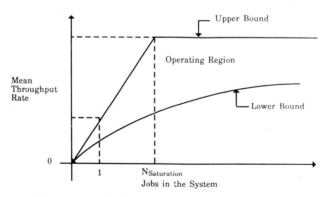

Fig. 5. The upper and lower bounds for the mean througput as a function of the number of jobs in
a system being processed. The upper bound is a linear function until a bottleneck is encountered.
The lower bound is an inverse function of the number of jobs in a system.

a message is transmitted into the system which is heard by everyone on the bus (multiple access). Once the transmission ceases, the signal rapidly dies away. The user transmits whenever desirable listening to all transmitted messages (carrier sensing). If no carrier is on the network, a node will transmit. If a collision is heard (collision detection), then all transmitting nodes cease and try again after a given time interval (CSMA/CD).

In the ring access method data is passed around the ring from one access point to another by repeaters. When a station receives a packet of data it can exercise one or more of the following options: read it, remove it, retransmit it, alter it, or add a new packet of its own. A 'token' (a short message) is passed around the ring. Only when a station receives a token can it transmit.

The most important measure of performance of a LAN is its mean throughput rate (fig. 5). As the jobs in a LAN increase, the throughput will increase linearly. If the completion of one job requires one second, then ten jobs will require ten seconds. However, as the number of jobs continues to increase a bottleneck will be encountered. A bottleneck occurs when too many images are transmitted requiring that a transmitting node queues its requests. Figure 5 illustrates that a bottleneck occurs when a specific number of jobs ($N_{saturation}$) are in the system. Actual throughput will be between the upper bound (linear until bottleneck is encountered) and the mean throughput lower bound.

3.2. Wide-area networks

A wide-area network (WAN) is a communication system that extends over large distances (covering more than a metropolitan area, Batnitzky et al., 1990). WANs often employ many different communication channel technologies such as copper wire cables, coaxial cables, fiber optic links, switched circuits, and microwave and satellite links. WANs which provide digital service are commonly implemented using circuit or message/packet switching. In circuit switching a complete set of connected links is established prior to transmission. These connected links are established by high-speed switches which keep the links intact until released at the end of the transmission. Message and packet switching use a store-and-forward means of transmitting data to a destination. Data is transmitted to nodes on the network and stored. The process is continued until data arrives at the destination node. In packet switching the data is also divided into small packets of 1024 bytes.

Wide-area networks are difficult to implement and maintain. The implementation of a WAN requires coordination between the local telephone carrier and the long-distance company. Reliability of a WAN network is measured by percent up-time (e.g., 99%) and the bit-error-rate (e.g., 1 bit error in 10^9 bits

TELERADIOLOGY SYSTEM

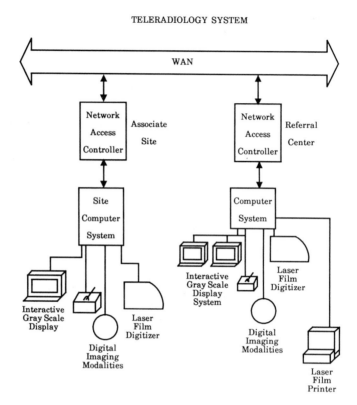

Fig. 6. A teleradiology wide-area network.

transmitted). Down-times are caused by disruptions such as electrical storms and accidental broken connections. Notification of down-time events is the responsibility of the WAN user. The maintenance of the equipment connected to the WAN is the responsibility of the user. Utilization management of the WAN is a difficult task. Computer software is required to both detect failures of the communication links and to manage high-demand peaks for use of the WAN.

Teleradiology requires the use of integrated LANs and WANs. A teleradiology system acquires radiographic images from one location and transmits them to one or more remote sites where they are displayed and/or converted to hard copy (fig. 6). The acquisition of digital image data may be from a laser film digitizer or interfaces to digital imaging modalities (CT, MRI, US, NM, DF, CR). The gray scale display workstations provide for the display and manipulation of $1 K \times 1 K \times 12$ bit or $2 K \times 2 K \times 12$ bit images. Laser film printers provide high-quality diagnostic reproductions of the transmitted image data. Archiving devices provide for storage and retrieval of the digitized and transmitted data.

4. Interactive gray scale display workstations

Interactive workstations are used to display and manipulate digital gray scale images (Arenson et al., 1990). Dedicated, technology specific, gray scale display workstations are attached to an imaging system and are provided by the manufacturer of the imaging modality. Image management network gray scale display workstations must be nonspecific and general purpose. They are used throughout the department. Clinical areas outside of the department can also be provided with gray scale display systems with limited display and manipulation functions. Such systems are less expensive.

The basic elements of an interactive gray scale display workstation are illustrated in fig. 7. The host computer is connected to the image management networks. Images to be displayed and manipulated are transmitted to an archive in the host computer. The display controller is a dedicated high-speed

A DIGITAL DISPLAY

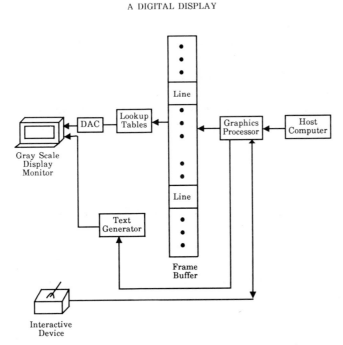

Fig. 7. The basic elements of a digital gray scale workstation.

microcomputer system which controls the display workstation. Image data is transferred by the host computer to the display controller. All requests for interactive processing is executed by the display controller in conjunction with the host computer. Image data to be displayed is framed by the frame buffer which is a dedicated high-speed image memory. Frame buffer image data is modified by selected look-up tables (LUTs) and converted to analog signals by the digital-to-analog converter (DAC) for display on the gray scale monitor.

User software for display workstations satisfies four functions. The presentation function provides for the interactive selection, positioning, and sequencing of image data on the display screen. Interactive manipulation functions provide for the manipulation of the pixel data contained in the digital image. These manipulations include window/level settings, contrast changes, region of interest selection, and generation of oblique and three-dimensional views. Quantification functions provide for the interactive analysis of digital images. These include, e.g., length and surface and volume measurements, histogram analysis, and texture analysis. Image processing functions include, e.g., image subtraction, data compression, edge enhancement, contour extraction, and volumetric displays.

The amount of digital image data to be displayed on departmental workstations is large. An estimate of the amount of time spent using gray scale display can be achieved by studying the check-out rates from the film library. In our department, the average retrieval demand for an inpatient film jacket is 10 retrievals in the first three days of the hospital stay, four retrievals for the remaining six days of the hospital stay, and three retrievals for the remainder of the first year. The retrieval rate is thus 17 times the digital image data generated. If 1.2 Gbytes are generated each day, then about 20 Gbytes per day will be displayed and manipulated. For a 12 hour day, this amount of daily displayed data will require an average network throughput rate of about

Table 2

Design goals for a digital gray scale display workstation.

Size	14 × 17 inches
Pixel size	0.2 mm
Spatial resolution	2.56 cycles/mm
Contrast range	12 bits (4096 gray levels)
Contrast ratio	50 : 1
Brightness	100 foot-lamberts
Screen refresh rate	72 Hz
Data transfer rate	$\frac{1}{2}$ s, full screen

4 Mbits/s. Multiple interactive gray scale display workstations will be required to maintain this mean throughput rate.

The efficient use of multiple gray scale display workstations on an image management network requires a well-conceived management protocol. Window system software was developed to provide users with a means of viewing multiple applications at the same time and of manipulating them in a user-friendly fashion. A popular means of accomplishing this task is the X-windows system. This software separates the windowing function into two distinct parts. The user interaction or display server is the program that controls each display and acts as the intermediary between user programs running on remote stations. The client applications program communicates across the network with the display server by means of calls to a low-level library of C-programming language subroutines.

The design goals set by our department for a gray scale display workstation are listed in table 2. The current level of CRT screen brightness is about 60 foot-lamberts. Radiographic films displayed on a light box provide a brightness of 400 foot-lamberts. This difference in brightness between the CRT and the light box requires careful gray level assignments for the CRT to render a display similar to film on a view box.

The use of interactive gray scale display workstations for consultative diagnostic digital image reading has encountered a number of problems. Spatial resolution and screen brightness are limited. Gray scale display monitors are readily available at 1280 × 1024 × 12 bits but of limited availability at 2048 × 2024 × 8 bits. The optimum choice of digital array size for digital radiography is not yet known. Screen fill times of the gray scale monitor must be one-half a second or less. The optimum number of display monitors for inclusion into a workstation is not known. The cost of interactive gray scale display workstations should not exceed $40 000 (1991).

5. Image archiving

Archived images provide the primary means of communication between radiologists and their referring physicians. Diagnosis can be improved by referring to previously archived images for purposes of comparison, correlation, and consultation. Archived images satisfy medicolegal and departmental management requirements. They facilitate research and teaching.

Image archiving can be divided into four, interconnected types of systems. An immediate image archive is provided with each imaging modality. This archiving capability is provided by the imaging equipment manufacturer. An on-line, high-speed 30-day archiving system is needed for handling the initial 30 days worth of examinations. An intermediate system handles examinations between 30 days and two years after the examination. Long-term archiving systems are needed for managing examinations between two to seven years. These four archiving systems are interfaced so that imaging data can be moved from one system to another. If the patient has a new examination, pointers to the patient's image file in the distributed database are generated. One strategy may be to generate pointers and also move the last examination image together with the new examination into the 30-day archive.

Technology available for immediate and on-line, 30-day, high-speed archiving are magnetic discs and optical discs. Winchester-type magnetic discs which store 600 Mbytes and more are readily available. Current fourteen-inch diameter optical discs, write once read many (WORM), provide 6.8 Gbytes of storage and transfer image data at 1 Mbyte/s transfer rates. It is estimated that a 30-day archiving system is required to manage 1400 Gbytes. Managing image data for a two-year system requires an optical disc library (juke box). It is estimated that a two-year archiving system is expected to manage approximately 23 500 Gbytes. An optical disc library as currently (1991) on the market can contain 150 disks, each disc being 14 inches in diameter and archiving 6.8 Gbytes (both sides together). Access times are 12 s and the data transfer rate is 1 Mbyte/s. The use of six optical disk library units and a 4-to-1 lossless compression will provide for two years of archiving at 47 Gbytes/day generation rate.

No technology is yet available for long-term five-year archiving. If an optical disk juke box is used for the two-year archiving system, then the optical discs can be stored off-line on shelves. A desirable technology for five-year archiving is optical tape cassettes. Each optical tape is sealed in a linear optical tape cassette. A 70 mm wide tape, 2400 feet in length, using a 5 μm laser spot size, archives 50 Gbytes per cassette. Two optical tape drives, using a 4-to-1 compression and 290 cassettes could archive five years of image data generated at 47 Gbytes/day.

Image data compression algorithms are used to increase the storage efficiency of archiving systems. There are three methods of image compression. Reversible compression (lossless) algorithms reduce the redundancy in an image and reinsert it on a pixel-by-pixel basis. Typical lossless compression ratios are between 1.5 and 2.8 to 1. Irreversible (lossy) compression algorithms reduce the redundancy in an image but image artifacts are generated during decompression. Typical lossy compression ratios are between 5 and 8 to 1 with no visually detectable artifacts. Clinical compression algorithms have also been attempted in which the radiologist discards images not deemed important to the examination.

Retrieval rates for archiving systems can be estimated by monitoring the film library. In our department an average of 2 000 patient film jackets are stored in the 10-day syspension file. In the two-year intermediate film library file, over 150 000 patient film jackets are stored. Over 410 000 patient film jackets are archived in the five-year long-term file. An average of 25 775 retrievals per month are requested by users of the department's film library. 71% of these retrievals are from the 10-day suspension file (18 300/month). 25% of the total retrievals are from the two-year intermediate file (over 6 000 retrievals/month) and 4% of the total retrievals are from the five-year long-term file (about 1 000 retrievals/month).

6. *Hard copy recordings*

Hard copy recordings are generated at the hard copy nodes on the image management system. Hard copy recordings of patient digital image data is used for inter-

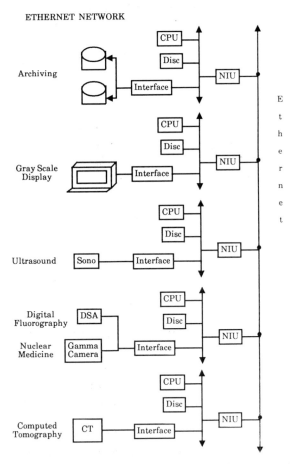

Fig. 8. A local-area network implemented by an Ethernet network.

HYPERCHANNEL NETWORK

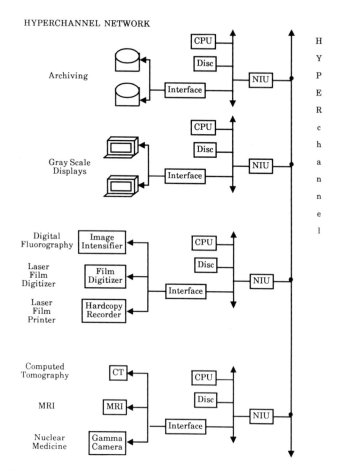

Fig. 9. A local-area network implemented by a HYPERchannel network.

pretation, consultation and treament planning. They are also used for teaching and research projects. Hard copy recordings are archived into the patient's film jacket. Technology used for hard copy recordings include video film camera units and laser beam scanning film printers. Digital pathways used in hard copy recorders include video pathways (the video signal is digitized and stored in the printer) and digital pathways (digital data is transferred directly into the printer). Laser film printers use a laser beam which is scanned across laser sensitive film. The laser beam is modulated by the digital image data to be printed. Generation of the two-dimensional laser scanned field may be accomplished by three different ways. One method pulls the film past a fixed optical stage. Another method moves the optical stage past a fixed sheet of laser sensitive film. A third method uses a slowly rotating drum to move the film past a fixed optical stage.

7. *University of Kansas experience with image management networks*

Our department has implemented and evaluated several prototype image management networks. From 1981 through 1985 we evaluated a system based on an Ethernet protocol network (fig. 8). Four imaging modalities were interfaced consisting of a CT scanner, a digital fluorography unit, a gamma camera, and an ultrasound scanner. Two interactive gray scale displays were implemented. A magnetic disc on-line archiving and a magnetic tape long-term archiving system were implemented. Each node contained a CPU using an INTEL 8086/8087 16 bit microcomputer and an IEEE-796 (MULTIBUS) internal bus. The CPU operating system was MP/M-86. 450 Mbytes of memory were provided at each node. More than 70 000 lines of application software was written by the department computer engineers. The maximum throughput rate of the Ethernet network and the INTEL 8086/8087 microcomputer system as measured in practice was 850 kbits/s. This was too slow to satisfy the requirements of an image management system. The gray scale display workstation used a $512 \times 512 \times 8$

BRIDGED NETWORK

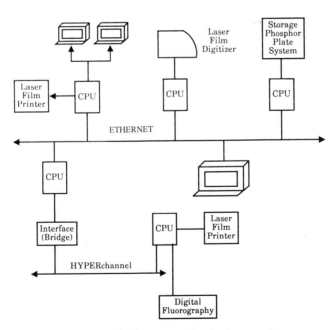

Fig. 10. A bridge between two local-area networks.

bit monitor. The image database system proved difficult to achieve reliable operation. This prototype was not capable of delivering clinical service.

A second image management network was implemented using a HYPERchannel network (fig. 9). HYPERchannel uses a carrier sense multiple access/collision avoidance networking protocol. Each node contained a CPU consisting of Motorola 68010 16 bit microcomputer. The internal node bus was IEEE 796 (MULTIBUS). The interactive gray scale display stations provided for the display of $1280 \times 1024 \times 12$ bits. Evaluation of the HYPERchannel – M68010 prototype image management network proved encouraging. The bottlenecks encountered were disc access times at each node. Throughput rates of the network were measured at 1.5 Mbits/s. The laser film digitizer and laser film printer proved to be highly acceptable. It would be desirable to upgrade the M68010 systems to the newer, higher-speed microcomputers.

Fiber optic wide-area networks will be capable of providing the backbone data rates for connecting multiple LANs. We have implemented an Ethernet network and a HYPERchannel network which is connected by a bridge device (fig. 10). Our intent is to study the requirements of bridging together two or more LANs.

8. Summary

The use of radiology image management networks is increasing. Increased patient examination throughput is made possible by using these networks. Improved patient care results from use of image management networks. Teleradiology wide-area networks require the use of these networks.

References

Arenson, R.L., D.P. Chakraborty, S.B. Seshadri and H.L. Kundel (1990) The digital imaging workstation, *Radiology* 176, 303 – 315.

Barnes, G.T., R.A. Sones and M.M. Tesic (1985) Digital chest radiography: performance evaluation of a prototype unit, *Radiology* 154, 801 – 806.

Batnitzky, S., S.J. Rosenthal, E.L. Siegel, L.H. Wetzel, M.D. Murphey, G.G. Cox, J.H. McMillan, A.W. Templeton and S.J. Dwyer III (1990) Teleradiology: an assessment, *Radiology* 177, 11 – 17.

Cox, G.G., S.J. Dwyer III and A.W. Templeton (1986) Computer networks for image management in radiology: an overview, *CRC Crit. Rev. Diagn. Imaging* 25(4), 333 – 371.

Cox, G.G. R.L. Arenson and H.L. Bosco (1988) Current status of radiology image management systems, *Invest. Radiol.* 23(9), 656 – 663.

Cox, G.G., A.W. Templeton J.H. McMillan, L.H. Wetzel and K.R. Lee (1990) Digital fluoroscopy and radiography systems: technical description and clinical examples, *Radiography* 10, 491 – 498.

Duerinckx, A.J. (Ed.) (1982) Picture Archiving and Communication Systems (PACS) for Medical Applications, First International Conference and Workshop, *Proc. SPIE* 318.

Huang, H.K. (1987) Elements of Digital Radiology: a Professional Handbook and Guide (Prentice-Hall, Englewood Cliffs NJ).

Oestmann, J.W., M. Prokop, C. Schaefer, S. Reichelt and M. Galanski (1990) Digital radiology in clinical use: review of current knowledge, *Electromedica* 58(4), 109 – 123.

Sonoda, M., M. Takano, J. Miyahara and H. Kato (1983) Computed radiography utilizing scanning laser stimulated luminescence, *Radiology* 148, 833 – 838.

Templeton, A.W., S.J. Dwyer III, J.A. Johnson, W.H. Anderson, K.S. Hensley, S.J. Rosenthal, K.R. Lee, D.F. Preston, S. Batnitzky and H.I. Price (1984) An on-line digital image management system, *Radiology* 152, 321 – 325.

Templeton, A.W., S.J. Dwyer III, J.A. Johnson, W.H. Anderson, K.S. Hensley, K.R. Lee, S.J. Rosenthal, D.F. Preston and S. Batnitzky (1985) Implementation of an on-line and long term digital management system, *Radiographics* 5(1), 121 – 138.

Templeton, A.W., G.G. Cox and S.J. Dwyer III (1988) Digital image management networks: current status, *Radiology* 169, 193 – 199.

Wandtke, J.C., and D.B. Plewes (1989) Comparison of scanning equalization and conventional radiography, *Radiology* 172, 641 – 645.

Integrated Diagnostic Imaging
Editor: J.P.J. De Valk
© *Elsevier Science Publishers B.V., 1992*

Chapter 2

Considerations for introducing digital image transmission into clinical medical practice

Glenn Forbes

1. Clinical issues

Computer-generated images with information in digital form have been performed in radiology for over two decades, beginning at a low volume in the 1960s with isotope studies and expanding through CT/MR (computed tomography/magnetic resonance) cross-sectional imaging in the 1970s – 1980s. During most of this time, little interest in the digital data could be found in clinical areas outside of the radiology department due to lack of both expertise and access to sophisticated equipment utilizing information in digital form. Requests for original computer image data were usually limited to research projects or the occasional need for measurements and three-dimensional reconstruction. During the mid 1980s, however, the success that imaging has had in influencing medical diagnosis began to see its counterpart in the sphere of therapy with the incorporation of images into direct treatment techniques such as stereotactic surgery, radiation therapy planning, and prosthesis development. Many of these activities require various forms of image reconstruction using the original digital data acquired in cross-sectional imaging and thus the modern radiology department is now often called upon to supply not only selected copy films of processed images but the original digital data sets as well. This has introduced concepts that are common to the computer world but less familiar to the medical imaging community such as archival, image management, data transmission, remote display, as well as data security, credibility, ownership and accessibility. Various terms have arisen to represent portions of this activity such as PACS (picture archiving communication systems), telecommunications, etc., but the overriding theme remains: the modern radiology department is becoming more responsible for providing and directing the transfer of digital image data to the rest of the medical community.

Several procedures and philosophical issues have arisen which do not current-ly have uniform understanding within all divisions of the medical community. Who owns or is primarily responsible for storage, security and credibility of the data? Where should post-processing best occur? What happens to processed data that becomes part of the medical record? Who pays for which part of the activity? These are all questions that are under debate and several years are like-ly to pass before uniform answers are obtained. Nevertheless, the technical issues and clinical requirements can be identified. These are fundamental to the approach and design of a system best suited to address the particular needs of each medical institution.

The first off-line use of the image digital data sets arose from post-processed images to extend diagnostic utility. These generally consisted of measurements and three-dimensional reformatted images to provide further perspective in diagnosis. A few centers developed methods of prosthesis and surgical implant design based on computer image data in the orthopedic and plastic surgery fields. Although stereotactic neurosurgery had been established for many years based on standard radiography, introduction of the more tissue sensitive CT and MR techniques expanded this operation into the biopsy and treatment of a host of small or deep-seated brain lesions that had previously been inaccessi-ble. Recent developments in radiation treatment based upon correlative CT/MR with predicted isodose curves are being introduced in many tertiary care institutions. Integration of data sets acquired from different modalities is in the investigative stage which may lead to new hybrid studies such as MR-positron emission tomography or MR-biomagnetism in the future.

In addition to clinical patient care, research and education have already benefitted from the availability of post-processing activity of digital image data sets. Investigative projects have long depended on analysis of original digital data or measurements in alternative reformatted image displays. Educational programs are just now beginning to take advantage of the accessibility to digital data files for purposes of image reconstruction and display in the fields of anatomy and pathology. The reader is referred elsewhere for a discussion of the extensive use of digital imaging in the research and educational spheres.

To appreciate the impact of digital image transfer in the clinical setting, it is necessary to have a basic understanding of the fundamental technical issues. Although each institution develops its own solution to the individual practice demands, the design of every system is based upon a similar approach to stan-dard operations of storage, retrieval, transfer and display of the image data.

2. Technical issues

The technical aspects of digital image data management are well known to computer workers in this field although their applications to clinical medicine create some new perspectives. This effort can be divided into five major steps: acquisition, archival, retrieval, transmission and display. These operations occur along a computer network which links multiple pieces of equipment and transfers the information. Each of these steps is a science in itself and interfaces closely with the others in creating a smooth flow of image data from the patient to the clinical physician. As in any series network, the steps act as a chain, the weakest link establishes the baseline for expediency measured by volume and rate of data transfer. A vast field of technology is associated with each of these steps. The integration of these components to provide random retrieval, transmission to remote sites, and expedient display is approached differently by each institution due to variable needs. Although most of these operations are transparent to the physician user, presentation of the final product at the end of the chain, the display station, is a very real and measurable commodity. Quality of image, time for display, and accessibility for image recall all become measurable standards by which the entire system is judged.

3. Acquisition

This operation is the part most familiar to radiologists and medical physicists and least understood by both the clinical physician and computer data management specialist. Diagnostic medical scanning with both computed tomography and magnetic resonance imaging is performed with manipulation of several parameters such as matrix size, field of view, and slice thickness which, among others, determine spatial resolution and image contrast. These parameters result in various levels of digital data that are necessary to transcribe to any system that intends to retain the ability to extract a full range of spatial and contrast image information. This includes research areas and workstations involved with off-line analysis such as three-dimensional reconstruction, stereotaxis, or radiation treatment planning. Simple prescribed images used only for review might otherwise be stored in only analog form.

Data acquisition, file storage, and file transfer are performed in different manners within systems of different commercial manufacturers. Several manufacturers involved in networking facilitate digital transfer utilizing their own software and source codes to interface units within a unique network. This obviously can become a limitation to the hospital or clinic user who may wish to link several units from different manufacturers to a generic network. To circumvent this problem, the American College of Radiology and the National Electronic Manufacturers Association have developed a joint interface specification called ACR-NEMA standard to convert commercial language to a common standard. Many scanning units and current PAC system components are now produced in an ACR-NEMA compatible form which expedites common networking.

It is imperative that end users of digital data understand and work in consort with those who have expertise in the theory and mechanism of the acquisition process. Without such fundamental understanding, erroneous steps are likely to be incorporated into the end use of the digital data. It is not sufficient to simply produce three-dimensional image reconstruction or plan stereotaxic measurements based on transported digital scanning data. Comprehension of potential measurement errors, boundary definitions that define true or false contrast and resolution, and computer artifacts inherent in the data acquisition process is necessary to avoid creating false computer images in off-line analysis. This is particularly true when the computer images are used for medical diagnosis or therapy.

4. Archiving

All medical images have been retained in the past in some form for variable periods of time depending upon the needs of the institution. In the precomputer image days, this was accomplished by film filing and storage in the X-ray department for a period of several years after which the films were destroyed, the silver recovered and images subsequently lost forever. With the advent of computer imaging in the early – mid 1970s, magnetic tape was used for recording data that might be later recalled for review or off-line analysis. For over a decade, few problems occurred with this process principally since very few areas outside of radiology had the capability or expertise or the need to manipulate raw digital scanning data. Several developments during the mid 1980s changed this and also exposed the limitations of data storage on magnetic tape. Off-line analysis for volume measurement, three-dimensional reconstruction for surgical treatment planning, prosthetic implantation, radiation therapy, and stereotactic surgery based on image-directed localization are just a few of the recent activities that require digital image data. Some of these activities may be performed near or at the time of acquisition and thus rely on short-term storage such as the hard discs of the scanning units. Other activities are performed at later dates requiring data from long-term magnetic tape storage including controlled storage environments, the need for compression algorithms, and bulk of storage medium have become more apparent as these off-line analysis operations have grown in the hospital environment.

The size of the data storage mechanism becomes a significant factor for the hospital as scanning volume grows beyond one or two units. One CT or MR unit typically will produce 150 – 500 Mbytes of data per day depending on patient volume and an institution can quickly enter the Tbyte (10^3 Gbytes or 10^6Mbyte) annual storage range if several CT and MR units are operating. These demands clearly point to optical media if any long-term storage needs are to be addressed.

As much as 10% of the examinations performed in a modern radiology department may produce information in digital form. This includes CT, MR, some angiography, ultrasound and isotope studies. It is neither practical nor desirable to consider at this time the remaining 90% of non-digitally acquired radiology examinations in terms of total storage, access, and transmission in digital form. The immense conversion of film to digital is seldom necessary and other mediums for transmitting analog images are usually more practical and cost effective.

5. Retrieval

Retrieval for clinical medical purposes can be anticipated from both within and outside the radiology department. Radiology retrieval needs will arise for review of selected diagnostic problems, comparison of old and recent examinations for diagnostic interpretation, and investigative projects. Retrieval from outside the radiology department will generally arise for off-line analysis for therapy, such as stereotactic surgery or radiation treatment planning. Retrieval may thus occur from any of three stages: immediate daily storage from hard discs, short-term storage (1 – 30 days) for active patients, and long-term storage (over 30 days) for comparison and investigation.

The type of retrieval will be dictated by the volume and expediency required in a clinical setting. Certain on-line therapeutic procedures, such as stereotaxic surgery may require immediate access to scanning data. Such patients are often scanned while in a surgical stereotactic frame and then moved to the operating suite for biopsy or treatment as soon as the off-line image data has been processed. The technical mechanism to provide such immediate access to image data should then be designed to address the issues discussed in Section 8 in this chapter such as security and lack of interference with data acquisition. Other off-line analysis operations such as volume measurement, or three-dimensional reconstruction may be performed during the course of patient care and require intermediate level access from short-term storage. Research activity utilizing long-term storage may seem to present the less expedient demand, but in fact may involve large volumes. Different level demands should be processed through a priority system under the image management program to avoid bottlenecks in image transport during peak loading time of the clinical day.

These data demands can usually be handled at flexible times when demands for clinical cases are least acute. Such investigative data is best downloaded to a separate file server which then provides access to an independent research network or workstation where data can be maintained and manipulated without interfering with the ongoing clinical work. Requests for data for educational purposes within a teaching institution are best handled in a similar fashion. In the latter case, selective stripping of header information such as patient identification might be performed while retaining interpretative information for teaching purposes. Programs to handle such selective operations need to be incorporated within the data management system that directs the archiving and retrieval of a teaching and research institution.

6. Transmission

The issues associated with transmission of digital image data within a network are usually transparent to the clinical end user involved with patient care. The effect most noticeable to the clinician will be the delay in data transfer during peak loading times if image data is transmitted over networks shared with other computer information users. Even then, delays in image transfer are usually due to bottlenecks at interfaces between stations and the network and not due to the transmission process itself.

The principle issue to be managed is related to the vast discrepancy in data volume between the transmission of digital image data and other medical computer information. As described in Section 4, the daily requirement to transfer data in the hundreds of Mbyte or even Gbyte range would not be unusual for a large hospital or a teaching institution whereas most laboratory, secretarial, transcription, billing, and non-image research activities operate at the kbyte or low Mbyte range. Although the image volume may be readily handled on a local area network solely designed for image transfer, daily downloading of hundreds of Mbytes or a Gbyte of image data on a generic institutional network shared by other computer facilities will have a noticeable impact on all data transmission. Thus such operations as routine archiving, off-line analysis, and expedient clinical review need to be separated and prioritized in order to distribute the data load efficiently throughout the system. In the current Mayo Clinic system under development, several hours of cross-sectional scanning archiving occur during evening hours or are deprioritized during the day when transmission between geographical scanning areas is necessary over a generic institutional network.

7. Display

The display parameters are those aspects that radiologists and medical clinicians are most familiar with and thus come under the highest level of scrutiny. Radiologists have become accustomed to working with computer screen display for medical diagnosis for over a decade and a half, and a fairly uniform standard of requirements has become established. Fast projection (screen paint) of single, multiple, and montage images, flexibility and optical display including adjustable level and window (pixel density and contrast), and capability of image magnification and measurement are basic operations that are expected in a standard workstation that would be used with most medical cross-sectional image devices (both CT and MR). These operations are used routinely on-line for manipulation of the digital image both to monitor the examination and prepare the diagnostic interpretation. Sample images are then pictured on film through a console camera interface and selected hard-copy images are sent to the medical record or clinical area similar to 'X-ray film' used in routine radiography. Any need for review is often performed on the original data set that may reside on either hard disc or recent storage while a patient remains in active care.

8. System requirements

The clinical requirements of a digital image management system relate to accessibility, security, lack of interference with data acquisition, display utility, and, finally, cost.

Demands for accessibility are considerably different in terms of both time and priority within the clinical medical environment. The most pressing need for expedient access to an image examination data set usually arises from on-line surgical procedures based on image-directed techniques. These include such things as CT-guided stereotactic biopsy, image-directed probe placement for biopsy or laser treatment, or three-dimensional radiation treatment (gamma knife surgical radiation). In these situations, the patient is placed within a rigid frame to allow correlation of image-calculated coordinates with direction of a biopsy or treatment probe. Digital image data may be obtained during angiography, CT, or MR and coordinates are derived from the processed image data while the patient is being transferred to the surgical suite. Somewhat less expedient transfer of image data may occur with standard radiation treatment planning or prosthetic design which can occur days after the image examination. The least expedient demand in terms of time may relate to diagnostic comparison or retrospective measurements used in follow-up diagnostic examinations.

The priority of data access may be highest for surgical cases undergoing immediate treatment, intermediate for consultation cases, and lowest for retrospective analysis on follow-up. For consultation, clinical physicians may find access to selective post-processed images with interpretative reports sufficient similar to receiving standard X-rays in a film jacket in the past. The advantages here relate to more immediate image display to remote areas. Retrospective analysis may occur in the investigative and educational activities where large batches of images might be accessed for review, for example, as in a research project or teaching session. For teaching, selective post-processed images may be sufficient whereas research work will require the original complete data set.

Confidentiality of patient information presents different levels of demand on the security of image data handled in a digital system. Well-established legal guidelines in the clinical world require that complete medical information becomes available only to those professionals directly involved in a patient's care. Thus, digital data transferred on a network that provides access to various areas such as research, education, billing, and system maintenance needs to be protected in terms of encoding or identification. In a similar fashion, archive data is best transferred to a type of relay station called a file server which then can be accessed by various users. This is sometimes referred to as a 'push system' in which selected data is pushed into the file server by data management and direct access to all archive data is prevented from being automatically pulled by any end user. It is also important to recognize that different cultural standards exist in the clinical and research spheres. Whereas the clinical users are guided by strict regulations in handling confidential patient information, researchers are accustomed to an environment of more open information exchange and research networks may provide access to terminals in collaborative projects often outside the parent institution that would not ordinarily be present in the clinical world. Thus, a worker in one institution might conceivably gain access to confidential medical information in another institution through an integrated network. These issues are usually approached by inserting file servers that act as gateways between different networks, such as a link between a clinical research network, or between the radiology and standard institutional network. The gateways are under the data management originally responsible for the integrity and confidentiality of the image data.

It is important that all operations of archiving and transfer be as transparent as possible to the operation of the acquisition of the original data itself. Since efficiency of patient care and revenue ultimately depend on patient throughput, such transmission activities should be designed to have as little interference on the CT/MR/angio systems as possible. Programs are designed to prioritize batch transfer data from a CT/MR hard disc intermittently during nonacquisition times, for instance, as patients are transferred on and off tables. Large transfer may occur during non-scanning times. Diagnostic display and the scanning operation itself should not be delayed by the archival process.

The utility of display depends upon the needs of the end clinical user. Diagnostic radiologists will require ability to window and level original data, to rapidly scan large sets of image files and perform such post-processing operations as reformatting and measurement. Clinicians may be satisfied with display of selected post-processed images with the diagnostic interpretation. They too, however, may require rapid scanning of a large data sets. It should be remembered that an experienced radiologist is accustomed to visually scanning 20 – 40 cross-sectional images on films within seconds to choose two or three images deserving closer scrutiny related to the specific clinical problem. This corresponds to the display of 10 – 20 Mbytes of image data per second any portion of which may be immediately used for in-depth analysis. Thus the demands on the display system in terms of disc storage, screen paint or display rate, and visual effects can be quite high. Montage displays may be used to offset a slower screen paint for some users. Terminals that are to be used by clinicians needing only post-processed selected image display may have less stringent demands in terms of screen paint and disc storage. They will, however, require integration of image and diagnostic interpretation as well as access to large index files to locate patient examinations. User friendliness becomes a more important issue for peripheral terminals in the non-radiology setting as the majority of clinical physicians are unfamiliar with the standard operations on the scanning display console.

An issue that is not always well recognized is the need to incorporate post-processed image data in the patient's medical record. All too often, image data undergoes off-line analysis for three-dimensional reconstruction or measurements used to direct treatment and the post-process data set is then discarded. Since critical decisions may be based on such data and potential errors may reside in a processed set, this data should be retained in a similar fashion as any other image data set. Historically, radiology departments have retained X-ray files for 5 – 10 years. Research departments may require longer retention and legal procedures (often supported by state legislation) will frown on any inability to reproduce patient data within at least five years. If the post-processed data set is created outside of radiology, a means of archiving such data under the institution's guidelines for retention and accessibility needs to be designed.

Evaluation of system costs is a complex but straightforward accounting analysis of hardware, software, and personnel management expense. A more obscure matter is determining the relative responsibility of cost sharing among the various providers and users of the hospital image transfer system. The majority of capital costs occurs in the initial establishment of the network, archival, and data management system. Later peripheral tie-ins, such as providing a link to a clinical area, then becomes a considerably less substantial cost. The original costs, however, should be clearly identified to determine appropriate billing of services among end users based on data volume and complexity of the image information access even as it all occurs within one institution. Usually, these costs are most easily identified within the center of image data management within radiology.

9. Mayo experience

A computer-based system for medical image archival and clinical review is under development jointly by the Future Development and Application Technology Group of IBM Applications Business Systems and the Radiology Department of the Mayo Clinic. A long-range plan entails a fully configured system for the efficient archival and review of digitized medical images covering over 25 MR/CT scanning modalities on three Mayo campuses across the United States (Rochester, Minnesota; Jacksonville, Florida; and Scottsdale, Arizona). A token ring network is used with a hardware platform based on an AS/400 computer with additional function provided by a series of system/36 minicomputers each connected to optical disc storage units. PS/2 microcomputers bridge the imaging modalities and the network and allow for image caching and routing as well as user interfaces for system management and review (see figs. 1 and 2).

Nine MR scanners, three CT modalities, three medical display stations, and three optical archive systems are operational in this archive network in late 1991. A pilot integrated system digital network telecommunications link is in place for wide-area network attachment of the Jacksonville, Florida, system to Rochester, Minnesota. Local image networks are linked to an institutional fibernet with minor impact on institutional daily data flow. As image data processing and transmission increase, scheduling and priority algorithms will be instituted to minimize the impact on other electronic data transfer.

Anticipated requests for digital data from outside radiology will be handled by a push system using a file server linked to an external workstation. In this way, data can be pushed by the computer management system in radiology after review and approval onto the file server which is then accessed by an external source. Security, confidentiality, integrity and appropriate use of the requested data sets can be assured prior to transfer to the file server. Source codes and proprietary commercial software on the imaging network can also be protected. Overall impact on archiving, retrieval and transmission operations within a large scale high-volume clinical practice are yet to be determined.

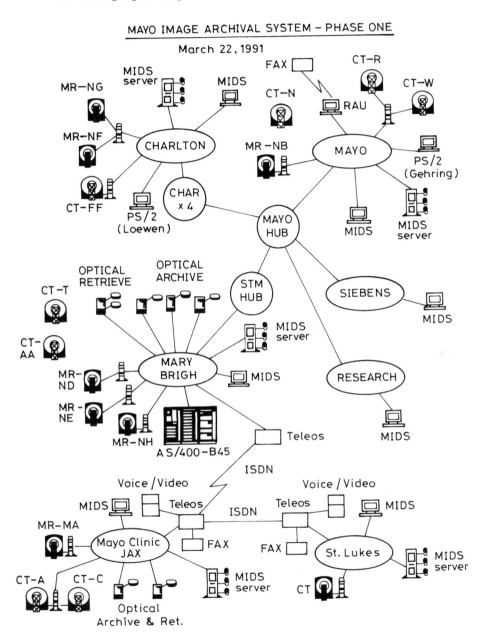

Fig. 1. Mayo image archival system, phase I.

Several lessons have been learned by the Mayo Community with PACS development and they need to be emphasized here:

(1) The same functions that have been performed for decades regarding image data prior to the computer age need to be performed in an analogous fashion before computer image data is electronically passed on for patient care. These include proper data acquisition, quality control, integrity of the data set before and after data transfer, interpretation of the original data set, archival of the data set, display and processing of the data set, and ability to record and retrieve the data set at a later date.

(2) Equipment that can be centralized can be maintained at a state of the art level at minimal cost. In a field where technical advances are made annually if not monthly, it will be extremely difficult and costly to attempt to maintain uniform software and hardware upgrades in numerous peripheral sites. Equipment that can be centralized to provide a necessary function can be more easily upgraded and maintained.

(3) Data formats of archived image sets (three-dimensional, four-dimensional, correlative techniques, radiation treatment, surgical planning, etc.) should be institutionally available and should be archived in a format that can be

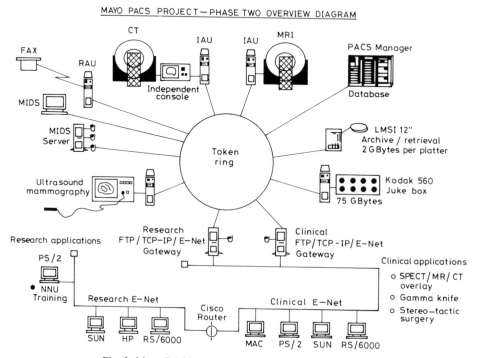

Fig. 2. Mayo PACS project, phase II, overview diagram.

reliably and easily retrieved. This requires central archiving and management.

(4) Quality control measures must be in place to ensure accurate computer-based information extraction and electronic image display. Off-line processing of image data may easily alter the credibility of the initial data set and if the physical principles are not properly addressed at either end, significant errors will occur. This will require close collaboration between those involved with the data acquisition (radiology) and those who may later manipulate or alter the data for specific needs (clinical peripheral workstation areas). Institutional standards are necessary to maintain uniformity of the data sets derived from the processed radiology examinations. Programs for image measurement and maintenance of credibility of the initial data set which are currently used in radiology should be extended to some level for data sets that are used in an altered form for patient care.

(5) Future plans for integration of digital imaging technology will compound many of these issues in the future. Programs under discussion such as the combination of MR and CT data sets with electrophysiological recordings and treatment planning techniques will require multidisciplinary efforts that will extend outside the scope of simply acquiring a computer workstation in the clinical area. These activities need to be understood at the institutional level so that the final impact in terms of personnel effort and later equipment requests are broadly recognized. These include programming efforts, maintenance and quality control personnel efforts, updating of hardware and software computer designs, network demands in information transfer, utilization of clinical time for activities that may be either central or peripheral to the direct patient care, and cost efficiencies related to the addition of new techniques.

10. Recommendations

(1) Requests from outside radiology for digital data are likely to increase in the coming decade. These will range from requests for processed digital data to simple image display without post processing capability. Radiology departments should evaluate the impact of such requests on the practice and prepare plans to respond.

(2) The most appropriate design of a system for medical digital image transmission is different for each hospital. The needs for digital image transmission are considerably different from the needs of other forms of digital information transfer.

(3) A digital image transmission system should be introduced in a series of

phases beginning with an archiving system, a retrieval system, a display system, a limited network linking a defined modality or area, and finally an expanded network interfaced with multiple modalities or areas.

(4) Costs of digital image transmission are significant and need to be clearly understood and analyzed with respect to potential benefit before designing a system. The cost of transmitting digital image data involve expenses beyond that immediately required to create a network. Hidden costs also involve modifications of hardware and software to interface with networks as well as personnel efforts to manage data retrieval and transmission.

(5) Transfer of clinical image information should occur only after acquisition, quality control assessment or monitoring, diagnostic interpretation, recording, billing, and archival have been completed. Direct links between the hard disks of image scanners and outside workstations are not recommended as they may provide external access to data before all of these operations have been completed. Transmission and external access should not adversely affect acquisition in terms of scanning delays or decreased throughput. Patient condifentiality and software integrity should be protected with computer security measures. All of these issues can be addressed in the overall system design.

11. Future

The issues discussed in this chapter are concepts to be used in approaching the integration of a digital image management system into a clinical environment. Technological advances will always impact the specifics of the system design but the underlying clinical operations are less likely to undergo dramatic change. The procedures of image acquisition, quality control, clinical interpretation, confidentiality, storage, and retrieval have all been part of medical practice since the dawn of X-ray work in the early part of this century. Technical advances that provide wider and more expedient information exchange in the future will only more forcibly return the user to a consideration of these fundamental principles.

References

Gehring, D.G., K.R. Persons, M. Rothman, J. Salutz and R.L. Morin (1991) Detailed technical description of the Mayo-IBM PACS project. In: Medical Imaging V: PACS Design and Evaluation, *Proc. SPIE* 1446.

Morin, R.L., G. Forbes, D.G. Gehring, J.R. Salutz and W. Pavlicek (1991) Present status and future direction of the Mayo-IBM PACS project. In: Medical Imaging V: PACS Design and Evaluation, *Proc. SPIE* 1446.

Myers, J.H., R.C. Murry, E.G. Brooks and D.G. Gehring (1990) MIDS: Multi-modality image display. In: Dwyer III, S.J. and G. Jost (Eds.), Medical Imaging IV: PACS System Design and Evaluation, *Proc. SPIE* 1234.

Integrated Diagnostic Imaging
Editor: J.P.J. De Valk   .
© *Elsevier Science Publishers B.V., 1992*

Chapter 3

PACS – a review and perspective

H.K. Huang

1. Review

1.1. History of PACS

The first international conference and workshop on picture archiving and communication systems (PACS) was held in Newport Beach, California, January 1982 (Duerinckx, 1982). The meeting was organized by André Duerinckx and sponsored by the SPIE – the international society for optical engineering. Thereafter, the PACS conference was combined with the medical imaging conference. The joint meeting became an annual event, always held in late January or early February in California. Sam Dwyer III and Roger Schneider took over the responsibility as co-chairmen of the conference as well as the editors of the proceedings in 1983 (Dwyer III, 1983; Schneider et al., 1989).

In Japan, the first international symposium on PACS and personal health data (PHD) was held in July 1982 (Medical Image Technology, 1986), sponsored by the Japan association of medical imaging technology (JAMIT). This conference, combined with the medical imaging technology meeting, also became an annual event. In Europe, the EuroPACS association (picture archiving and communication systems in Europe) has held at least annual meetings since 1984 and is the driving force for European PACS information exchange.

One of the most concentrated efforts in dedicated PACS meetings so far was the NATO ASI (advanced study institute): 'PACS in medicine' held in Evian, France, from October 12–24, 1990. In this meeting approximately 100 scientists from over seventeen countries participated. The ASI proceedings (Huang et al., 1991) summarize the most up-to-date information in PACS research and development at this moment.

One of the earliest research projects related to PACS in the United States is the teleradiology project funded by the U.S. Army (Curtis et al., 1983). A follow-up project is the 'installation site for digital imaging network and picture archiving and communication system (DIN/PACS)' funded by the U.S. army and administered by the MITRE corporation. Two university sites were selected for the implementation; the university of Washington in Seattle, and Washington and Georgetown university/George Washington university Consortium (The MITRE Corporation, 1985). The national cancer institute in the U.S. funded one of its first PACS-related research projects under the title 'multiple viewing stations for diagnostic radiology' to UCLA in 1985 (Multiple Viewing Station for Diagnostic Radiology, 1985).

1.2. Methods of PACS research development and implementation

Most PACS research development and implementation efforts are initiated by university hospitals and academic departments and by research laboratories in major computer imaging manufacturers. There are generally three methods of approach (Huang et al., 1991). In the first approach, a multidisciplinary team, with technical know how, is assembled by a radiology department. The team becomes a system integrator, selecting PACS components from various manufacturers. The team develops system interfaces and writes the PACS software according to the clinical requirement. In the second approach, a team of experts is assembled to write a detailed specification of PACS for a certain clinical environment. A manufacturer is contracted to implement the system. In the third approach, the manufacturer develops a turn-key PACS system and installs it in a department for clinical use.

There are advantages and disadvantages in these approaches. The advantages of the first approach is that the PACS system can be continuously upgraded by the research team using state-of-the-art components and therefore it will not become obsolete. The system so designed is geared to the clinical environment and the system is not at the mercy of the manufacturer. The disadvantages are that it requires a substantial commitment by the department to assemble a multidisciplinary team. The system developed will be one of a kind, therefore service and maintenance will be difficult because it consists of components from different manufacturers.

The advantage of the second approach is that the PACS specification is written for a certain clinical environment and the responsibility of implementation is delegated to the manufacturer. The department acts as a purchase agent and does not have to be concerned about the installation. The disadvantage is that the specification tends to be over-ambitious because some outside experts might underestimate the technical and operational difficulties. The designated manufacturer, lacking the learning experience of some components in a clinical environment, may tends to over-estimate the performance of each component.

As a result, the total PACS may not meet the complete specification. The costs of contacting the manufacturer to develop a specified PACS is also expensive due to the manufacturer's profit margin of building only one system.

The advantage of the third approach* is that it is a generalized production system, and the cost tends to be lower. In this approach, since it is a production, the manufacturer needs a few years to complete the production cycle. By the time it is commercially available, some components already become obsolete because of the fast pace in high-technology development. Also, we are still doubtful whether a generalized PACS can be used for every specialty in a department and be used for every radiology department. We foresee that these three approaches will gradually merge as additional clinical PACS data become more available.

Due to various operating conditions, PACS research and development emphasis is different in North America, European countries and Japan. In the United States, PACS research is mostly supported by government agencies and manufacturers. In the European countries, PACS research is supported either through a national or a regional resource. European research teams tend to work with a single major manufacturer, and since most PACS components are developed in the United States and Japan, they are not as readily available. European research teams emphasize PACS modeling and simulation, as well as investigate the image processing component of PACS. In Japan, PACS research and development is a national project. The national resources are distributed to various manufacturers and university hospitals. A manufacturer integrates a PACS system and installs it in a hospital for clinical evaluation. The manufacturer's PACS specification tends to be rigid and leaves little room for the hospital research team to modify the technical specification.

1.3. PACS and related research in various countries (Huang et al., 1991)

In this section, we summarize PACS and related research in eleven countries. The summary is extracted from the respective country's presentation during the 1990 NATO ASI meeting. The eleven countries are Austria, Belgium, France, Germany, Italy, Japan, the Netherlands, Sweden, Switzerland, Turkey and the United Kingdom.

Austria is planning a large scale PACS project at the social and medical center East (SMZO) being constructed. Further detail of this will be presented in Section 2.2.

In Belgium, three institutes are active in PACS research: the University of

---

* The fourth (mixed) approach is one of system integration: Many (smaller) manufacturers involved in one big contract under responsibility of a (bigger) manufacturer.

Leuven (KUL), the University Hospital of Brussels (ULB), and the Pluridisciplinary Research Institute for Medical Imaging Science (PRIMIS) at the University of Brussels. At the KUL the PACS project's main application is to support research activities in acquisition techniques and image processing methods. The ULB, together with the PRIMIS group, started a multi-vendor installation PACS project in 1986. In addition, the ULB is also working on an evaluation project in teleradiology. In France, there are six PACS projects from Grenoble, Lille, Montpellier, Nantes, Rennes and Villejuif. In Grenoble and in Rennes, PACS is in the university hospital with a special connection to neurosurgery. In Lille and in Villejuif, PACS are designed in the university hospital under the framework of a hospital information system (HIS) project. In Montpellier, it is inside the university hospital. In Nantes, the PACS is within the nuclear medicine area.

In Germany, there are two PACS-related projects, one from the university of Hamburg and the other from the university of Berlin. The Hamburg project is related to the use of computed radiography (CR). The Berlin communication system (BERKOM), initiated in 1986, serves as a test bed for future developments of broadband communication services, terminal devices, and applications. The project is shared by a spectrum of partners comprising 40 scientific institutions, 17 industrial companies and 5 users.

PACS and related research in the Netherlands concentrates in radiology and hospital information systems, ROC analysis, image quality evaluation, and modeling. A consortium completed a first phase study (1986 – 1989), which was a cooperative effort between Utrecht University Hospital (AZU) BAZIS, and Philips Netherlands.

Japan is very active in CR, more than 250 CR systems are in clinical use. As for PACS, about 100 hospitals have already installed systems of various complexity. In Section 2.2, we will describe a very large scale PACS project at the Hokkaido university.

In Italy, there are nine hospitals installed with the turn-key CommView PACS system from AT&T and Philips. These hospitals are Mater Dei Clinic, Bari; Maggiore Hospital, Bologna; Castelfranco Hospital, Castelfranco; Sant'Anna Hospital, Ferrara; Messina Hospital, Messina; S. Gerardo Hospital, Monza; Cattinare Hospital and Maggiore Hospital, Trieste; and S. Paolo Hospital, Milano. The Collemaggio Hospital, L'Aquila, on the other hand, develops its own PACS. Research activities in Italy includes economic evaluation, metropolitan PACS, operational analysis, RIS/PACS integration, and teleradiology.

Large-scale PACS installations do not exit in Sweden; however, at present there are two hospitals, in Karolinska and Lund, which have experience of limited PACS activities. Also, about 12 teleradiology systems are in use.

In Switzerland, a hospital-wide PACS project integrated within a HIS is in progress in the university hospital of Geneva. In the United Kingdom two government-supported PACS projects are planned at Leeds general infirmary and at Hammersmith hospital. The Leeds' groups are carrying out an assessment of CR, and developing image processing algorithms. The Hammersmith group will be installing a large scale whole hospital PACS, the details of which will be presented in Section 2.2. In Turkey a PACS project is being designed with the cooperation of two universities. The system will be designed and implemented by Bilkent university. It will then be deployed at the Radiology Department, Hacettepe university. Both universities are in Ankara.

1.4. PACS program direction by various manufacturers (Huang et al., 1991)

This section summarizes the PACS research, development, and implementation of five major medical imaging manufacturers: AT&T and Philips, General Electric Medical Systems (GEMS), Siemens Medical Systems, Hitachi Medical Corporation, Toshiba Medical System, and NEC. Philips Medical Systems and AT&T have been involved with various PACS projects for over five years. They have provided PACS products with a trade name CommView in a range of configurations to meet various applications. These products have been based on technology and design requirements which centered on a common core architecture and network configuration. The CommView is based on a distributed processing architecture with a central data management system supporting various size magnetic storage sub-systems, optical archives, network management subsystems and external interfaces to the information system. Both acquisition and display components are interfaced to the data management system via a fiber optic link. The first generation CommViews have several weaknesses in slow image transfer speed, slow display speed, 1-K display monitor, and the lack of a direct digital interface to CT/MR scanners. The newer generation system is supported to minimize these drawbacks and improve the display monitor from 1-K to 2-K.

GEMS invested in PACS as early as 1983 in the worldwide research and development centers – in the USA (Milwaukee), Europe (Buc-France, GE CGR Company, previously owned by Thomson), and at the YMS Headquarters of Tokyo, Japan.

The work started with a 1-K workstation, network and standard interface. First generation systems were installed in 1987. Clinical feedback showed the necessity of a 2-K display for diagnostic display, and better integration at users level. Having defined the development and marketing strategy of the three poles, GEMS together with IBM, for which there is a marketing and development agreement addressing the US market thus far (1991), is now ready to launch the ID-System concept. This concept handles diagnostic workstations

(2 – 4 screen, 2048 × 1536) fully integrated in PACS environment with archiving and communication access, including HIS/RIS integration.

GE PACS research and development effort is committed on both product integration (standard ACR-NEMA, standard modalities CPU, peripheral, user interface) and multimodality workstation application such as CT/MR three-dimensional visualization, and digital X-ray diagnostic/therapy applications such as cardiac and angiography workstations.

Siemens has been working in PACS for several years. One of its first PACS efforts was to introduce the ACR-NEMA standard interface card to its CT/MR scanners. In 1988, Siemens acquired the licensing agreement from Fuji to introduce the Digiscan, a product line which is a modified version of the Fuji CR systems. In the same year, it introduced the diagnostic reporting console (DRC) with eight 1-K monitors. Its latest product is the digital light box concept using a Macintosh computer as host. Siemens started to introduce the whole hospital PACS concept in 1989 and will install the first such system in the SMZO, Vienna, Austria (see Section 2.2).

Hitachi Medical Corporation, with close cooperation on several research and development institutes of Hitachi group, is responsible for the PACS development. Hitachi's strategy in PACS is based on an open architecture. It allows the Hitachi PACS to be integrated with modalities from other manufacturers. Two major clinical partners are Kyoto university and Kobe university hospital. There are a total of ten systems installed. The largest system is composed of a star and ring architecture in which three workstations, three CTs, two laser printers, one MR, one DSA, one FCR, one film digitizer, two optical disk libraries and an image database management system are connected. The smallest system consists of two CTs, one workstation, and an optical disk unit. The future plan of Hitachi PACS is to integrate the personal health data recording system and the diagnostic reporting system to PACS as well as implementing a hospital-wide PACS in the Tokyo Hitachi hospital.

Toshiba hospital systems' PACS development is very extensive. Its input includes Toshiba CT and MR scanners and the TCR (Toshiba computed radiography). Its file management system and the display unit is called TDIS-FILE. It consists of multiple 1-K display monitors and an optical disk library. It has more than 30 installations in Japan. Its two major clinical partners are Nagoya university and the national defense medical college, Japan (Huang et al., 1990a). In the United States, it is the university of Arizona, Tucson.

NEC, the Japanese electronic company, has an extensive collaborative project with the Hokkaido university (see Section 2.2). However, NEC is not offering any commercial products at present.

1.5. UCLA experience

At UCLA, we started PACS research and development in 1984 by first establishing the medical imaging division in the department of radiological sciences. Our research and development efforts can be generalized in three phases. Phase I, from 1984 – 1990, is for demonstration of the concept and the design of PACS infrastructure. Phase II, from 1990 – 1991, is for clinical implementations of several PACS modules. Phase III, from 1992 on, is for clinical implementation of other modules and PACS applications.

Phase I – demonstration of concept and PACS infrastructure

Demonstration of concept. To demonstrate the concept, in 1987 we implemented two PACS modules, one in pediatric radiology (within the department) (Taira et al., 1988), and the other in coronary care unit (CCU) (Cho et al., 1988). The pediatric radiology section was selected because it operates independently and resembles a mini-radiology department. It is an excellent model with which to study the total PACS implementation for the radiology department. In this module, images are displayed on six 1024-line monitors and on two 2048-line monitors. The module is used for daily conference and case review. The CCU was chosen for the second PACS module because a viewing station in this unit is convenient for clinicians who need to stay near their patients. It is a model of the PACS outside of the radiology department. In this module, images are displayed on three 1024-line monitors. Both modules are in clinical operation 24 hours a day, 7 days a week. The reaction from both radiologists and clinicians of using these two systems is very positive. The results were documented (Cho et al., 1988; Taira et al., 1988).

Now that we had demonstrated the PACS concepts, we were ready for planning a digital radiology department. However, we faced a problem in that the two systems implemented were actually not modules but isolated islands. The earlier design did not consider the connectivity. This mistake was partially due to the lack of understanding of the complexity of a total PACS at that time.

PACS infrastructure. From 1988 – 1990, we concentrated on the design of the PACS infrastructure. The critical components in the infrastructure are the communication systems, cluster controllers, database, fault tolerance design, and system integration software (Huang et al., 1990b). This infrastructure will support a digital-based radiology operation.

Communication system. We designed a three-tier fiber optic communication system with Ethernet, FDDI, and Ultranet (Huang et al., 1990c; Stewart, 1991; Stewart et al., 1991). Ethernet is used to transmit images from acquisition devices to the acquisition computer where the speed of transmission is not critical. This is because the acquisition device is slow in generating images. Images are reformatted at the acquisition computer and sent to the cluster controller with FDDI. Images are archived onto the optical disk libraries and distributed to the image display stations with the one Gbitps (Gbit/s) Ultranet. The three communication networks are coexistent in the infrastructure and they serve as the backup of the others.

Cluster controller.   There are multiple cluster controllers in the infrastructure. Each cluster controller is composed of a Sun 4/490 SPARC Image Server with 4-Gbyte magnetic disk storage, and a 1-Tbyte optical disk library for images, and a SUN 4/490 SPARC Server running the Sybase database for patient directory and text information. The architecture of each cluster controller is identical and can be used as the backup of the others. Cluster controllers are connected with the Ultranet. Images can be transmitted between cluster controllers at 4 – 8 Mbyteps. Figures 1, 2 and 3, show the hardware configuration, the communications software, and the data flow in the cluster controller, respectively.

Database.   An identical Sybase database exists in each cluster controller. Current patient image information is updated continuously on the database of even cluster controllers.

Fault tolerance design.   In the infrastructure, every component has a backup. The database exists in multiple copies, one in each cluster controller. Each cluster controller is located in a separate room to avoid potential disaster. The

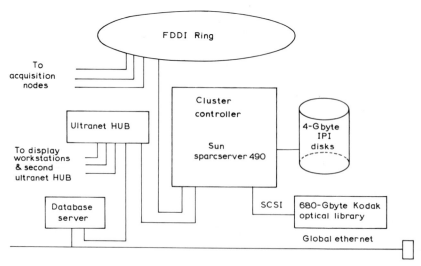

Fig. 1. Hardware configuration of cluster controller.

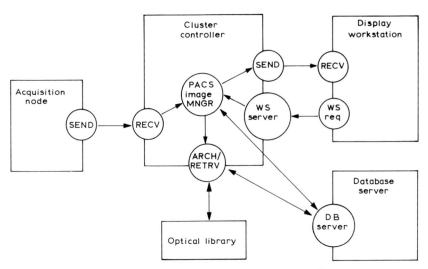

Fig. 2. Communication software in cluster controller.

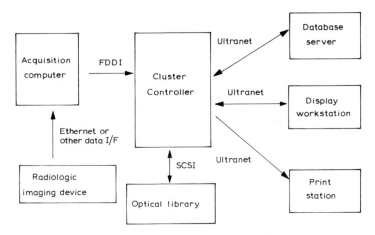

Fig. 3. Data flow in a cluster controller.

three communication networks backup each other and all active fiber optic cables have a duplicate. Each cluster controller is powered by an uninterruptible power supply (UPS) with up to 20 min of uninterrupted power.

From 1990 to 1991, we implemented the infrastructure. There are 64 multimode and 48 single-mode fibers connecting three buildings (Center for Health Sciences, Medical Plaza, and Taper building) housing the radiology department. There are two cluster controllers, one at the Center for Health Sciences

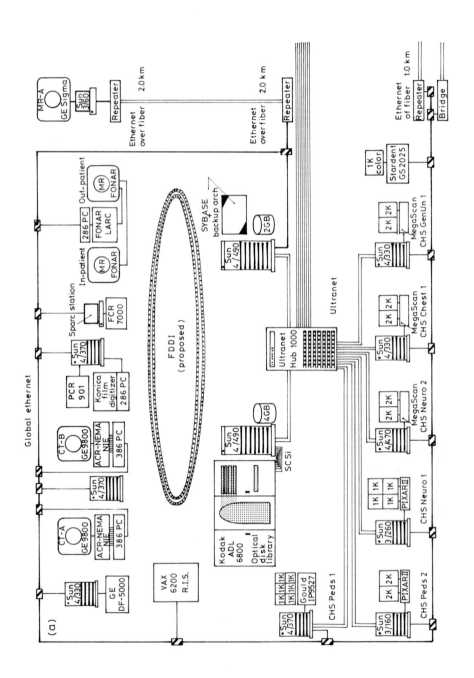

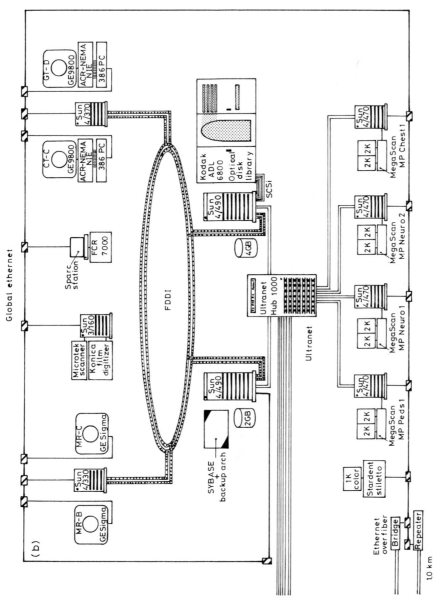

Fig. 4. UCLA PACS intrastructure, image acquisition, and display stations (adopted from Stewart, 1991). (a) The network at the Center for Health Sciences and the remote MR site, (b) the network at Medical Plaza.

and one at the Medical Plaza. The infrastructure has been on-line since the beginning of 1991.

Phase II – image acquisition and display station

For phase II, two tasks are defined. The first task is to connect image acquisition devices to the cluster controller through the infrastructure. The second is to design and implement display stations in the department and clinics. We have successfully connected three CT and three MR scanners with direct digital interface to acquisition computers and to two cluster controllers. Also, three CRs and three film digitizers are connected. The establishment of the infrastructure makes these connections possible. Future connections of new acquisition devices will become a routine engineering exercise.

We are developing standard 2-K- and 1-K-monitor display stations. The 2-K station consists of a Sun 4/470 host computer, a two-monitor Megascan 2-K display system, a 2.4-Gbyte parallel transfer disk storage, and an X-window standard display software. The 1-K station is comprised of a Sun 4/E host computer, a three-monitor or six-monitor 1-K display system, a 1-Gbyte magnetic disk, and an X-window standard display software. The 2-K-monitor stations are for the radiology department and for use in primary diagnosis. The 1-K-monitor station is for the hospital wards and for conference and case reviews. We have two 2-K-monitor stations, one in pediatric radiology and the second in genitourinary radiology for clinical evaluation. The 1-K-monitor station is designed and built in our laboratory. Three stations in the pediatric ICU, neonatal ICU, and CCU will be on-line in the later part of 1991. Phase III will be described in Section 2.3. Figure 4 shows the UCLA network as of today.

2. Perspective

2.1. PACS modules and components

Modules

PACS has many definitions depending on the user's perspective. It can be as simple as a CR connected to a display station with an image management system ('mini-PACS' for example), or it can be as complex as a total hospital imaging system. We believe two types of PACS modules, in teleradiology and for ICU, will be among the first to proliferate.

Teleradiology has two major applications. It can be used to connect peripheral imaging centers to a major radiology consultation center. In this scenario, an imaging center is equipped with diagnostic modalities, technologists, and a general radiologist. Routine radiologic diagnosis will be done at the imaging center; cases required the attention of a specialist will be transmitted through teleradiology to the consultation center for interpretation. An example is the Mayo Clinics with peripheral imaging centers in Florida and in Arizona, whereas the consultation center is in Rochester, Minnesota. The reason for such a set-up is to deliver the best possible radiology service to the patient. The peripheral imaging centers provide a convenient examination site so that the patient does not have to travel extensively for the examination. The remote diagnosis by the specialist provides the patient examination with the expert opinion.

The second application in teleradiology is to serve remote and rural areas where radiologist are scarce. A radiologist receives contracts from various imaging centers within a radius of a few hundred miles to review images. He/she travels among these centers to review images at certain days of the week. It is not uncommon for a patient in a rural area to wait for a radiologist to drop by to review the images a couple of days after the examination has been done.

Teleradiology becomes very useful in this situation. Each imaging center can transmit images to a preferred location for the radiologist to make the diagnosis. Or images can be transmitted to a metropolitan area where a consultation center is located. To fully utilize the capability of teleradiology is an important strategic planning in the U.S. Army because of the many remote army health care stations.

In the case of ICU application, the important factor is the timing required in providing the necessary radiologic services. In a couple of clinical evaluation sites (Arenson et al., 1988; Cho et al., 1988), results clearly demonstrate that PACS will improve the efficiency as well as the clinical services in the ICUs. In applying teleradiology in ICU, there are two possible system designs. The first method is to have the digital imaging system including the transmission component located in the radiology department, and the display component in the ICU. Examinations are performed at the ICU and brought to the radiology department for processing either in the analog or the digital mode. If the analog mode is used, a film digitizer is necessary to convert it to a digital image. A radiologist can perform the wet reading, the digital image along with the digital voice dictation are transmitted to the ICU for the referring clinician. The second design is to have the imaging system, transmission component, and the display component in the ICU. A high-resolution display system is also placed in the radiology department. In this arrangement, the digital image from the radiologic examination is generated at the ICU. Images are transmitted to the radiology department to be read. Digital voice dictation is transmitted from the radiology department to the ICU which is appended to the image. Both architectures have some advantage and disadvantage. In the first design, the technologist is still required to bring the exposed film cassette or CR plate to the department for processing. A trip normally takes 30 min. In the second design, it requires the department to place a digital imaging system, e.g., a CR, in the ICU as well as a high-resolution display system in the department. The requirement of two additional components will increase the cost of the system.

Components

Three major components essential for PACS are: compact and inexpensive CR, high-quality daylight and a 'dry' hard copier, and inexpensive high capacity media for personal imaging file. A film digitizer is only an intermediate step before CR becomes commonly affordable. We anticipate compact and inexpensive CR with high image quality will become available in the next couple of years. This component is essential for the teleradiology and the PACS module in ICU. A compact CR system is analogous to a remote film processor except that it is an electronic processor and it does not require water. The installation of such a system should be lower in cost and easier than that of a remote film processor.

Although PACS is a digital-based system, we believe that some form of hard copy is still necessary in a radiology operation. A new type of high image quality hard copy system which is straightly electronic and does not require wet processing will emerge. This component can be attached to the PACS as a printing station. It is used when a hard copy becomes necessary, e.g., for an outside referral physician who has no access to the PACS.

Another component which is important for a successful PACS operation is a low cost media for storing personal images. The concept of a personal imaging file system is not new (Huang et al., 1989). However, it has not materialized because of the expensive media. We expect an inexpensive media, 100 Mbyte capacity costing a few dollars will become available in two to three years. With this type of media, the patient can easily possess his/her own images in a very compact form. This arrangement will alleviate a major problem of image storage in the radiology department. We have seen a demonstration of prototypes of these three components in research laboratories. The chance of seeing them in the market is very high.

2.2. Large-scale PACS projects

We anticipate a few large-scale PACS projects will materalize. Large-scale PACS is a necessary stimulus for the radiology community to accept PACS. In this section we discuss four large-scale PACS projects which have the potential to be clinically operable in the next few years. All these four projects select the second approach described in Section 1.2.

Hokkaido university medical information system project

Hokkaido university PACS project (Irie, 1991) in Japan is probably one of the largest scale projects in medical information systems. It integrates PACS, hospital information systems, and medical records together. There are three networks, one for each system. The project, started in 1989, adopts a top-down approach and is a whole hospital information system, connected together through a PACS loop. The system is designed and implemented by NEC. The department used CR exclusively and all CR are connected to the network. Currently, there are twenty 1-K-monitor display stations, each equipped with look-up-table, rotation, inverse, zoom and scroll, subtract, edge enhancement, and linear and angular measurement function software. The system handles 30% CR images (300 films/day), 100% CT, MR, DSA (500 films/day). Images stay in magnetic disks for one week and older images can be retrieved from the optical disk library in 40 – 60 s. As of today, clinical evaluation concludes that:

(a) 75% of the orthopedics feel that the quality on CRT is as good as on film;
(b) all users feel that it takes too long to use the CRT;
(c) radiologists feel CT/MR images are good on the CRT;
(d) two monitors are not sufficient for radiologists to make diagnoses.

The system is continuously upgraded by NEC. Its final target date integrating the medical records is in 1993. The medical records will include images from echography, endography and microscopy, as well as charts from EEG, ECG and EMG. The number of terminals will be approximately 200.

Vienna SMZO social and medical center East project

The SMZO in Vienna, Austria (Masser et al., 1991) is a 1400 bed teaching hospital with nurse training and a geriatric center. It will start operation in 1991 and serve 100 000 people. The planning of PACS started in November 1989, with a team with members from the hospital and the vendor. It adopts a top-down approach integrating PACS, RIS, and HIS together. The data include organization, information production, and communication links. The planning is based on a two-level approach: macro and micro. The computer science department in the hospital and the development group from Siemens are in charge of the macro planning whereas the radiology department is in charge of the micro planning. The system architecture is based on a token ring topology with the 100 Mbitps FDDI, its database and network adheres to the ACR-NEMA standard.

There are two optical disk libraries with on-line access of 2×179 Gbytes. The system has a fault tolerant control image management system including storage and archiving. In the radiology department the workstation will be $2 - 8$ monitors whereas in the hospital it will be a PC-based inexpensive display station. The system anticipates data volume about 9 Gbyte per day in the first two years of operation. The system installation is expected in late 1991. Opening will be in March, 1992, with continuing modification and fine tuning. The project has a built-in five year upgrade and update program.

Hammersmith hospital project

The Hammersmith hospital in London, England (Glass and Slark, 1991) is building a new radiology department. A committee chaired by the hospital director of finance and information is planning a top-down whole hospital PACS project. The hypothesis of the project is that cost savings arising from PACS will be due to increases in the efficiency in the hospital. The Hammersmith hospital includes the royal postgraduate medical school and the institute of obstetrics and gynecology. It consists of 543 beds and serves 100 000 people. The specification is based on the medical diagnostic imaging support system (MDIS, see next section). The justification of the project is based on the direct cost/saving and the indirect cost/saving components. In the direct cost/saving, the following components are considered: archive material and film use, labor, maintenance, operation and supplies, space and capital equipment and buildings. The indirect cost/saving is comprised of junior medical staff time, reductions in unnecessary investigations, saving in radiologists, technologists and clinician time, re-designation and change of use of a number of acute beds, and reduction in the length of stay. The target dates of the project are: installation in end of 1992, amendment in August, 1993, and evaluation in January, 1994.

Medical diagnostic imaging support systems for the military medicine project

The MDIS project in the U.S. (Goeringer, 1991) tries to achieve the objective of implementing filmless medical imaging systems at several military medical treatment facilities over the next four years. The surgeon general of the military services created the MDIS project to exploit the results of extensive imaging research efforts over the past ten years. These filmless MDIS systems will be required from industry through a contracting approach that (a) functionally describes subsystem and system performance for acceptable clinical operations, (b) validates proposed systems in performance evaluation, and (c) makes a system selection and contract award on the basis of best value to the U.S. government. The first four sites of the MDIS project will be Madigan army hospital, Washington; Brooks air force – army hospital, Texas; Wright – Patterson air force hospital, Ohio, and Luke Davis – Monthan air force hospital, Arizona. The target dates of the first four sites are as follows: Phase I, six months after the contract awarded, basic MDIS for inpatients should be operational (40% digital). Phase II consists of a graceful MDIS transition including the high volume outpatient examinations (65% digital). Finally,

Phase III is for refinement and to include low volume outpatient examinations (90%). The contract was awarded in late 1991. The MDIS technical specifications are considered as one of the most comprehensive PACS requirements and implementation plan. It could become an industry standard.

These four large-scale PACS projects have past the first few hurdles of system design, fund raising, and site selection. The success of their clinical operation will demonstrate that the vendor can provide a PACS for a specific site. It will also provide the medical community solid data for future PACS planning and implementation.

2.3. UCLA perspective

UCLA PACS research and development is comprised of three phases. The first phase is the demonstration of the concept and PACS infrastructure and the second phase is the implementation of image acquisition and display station. Phase III is comprised of three stages. Stage one is the continuing development of display stations and their clinical implementation. Stage two is on system refinement, display stations software upgrade and the establishment of training, maintenance and service. Stage three is on PACS applications.

Stage one – display station and clinical implementation

In this stage, five 2-K-monitor stations will be implemented in the pediatric (two stations), neuroradiology, chest and bone radiology section. In addition, one printing station will be implemented as a hard copy device with the new technology described in Section 2.1. Additional 2-K-monitor stations will be added as required after stage two. Additional 1-K-monitor stations will also be implemented in hospital wards as needed. Implementation of additional 2-K- and 1-K-monitor stations will not be in the research and development category and will be purely engineering. Figure 4 shows the UCLA PACS infrastructure image acquisition and display stations.

Stage two – system refinement and training, maintenance, service

The five 2-K-monitor stations and three 1-K-monitor stations will go through system refinement in the clinical environment during stage two. System refinement will include hardware and software upgrade. Both hardware and software upgrade will be identical for all stations. These upgrades include all basic operation functions for primary diagnosis, conference and review.

During clinical implementation, we will also set up procedures for training, system maintenance and service. Training is in three categories: the first category is radiologists and clinicians. Training for this category is simple and should be no more than 15 min since the display station is designed as simple to use and user-friendly. The second category is for PACS coordinator, technologists and clerical personnel. This training is extensive, it includes quality assurance, patient directory update, and first-line trouble shooting. The third category is for PACS engineers. This training is most elaborative, it includes all operational aspects of PACS. We currently (1991) have two PACS coordinators and engineers in training. They are integrated in the PACS research and development team to gain experience. We are planning to shift the department radiology engineering service staff and some technologists gradually to the PACS service and engineering for long-term service and maintenance.

Stage three – PACS applications
We are now convinced that PACS is not just a management tool; PACS is a vehicle for future radiology practice and research. For this reason, we have planned three research areas in PACS applications. The first research area is in image quantification which includes the conventional image measurement methods, image reformatting and registration, and deriving parameters from images. This research area is to explore the potential of extracting information from digital images to facilitate radiologic diagnosis. The second area of research is interactive teaching. Traditional radiology teaching is passive in the sense that learning is through teacher and textbook. PACS can be used as an interactive teaching tool for diagnostic radiology through the rich PACS database. The third area of research is on knowledge base. Information science has taught us to derive knowledge from a database. However, so far the database has been limited to text information since no large radiologic (digital) image database has ever been in existence. The PACS database is the hidden treasure which awaits the probing by the hunters. We anticipate the knowledge base will open a new horizon for radiologic research.

3. Conclusion

We have given a brief review on the history of PACS and the three basic methods of PACS research, development and implementation. Based on the information acquired during the 1990 NATO ASI 'PACS in Medicine' held in Evian, France, we summarized PACS research in various countries and by imaging manufacturers.

We anticipate teleradiology and ICU modules will be the first two useful products of PACS. Three important components in PACS' future development are compact CR, daylight 'dry' image printer, and compact, high-density, inexpensive optical media for personal image archival. The three large scale hospital

PACS projects in Hokkaido, Vienna social and medical center East and Hammersmith hospital as well as the MDIS for the U.S. military medical project will influence the future progress and approach in PACS research, development and implementation.

We also discussed the UCLA PACS research, development and implementation plan. It is important to realize that PACS is more than an image management system, PACS is a tool which will revolutionize the practice and research of radiology.

Acknowledgement

This work was supported in part by Public Health Service Grant No. RO1 CA39063, RO1 CA40456, and PO1 CA51198, awarded by the National Cancer Institute, Department of Health and Human Services; by Konica Corporation, Philips Medical Systems, Inc., GEMS, Kodak, and Lumisys; and by the UCLA Department of Radiological Sciences Research Fund. Some material is extracted from the NATO ASI 'PACS in Medicine' held in Evian, France, October 1990. I appreciate the contribution by the staff in the Medical Imaging Division, Department of Radiological Sciences, UCLA during the past eight years.

References

Arenson, R.L., S. Seshadri, H.L. Kundel, D. DeSimone, F. Van der Voorde, W.B. Gefter, D.M. Epstein, W.T. Miller, J.M. Aronchick, M.B. Simson, P.N. Lanken, S. Khalsa, I. Brikman, M. Davey and N. Bribon (1988) Clinical evaluation of a medical image management system for chest images, *Am. J. Roentgenol.* 150, 55–59.

Cho, P.S., H.K. Huang, J. Tillisch and H. Kangarloo (1988) Clinical evaluation of a radiologic picture archiving and communication system for a coronary care unit, *Am. J. Roentgenol.* 151, 823–827.

Curtis, D.J., B.W. Gayler, J.N. Gitlin and M.B. Harrington (1983) Teleradiology: results of a field trial, *Radiology* 149, 415–418.

Duerinckx, A.J. (Ed.) (1982) Picture Archiving and Communication Systems (PACS) for Medical Applications, First International Conference and Workshop, *Proc. SPIE* 318.

Dwyer III, S.J. (Ed.) (1983) Picture Archiving and Communication Systems (PACS) for Medical Applications, Second International Conference and Workshop, *Proc. SPIE* 418.

Glass, H.I., and N.A. Slark (1991) PACS and related research in the U.K. In: Huang, H.K., O. Ratib, A.R. Bakker and G. Witte (Eds.), Picture Archiving and Communication Systems (PACS) in Medicine, *NATO ASI Series F* 74, 319–324 (Springer, Berlin).

Goeringer, F. (1991) Medical diagnostic imaging support systems for military medicine. In: Huang, H.K, O. Ratib, A.R. Bakker and G. Witte (Eds.), Picture Archiving and Communication Systems (PACS) in Medicine, *NATO ASI Series F* 74, 213–230 (Springer, Berlin).

Huang, H.K., P.S. Cho, O. Ratib, B.K. Ho and C. Morioka (1989) Personal digital image filming system, *Radiology* 173 (P), 292.

Huang, H.K., P.S. Cho, R. Taira, B.K. Ho and K.K. Chan (1990a) Picture archiving and communication systems in Japan: 3 years later, *Am. J. Roentgenol.* 154, 415–417.

Huang, H.K., H. Kangarloo, P.S. Cho, R. Taira, B.K. Ho and K.K. Chan (1990b) Planning a total digital radiology department, *Am. J. Roentgenol.* 154, 634–639.

Huang, H.K., S.L. Lou, P.S. Cho, D.J. Valentino, A.W.K. Wong, K.K. Chan and B.K. Stewart (1990c) Radiologic image communication methods, *Am. J. Roentgenol.* 155, 183–186.

Huang, H.K., O. Ratib, A. Bakker and G. Witte (Eds.) (1991) Picture Archiving and Communication Systems (PACS) in Medicine, *NATO ASI Series F* 74 (Springer, Berlin).

Irie, G. (1991) Clinical experience – 16 months of Hu – PACS. In: Huang, H.K., O. Ratib, A.R. Bakker and G. Witte (Eds.), Picture Archiving and Communication Systems (PACS) in Medicine, *NATO ASI Series F* 74, 183–188 (Springer, Berlin).

Masser, H., A. Mandl, M. Urban, H. Hradil and W. Hruby (1991) The Vienna project SMZO. In: Huang, H.K., O. Ratib, A.R. Bakker and G. Witte (Eds.), Picture Archiving and Communication Systems (PACS) in Medicine, *NATO ASI Series F* 74, 247–250 (Springer, Berlin).

Medical Imaging Technology (1986) The Fifth MIT and the Third PACS/PHD Symposia, Vol. 4, No. 2.

Multiple Viewing Station for Diagnostic Radiology (1985) RO1 CA39063 National Cancer Institute, Department of Health and Human Services.

Schneider, R.H., S.J. Dwyer III and R.G. Jost (Eds.) (1989) Medical Imaging III, *Proc. SPIE* 1090, 1091, 1092 and 1093.

Stewart, B.K. (1991) Three-tiered network architecture for PACS cluster. In: Huang H.K., O. Ratib, A.R. Bakker and G. Witte (Eds.), Picture Archiving and Communication Systems (PACS) in Medicine, *NATO ASI Series F* 74, 113–118 (Springer, Berlin).

Stewart, B.K., S.L. Lou, W.K. Wong and H.K. Huang (1991) An ultrafast network for communication of radiologic image, *Am. J. Roentgenol.* 156, 835–839.

Taira, R.K., N.J. Mankovich, M.I. Boechat, H. Kangarloo and H.K. Huang (1988) Design and implementation of a picture archiving and communication system for pediatric radiology, *Am. J. Roentgenol.* 150, 1117–1121.

The MITRE Corporation (1985) Installation Site for Digital Network and Picture Archiving and Communication Systems (DIN/PACS), RFP B52-1545.

Integrated Diagnostic Imaging
Editor: J.P.J. De Valk
© *Elsevier Science Publishers B.V., 1992*

Chapter 4

Clinical integration of image management and communication (IMAC) network

Seong K. Mun

1. Introduction and problem definition in radiology operations

An image management and communication (IMAC) system is a computer network supported by imaging devices, archive, temporary on-line storages, communication capabilities, workstations and other peripherals to provide diagnostic decision support functions in a radiology service. IMAC, also known as picture archiving and communication system (PACS), has been a topic of growing interest in the medical community, especially in radiology. The Georgetown project and other similar projects have demonstrated that radiological images can be archived, communicated and displayed electronically. However, the general goal of improving the global efficiency of the radiology image management service by means of IMAC technology has not been fully achieved. This paper reviews the progress of the IMAC project and its clinical integration and suggests possible future directions.

IMAC is important because the current film-based system has major flaws that result in less than optimal patient care in spite of a high cost of operations. Radiologists are so accustomed to and comfortable with films, as far as image quality itself is concerned, that they are reluctant to accept other image display media even though the new media could solve many of the image management problems except in crisis situations. When crises occur, the common response is to increase the use of film and the number of people to manage films, for example, intensive care unit (ICU) physicians complaint about access to relevant images and request to copy all ICU images. The paradigm is that in an information age it is the two-way flow of information in a timely manner that determines the quality of a process. Among radiologists, there is very high degree of satisfaction in the technological developments of individual diagnostic imaging devices in the 1970s and 1980s, but radiology does not yet provide integrated information easily and rapidly to the referring physicians and radiologists. Radiologists often work with information distributed throughout a department. Portions of this information are available in the subspecialty areas, but this specialization and the associated work patterns may serve to inhibit the collection of these information segments into an integrated multimodality diagnosis.

Chronic problems in the management of X-ray films call for significant improvements and rethinking the handling of radiological films. These problems are met currently using a variety of methods that tend to be labor intensive and unreliable. As many new digital modalities are introduced in radiology, more labor intensive and specialized fragmented manual activities are patched into the existing system, making the entire radiology operation more cumbersome and expensive.

At Georgetown University Hospital (GUH) we have surveyed 826 jackets that were requested by referring physicians. Initially the data showed a rather large failed retrieval rate of 36% (293 out of 826). However, a majority of missing cases were due to new patients who had never completed the requested study. Excluding these cases the failure rate is 13%. Twenty-two requests were not fulfilled because they were assigned to other 'competing users'. This leaves 84 cases (10%) that cannot be retrieved due to the failure of the current film-based system. The cases with data problems involve wrong birth dates, duplicated ID's or imcomplete information. This 10% may be considered as the true failure rate. This is a significant rate of loss familiar to many of us but it should not be the norm.

The current manual image management in radiology is a complex and expensive task and a conventional approach has not proven satisfactory in terms of efficiency, productivity, cost and quality of service. Furthermore, an increase in resources alone has not provided adequate solutions to the rapidly changing radiology environment. It is doubtful that one can afford to continue operation in a manual mode for many more years.

For radiologists, a great deal of time is spent collecting clinical data and images for diagnosis and communicating with referring physicians through a long list of manual operations. Often this process breaks down. One should seek an improved method of managing radiology service using available computer technologies. Advances in computer technology and image processing and display make it possible to develop a film-independent radiology service for the entire hospital.

2. A potential solution: IMAC

The IMAC network is a functional single entity that provides radiologic image and data management support within a hospital or between supporting and supported hospitals. While performance of each IMAC network component and subsystem is important, the integrated performance of the entire system is the most meaningful measure of clinical acceptability in providing a quality patient care solution.

A comprehensive IMAC network (as shown in fig. 1) consists of the following major functional capabilities:
- image and data capture (input imaging device);
- storage of images throughout the network (database and archive);
- image and data retrieval and distribution (communication);
- image handling and processing (workstation group);
- special applications and research and educational support;
- communication with external system;
- interface to a radiology information system (RIS).

Input devices can be a computed radiography (CR) for projection radiographs, a film digitizer to convert films to digital images, interfaces to digital imaging systems such as MRI and CT. Databases consist of data manager, image storage and archival storage and interface to radiology information system for patient demographics and diagnostic report. The communication system can be any combination of media and configuration depending on the required performance. A link to teleradiology may be needed to support long-distance diagnostic support capabilities. Images can be displayed on either reporting workstations or review workstations. There must also be a laser film printer to make hard copies for other facilities without a compatible system. A special application platform is needed to support research and education efforts. Communication with external system can be a teleradiology support function.

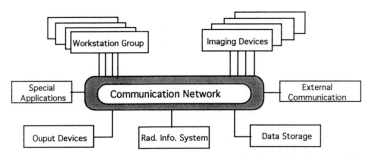

Fig. 1. Conceptual image management and communication (IMAC) network.

The IMAC network system should support the following operational scenario for radiologic practice.

Exams are ordered in the radiology information system (RIS) environment. This order entry information is sent to IMAC network through the RIS – IMAC network interface. The IMAC network system checks its database for previous exams and, if appropriate, automatically restores them from the long-term archive to the short-term storage for autorouting to the primary reading diagnostic workstation.

When a patient reports to the radiology department for an exam, a radiology technologist logs the order request data on the IMAC network and verifies the accuracy. Next, the patient demographics and particulars of the radiologic exam order will be transmitted from RIS to IMAC network automatically. This verification action should require a minimum of typing (patient name or medical record number), barcode reading or equivalent. If information, such as examination type, is incorrect, the technologist will correct it at this time. The new radiology exams are acquired and, following an image quality control check at the image acquisition site, the image or examination is presented to the network. These images and associated data are routed on the network to the database storage. They are then available on short-term or workstation local storage for viewing at appropriate workstations.

The network shall support routing of images from one workstation to a selected second workstation (diagnostic or clinical for either workstation) at the request of the sending workstation user.

Diagnostic workstation storage receives images and text from image storage or directly from imaging devices. By the time a radiologist goes to a workstation for a clinical session, all the necessary images shall be pre-loaded in workstation local storage. Based on the preselected protocol, the worklist of images shall be presented to the users for diagnosis and review. In some cases – e.g., emergency exams – images are immediately routed so that they are available at a particular workstation or hard copy device as they are produced. The selection and presentation variables are orientation of image, display order by image modality, time of image acquisition, and image acquisition paremeters.

The radiologist selects exams from the worklist and performs interpretation. The required method of operation is to have the worklist updated automatically with new images. Associated images and reports from previous exams are available on the workstation for review with the new examination. Reports are dictated at the workstation and transcribed into the RIS. Subsequently, the reports are introduced into the IMAC network system along with appropriate patient data elements so that they are logically matched with the examinations in the patient image exam folder. If a report has been received by IMAC network from the RIS, it is displayed when the corresponding examination is displayed.

Images that are in the short-term storage (STS) or long-term archive (LTA) are available for viewing at various workstations on demand.

The database autoroutes radiographic and other digital images (i.e., CT, MR, US, etc.) and exams to appropriately identified clinical review workstations located throughout the hospital. Short-term storage and/or local workstation storage holds images which are available for review at the clinical workstation. A local list of available images is present. On an hourly basis or as expedited for emergencies, autorouted images are available at the workstation based on: (1) RIS appointment schedules or (2) radiologic exam orders placed by the referring physician. Additionally, on-demand interrogations of storage devices to retrieve images to a particular workstation are possible.

3. IMAC network at Georgetown University Medical Center

A brief description of the IMAC network system at Georgetown University Hospital is presented. Georgetown University has installed a comprehensive IMAC network. Figure 2 depicts the general system configuration of the Georgetown network as operational in 1991. The primary network topology used in the CommView® system is a star based on 40 Mbps (Mbits/s) optical fiber. The central data management system (DMS) is connected to: (a) acquisition modules (AM) which collect images from imaging devices, (b) high-speed workstations located throughout the hospital, (c) an archival juke box of 89 optical platters, (d) an interface to a RIS through a PC, and (e) gateways that support PC-based workstations and a research environment on an Ethernet.

The central node is equipped with storage capacity of 7.5 Gbytes in a mirrored magnetic disk configuration that reduces the amount of on-line storage, but significantly increases system reliability. The long-term storage medium is a two-sided write-once/read-many (WORM) optical disk with a storage capacity of 2.0 Gbytes. A Cygnet juke box holding 89 optical platters and 2 disk drives supports an average disk exchange time of less than 8.7 s with a data transfer rate of 262 Kbytesps.

The acquisition modules (AM), connected to the DMS by means of high-speed optical fibers that operate under AT&T's communication protocol, are interfaced to imaging systems and film scanners. Each AM has 800 Mbytes of magnetic storage and can acquire images automatically and send them to the DMS. Several AMs are used to avoid bottlenecks on the acquisition side. Seven imaging systems (a Siemens MRI, two GE 9800 CTs, and four ultrasound) and two laser film digitizers are supported by the AMs. A new Agfa ADC computed

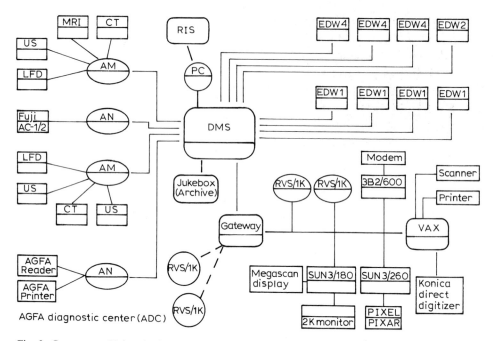

Fig. 2. Georgetown University image management and communication system. LFD: laser film digitizer; AM/N: aquisition module/node; DMS: database management system; EDW4: four screen high-speed workstation; RVS: result viewing system; AGFA reader: phosphor plate reader; AGFA printer: laser printer; Fuji AC 1/2: phosphor plate reader and laser printer.

radiography system is supported by a separate AM. A Fuji CR system, AC-1, has been installed and is to be upgraded to AC1-Plus to accomodate a digital interface to the network.

The IMAC network supports three categories of workstations: (a) high-speed display workstations, (b) results viewing stations (RVS), and (c) special workstations such as SUN3 and 4, SUN SPARC, PIXEL, and PIXAR. The high-speed workstations, enhanced display workstation (EDW), are supported by 40 Mbps optical fiber links. EDWs can be configured with four, two, or a single screen in portrait mode. Each EDW has 760 Mbytes of image and data storage.

The image data matrix size is 2 K × 2.5 K × 12 bits for digitized 14 × 17 inch chest images on the network. The workstation displays 1 K × 1.2 K images, or a full data set can be accessed using the pan or magnification features. Workstations can display 80 MR or CT images in less than 20 s across the four screens. Many PC-based and Macintosh workstations are supported on Ethernet or over a 19.2 K modem.

The GUH network collects approximately 2 500 – 3 000 images per day and provides high-speed four screen workstations to neuroradiology, ultrasound imaging, and general radiology. Single or dual screen high-speed workstations are located in nuclear medicine, the cardiac surgical intensive care unit, the intensive care nursery, and the pediatric intensive care unit. Additional workstations are placed in various locations in the hospital.

The IMAC network is interfaced with a hospital information system (HIS) that contains a RIS. Selected patient information is pushed unidirectionally from the RIS to the IMAC. Radiological reports managed by RIS are also pushed to the network.

A research environment for a developmental network is based on Ethernet and it is connected to the Comm View® network through a gateway. Image and information exchange between the clinical and developmental environments is supported by DECSTATION 5000, SUN computers, PIXEL, PIXAR, Mega-scan 2 K display monitor, Macintosh II workstations, and PC workstations.

4. Clinical integration and experience with an IMAC network at Georgetown

The IMAC network at Georgetown has been operational for four years. Our experience, including successes and disappointments, is summarized in this section.

The areas of IMAC technology that have been highly successful at Georgetown are:
- provision of portable ICU images over a high-speed network;
- teleradiology applications with distant locations;
- archiving of a large number of multimodality diagnostic images;
- rapid retrieval and display of multimodality images;
- multiple simultaneous access to images;
- sharing of data through an interface with RIS;
- diagnostic image quality in the case of ultrasound and MRI.

A number of major remaining problems preventing us from moving to filmless radiology operations are:
- incomplete image and data presentation;
- limited workstation functions beyond image display;
- limited database operations;
- no immediate and obvious advantage to change;
- poor image quality in the case of chest imaging and CT;
- lack of hard copy capability off the network;
- unresponsiveness;
- poor reliability and dependability;
- high cost of the system.

Portable films have been digitized and transmitted to high-speed workstations located in intensive care units with a great deal of success. For referring physicians, GUH has shown that the time saved results in more time spent by the physicians with critically ill patients. While this may not mean improved productivity, the physicians agreed that this does translate into better patient care. Referring physicians welcome the use of soft copy workstations in the pediatric intensive care unit (PICU) and intensive care nursery (ICN), because the workstations provide reliable and convenient access to critical images and the point has been reached where those clinicians are heavily dependent on the system.

Teleradiology has been an important extension of our digital imaging network system (DINS) project because of the interest of our funding agency, the US Army. Teleradiology can be seen as a subsystem of a larger IMAC network. In the military medicine, expert radiology service must be provided to many remote medical treatment facilities (MTF) that are a long distance away from radiologists.

We have done a number of teleradiology projects using T-1 lines, telephone lines, and satellite links. Neuroradiology images of MRI and CT at an outpatient imaging center located 13 miles away from GUH were sent over a dedicated T-1 line (1.5 Mbps) to GUH for radiological consultation for two years.

A temporary off-shore National Guard Hospital facility was established in St. Croix in the Virgin Islands after a permanent hospital was destroyed by hurricane Hugo. Chest films were digitized using a DuPont laser digitizer. Using an AT&T teleradiology system the images were sent first to a satellite link using a portable radio at 19.2 Kbps rate and the signal was sent to an earth station and then to Walter Reed Medical Center, Georgetown University in Washington, D.C. and Eisenhower Medical Center in Georgia. Often, poor communication interrupted image transmission and required lengthy retransmission. Automatic recovery routing had to be developed so that retransmission could start from where the line drop occurred. While it was possible to send over 70 images over the 19.2 Kbps modems, long transmission makes routine clinical operations impractical for chest images without significant data compression.

Currently two radiologists have workstations at home for on-call coverage. Images are communicated over regular telephone lines. These on-call workstations have proved to be very useful and effective in providing timely radiology service at all times.

Approximately 3000 frames of images (all MR, CT, ultrasound, and most of the ICU images) are acquired daily on our IMAC network. They are then stored in magnetic storage for two days and subsequently archived onto optical disks managed by an 89 platter juke box. While no film processors or film libraries have been replaced by IMAC technology, IMAC storage is serving as a dependable image archive. The use of the network as a film archive has increased significantly as the archive has been growing in its 'collection'.

Since all images and related data are stored electronically, several users of the IMAC network at different locations can examine a given case at the same time, improving the convenience and effectiveness of consultations among busy clinicians. When images are acquired on the network they are automatically directed to the central database and then to targeted workstations. The workstations are loaded with the desired images before a user demands these images at the workstation. This automatic routing feature reduces the peak load demand on the network and dramatically improves the image display time. An image can be 'copied' to multiple workstations so that the network can facilitate simultaneous viewing at a number of workstations.

We have developed a one-way interface between our radiology information system and the IMAC network to 'push' patient demographics. This interface has demonstrated both (a) significant reduction in technologists' work loads and (b) improved database integrity.

Image quality in the digital network environment is determined in part by the quality of the interface to imaging systems and the quality of display. In the case of CT, we are in the process of installing digital interfaces to two GE 9800 CT scanners. We have been operating with a video interface which limits the dynamic range of CT images to 8 bits. This is not adequate for clinical diagnosis because 8 bits do not fully cover the entire dynamic range of CT images of 12 bits.

In the case of ultrasound imaging and nuclear imaging, the image quality is not seen as a road block to a filmless environment. Nuclear medicine images have been routinely reviewed on display monitors for some years. Ultrasound image quality on video monitors has been reported to be acceptable.

In the case of chest images, significant degradation of image quality was noted when they were digitized using a laser film digitizer. The changes in the noise characteristics and dynamic range were especially significant. When the images are displayed in video displays we have found a dramatic change in contrast characteristics.

Currently, only about 20 – 30% of medical images (in terms of data volume) are obtained in digital form; the remainder must be converted for filmless operations. Plans for an IMAC network must include some form of digital replacement for film/screen radiography. At present, computed radiography (CR) systems based on photostimulable phosphor plate readers are best suited for Georgetown. Several computed radiography systems (Konica Direct Digitizer, Fuji AC-1, and Philips prototype CR and AGFA CR unit called

ADC) have been studied. A direct digital interface between the AGFA CR system and our IMAC network has been developed and the interface is under final testing. A number of projects are underway to develop optimized image quality and image management methods with CR images.

There will always be a need for hard copy of images, even if they are not needed for use within the radiology department and the hospital. Images need to be sent to other institutions. Dry hard copy devices will be used.

The Georgetown IMAC network has been evolving over the past several years in the area of network response. When a user requests certain actions at a workstation, it should provide some response informing what the network is doing or not doing so the user can adjust his or her work flow. This type of issue is generic to any computer system design. We believe that such enhancements are outside the scope of the proposed project and we expect they will be made available to us by the vendor.

Over the past several years, we have enjoyed relatively good reliability and dependability with our network. However, the last software and hardware upgrade resulted in down time of approximately 30% over a four month period. This created a serious problem in clinical acceptance. Every time there is a problem, users go back to their old routines and it becomes exceedingly difficult to move them back to a digital environment. This problem is not viewed as scientific in nature and it will not be studied in the program project. As the IMAC technology matures, we expect that such problems will be addressed.

Costs must be examined in a larger picture of conventional methods versus the digital approach. While it is true that IMAC equipment is expensive to acquire, install, and operate, GUH (and other) financial models have shown possible net savings over the continued use of film-based technology.

The experience at Georgetown provided us with a rare opportunity to see the future of a fully automated radiology service. There are a number of obstacles. Technical system integration has been possible, but functional integration will take more time.

5. MDIS project

Based largely on the result of the DINS project at Georgetown University and University of Washington, the US Army and Air Force developed a medical diagnostic imaging support (MDIS) system project to implement IMAC technology at a number of hospitals. The first large hospitals to recieve MDIS technology are the Madigan Army Medical Center (MAMC), Fort Lewis, Tacoma, Washington; the Wright–Patterson Air Force Base, Dayton, Ohio; and Brooke Army Medical Center, Fort Sam Houston, San Antonio, Texas.

The smaller hospitals projected to receive this technology initially include an inter-hospital system link from Luke Air Force Base to Davis-Monthan Air Force Base in Arizona.

The Madigan Army Medical Center is a completely new hospital currently under construction and scheduled to open at the end of 1991. It is projected to be the first 'filmless hospital' by the time full-scale MDIS is implemented. The IMAC systems will be put into operation in a time-phased implementation plan over a period of twelve to thirty-six months as shown in table 1. Each phase represents a 'critical mass' that focuses on a specifically defined portion of radiology service. In phase II, interface with the composite health care system (CHCS) military hospital information system is planned.

Teleradiology (TR) is an important component of the MDIS program because in the military often radiology service must be provided to many remote medical treatment facilities (MTF) scattered around the world. A major teleradiology project is underway in Korea where over 40 000 US troops and their dependents are stationed. The 18th Medical Command, headquartered in Korea, has 3 army radiologists at the 121 Evacuation Hospital and 1 airforce radiologist at the 51st Medical Group to provide radiology service for the troops and their dependents stationed throughout Korea. The total of 17

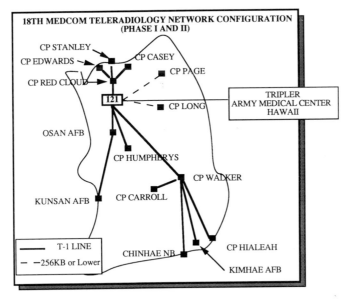

Fig. 3. Proposed teleradiology network for USAF in Korea.

Table 1

Phased implementation summary for a large MTF.

Work-load	Annual: 100 000 radiographic images for inpatients, 300 000 radiographic images for out patients, 900 000 digital images. Clinical days: 250 days per year. 400 inpatients and 1200 outpatients radiographic images/day. 3600 digital images day.		
Phases	Phase I	Phase II	Phase III
Image input devices	All digital modalities: 2 CT, 1 MRI, 2 Angio, 5 Fluoro, and 3 Ultrasound devices CR's images per day (IPD) 1380 IPD for radiology 100 IPD for critical care 120 IPD for orthopedics LFD's for 475 films per day	Nuclear medicine imaging systems CR reader at TMC for teleradiology	CR's for urology and operating room suppport
Diagnostic workstation	Bone radiology - 1 Chest radiology - 2 ER radiology - 1 MR/CT - 1	Workstations in radiology-6 Orthopedic clinic nuclear medicine	Workstation in urology clinic Pulmo, clinics ICU
Clinical workstation	Intensive care units - 5 Emergency room - 3 Nuclear medicine - 1 Radiology - 4	Patient care unit Team center - 12 Operating rooms - 7 Orthopedic - 5 Other clinics - 16	Operating rooms - 7 Other clinics - 29

Table 1
(Continued)

Work-load	Annual: 100 000 radiographic images for inpatients, 300 000 radiographic images for out patients, 900 000 digital images. Clinical days: 250 days per year. 400 inpatients and 1200 outpatients radiographic images/day. 3600 digital images day.		
Phases	Phase I	Phase II	Phase III
Imaging operations	Primary focus in Phase I is to cover inpatient radiology	Phase II MDIS expands to other outpatient services	Phase III expansion covers the rest of the hospital
	All plain radiographs except urology are acquired by CR's	Ultrasound images are read on MDIS workstations	CHCS interface matures*
	For inpatients, selected old films are digitized	Orthopedics start reading on MDIS workstations	
	Laser printers and a 35 mm slide maker are used		
	RIS interface	RIS interface conversion to CHCS*	

* May be implemented in an earlier phase if CHCS is present.

military medical facilities, 12 army, 3 airforce and 1 navy medical facilities in Korea will be covered by this projects in two phases.

The present method of providing diagnostic radiology support to clinics scattered throughout Korea is inadequate. Films are bused in daily or weekly from these remote clinics to the 121 Evacuation Hospital for radiologist reading. Once the diagnosis is made the images and reports are bused back to clinics. In many cases, especially for the army, radiology service turnaround time is as long as two weeks. In emergencies, since proper diagnosis cannot be obtained, air evacuation is carried out to be safe. These unnecessary evacuations are very costly.

The TR system in Korea will provide the ability to acquire diagnostic medical images at remote sites and electronically transmit them to the central site – either the 121 Evacuation Hospital in Seoul or the 51st Tactical Fighter Wing (TFW) Hospital at Osan AFB for clinical diagnosis and consultation. The system will improve the speed and quality of radiology service and reduce the dependency on radiographic films that requires expensive logistical support.

Figure 3 shows locations of medical facilities in Korea and two types of high-speed communication lines to move diagnostic images. The digital form of chest or bone films can be acquired either by laser digitization of a radiographic film or by use of computed radiography (CR). The CR system acquires X-ray images by placing a reusable phosphor plate in place of a film. Exposed plates are scanned electro-optically to extract images in a digital format. The TR network can also acquire images from existing imaging systems. CT, MRI and ultrasound images can be acquired for the network for transmission and management. The remote display station is used for a quality check before transmitting the image to the central site (either the 121 Evacuation or 51st Tactical Flight Wing Hospital).

Image transmission occurs over an in-country dial-up phone line using 512 Kbytes or T-1 line for high work load sites. The communication system will use existing capabilities and the TR system will access them through high speed interface.

The MDIS project has a long history of careful and comprehensive assessment of the needs and availability of technical solutions to the management of diagnostic images in military hospitals. The technical section of the MDIS document details the system specifications and functional requirements of subsystems and the entire network. It also contains a phased operational scenario. The document is the first of its kind in the IMAC arena. It is technically comprehensive and contains clear operational and clinical objectives, making it a fine platform upon which other related projects can be built. Table 1 summarizes the phased implementation plan as described in the request for proposals.

6. Conclusion

Filmless radiology service faces many difficulties. Films are the preferred choice of diagnosis for fine detail and above all familiarity. The use of IMAC technology will make a significant contribution in improving the quality of radiology service, but on the other hand there is a great deal of resistence in the radiology community for the change. In the past, many of the IMAC projects tried to mimic the use of films. The use of IMAC technology must demonstrate a significant advantage over the film system in two ways: diagnostic and operational.

Diagnostic advantages can be achieved through the use of various image processing and display technologies. Computer processing of digital images may provide additional accuracy to diagnosis. Radiologists do not always interpret images with the same level of skill or same level of consistency. A single radiologist has good days and bad days. There are biases in diagnosis based on what the radiologist has seen recently, compared to those things to which s/he is seldom exposed. Computer-assisted diagnosis (CADx) techniques could provide the ability to bring the less skilled radiologist up towards the skill level of the more skilled radiologist and could help correct the intermittent lapses of perception of the more skilled. CADx could also improve the consistency of diagnosis.

The electronic workstation must be a single point of contact (SPOC) for all necessary images, medical records, lab results, new and old reports and patient data. Getting images rapidly to a workstation is not enough. The workstation and network must be comprehensive to support availability of images and data in a dependable and predictable manner.

The growing complexity of imaging service and the demand for efficiency will further highlight the need for IMAC technology. Rapid development of the necessary technology in the commercial and consumer market place will bring down the cost of IMAC technology. Many challenges remain but they will be met soon if the history of computer applications in other areas is our guide.

Acknowledgment

The author is grateful to the following colleagues who made significant contributions in Georgetown IMAC project: S.C. Ben Lo, Ph.D., Steve Horii, M.D., Matthew Freedman, M.D., Betty Levine, M.S., COL Fred Goeringer, Brian Krasner, Ph.D., Harold Benson, Robert Fielding, Mitate Matsui, George Brys, Ed Nilges, Bill Proetta, John Giunta, and Bruce Majors.

References

Benson, H.R., S.K. Mun and P.L. Choyke (1985) Integration of clinical reporting system into PACS, *Proc. SPIE* 536, 214 – 228.

Benson, H.R., G. Plumlee and S.K. Mun (1989) Cost analysis of an image management and communication system. In: Schneider, R.H., S.J. Dwyer III and R.G. Jost (Eds.), Medical Imaging III: PACS System Design and Evaluation, *Proc. SPIE* 1093, 448 – 456.

Braudes, R.E., S.K. Mun, J. Sibert, J. Schnizlein and S.C. Horii (1989) Workstation modeling and development: clinical definition of a picture archiving and communication system (PACS) user interface. In: Schneider, R.H., S.J. Dwyer III and R.G. Jost (Eds.), Medical Imaging III: PACS System Design and Evaluation, *Proc. SPIE* 1093, 376 – 386.

Davros, W.J., J.W. Gaskil and S.K. Mun (1989) Quality assurance protocol for display monitors used in a hospital-wide IMAC network. In: Scheider, R.H., S.J. Dwyer III and R.G. Jost (Eds.), Medical Imaging III, *Proc. SPIE* 1091, 301 – 304.

Goeringer, F., S.K. Mun and B.D. Kerlin (1989) Digital imaging needs of the US military diagnostic imaging service. In: Schneider, R.H., S.J. Dwyer III and R.G. Jost (Eds.), Medical Imaging III: PACS System Design and Evaluation, *Proc. SPIE* 1093, 429 – 437.

Horii, S.C., H.N. Horii, S.K. Mun, H.R. Benson and R.K. Zeman (1989) Environmental designs for reading from imaging workstations: ergonomic and architectural features. In: Schneider, R.H., S.J. Dwyer III and R.G. Jost (Eds.), Medical Imaging III, *Proc. SPIE* 1091, 172 – 183.

Levin, K., S.C. Horii, S.K. Mun, M. Freedman and C. Leftridge (1990) Analysis of data gathering for radiologists and its implications to the clinical acceptance of PACS. In: Dwyer III, S.J., and R.G. Jost (Eds.), Medical Imaging IV: PACS System Design and Evaluation, *Proc. SPIE* 1234, 670 – 675.

Levine, B.A. and S.K. Mun (1989) Image management & communication systems: a new challenge in radiology, *Med. Prog. Technol.* 152, 199 – 216.

Levine, B.A., M. Meissner, H.R. Benson, C. Bozarth, S.K. Mun (1989) Integration of a radiology information system (RIS) with an image management and communication system (IMACS): a comparative analysis. In: Schneider, R.H., S.J. Dwyer III and R.G. Jost (Eds.), Medical Imaging III: PACS System Design and Evaluation, *Proc. SPIE* 1093, 183 – 192.

Levine, B.A., K. Randall, S.K. Mun, H.R. Benson, M. Meissner, A.B. Sherman (1989) Optimization of picture archiving and communication systems (PACS) network performance: simulation and validation. In: Schneider, R.H., S.J. Dwyer III and R.G. Jost (Eds.), Medical Imaging III: PACS System Design and Evaluation, *Proc. SPIE* 1093, 330 – 344.

Lo, S.C. and S.K. Mun (1988) Data compression for a radiology image display system with visual directory. In: Schneider, R.H., and S.J. Dwyer III (Eds.), Medical Imaging II, *Proc. SPIE* 914, 1203 – 1208.

Lo, S.C., J.W. Gaskill, B.H. Krasner and S.K. Mun (1989) Image information in film digitization and display monitor – implication for teleradiology. In: Schneider, R.H., S.J. Dwyer III and R.G. Jost (Eds.), Medical Imaging III: PACS System Design and Evaluation, *Proc. SPIE* 1093, 252 – 258.

Lo, S.C., J.W. Gaskill, S.K. Mun and B.H. Krasner (1990) Contrast information in film digitization and display monitor, *J. Digital Imaging,* May, 119 – 124.

Lo, S.C., S.C. Horii, S.K. Mun, R. Braudes and B. Garra (1989) Development of pictorial directory workstation for rapid image presentation. In: Schneider, R.H., S.J. Dwyer III and R.G. Jost (Eds.), Medical Imaging III, *Proc. SPIE* 1091, 234 – 239.

Lo, S.C., B.H. Krasner and S.K. Mun (1990) Noise impact on error-free image compression, *IEEE Trans. Medical Imaging,* June, 206 – 211.

Lo, S.C., E. Shen and S.K. Mun (1990) An image splitting and remapping method for radiological image compression. In: Dwyer III, S.J., and R.G. Jost (Eds.), Medical Imaging IV: PACS System Design and Evaluation *Proc. SPIE* 1234, 300–311.

Mun, S.K., H.R. Benson, B.D. Kerlin, F. Goeringer and T. Gore (1989) Completion of a hospital-wide comprehensive image management and communication system. In: Schneider, R.H., S.J. Dwyer III and R.G. Jost (Eds.), Medical Imaging III: PACS System Design and Evaluation, *Proc. SPIE* 1093, 204–213.

Mun, S.K., H.R. Benson, S.C.B. Lo, B.A. Levine, R. Braudes, L.P. Elliott, T. Gore and M.L., Mallon-Ingeholm, Development and technology assessment of a comprehensive image management and communication network, *Med. Inform.* 13, 315–322.

Mun, S.K., H.R. Benson, C. Welsh, L.P. Elliott and W.J. Davros (1988) Baseline study of radiology services for the purpose of PACS evaluation. In: Schneider, R.H., and S.J. Dwyer III (Eds.), Medical Imaging II, *Proc. SPIE* 914, 978–987.

Mun, S.K., M. Greberman, W.R. Hendee and R. Shannon (1989) *IMAC 89,* The First International Conference on Image Management, IEEE Publications.

Mun, S.K., S.C. Horii, H.R. Benson, S.C.B. Lo, Y. Kim, D.R. Haynor, A. Sarrinen, J. Loop, M. Greberman and R. Allman (1989) Experiences in implementation, clinical acceptance and operations of comprehensive radiology networks. Is the PACS cup half full or half empty? In: Schneider, R.H., S.J. Dwyer III and R.G. Jost (Eds.), Medical Imaging III: PACS System Design and Evaluation, *Proc. SPIE* 1093, 194–201.

Integrated Diagnostic Imaging
Editor: J.P.J. De Valk
© *Elsevier Science Publishers B.V., 1992*

Chapter 5

PACS – clinical evaluation and future conceptual design

Alan H. Rowberg and Gregory L. Zick

1. Introduction and background

Although several faculty members at the University of Washington had a long-standing interest in technology assessment (Loop and Drui, 1971), the history of the involvement of the Department of Radiology at the University of Washington in areas related to PACS really began in 1978, with the development of a proposal for teleradiology with a remote site in Alaska using the ATS/7 communication satellite. Although this proposal was not funded, the interest in using digital computers to communicate images remained strong, and in 1980 a local area network (LAN) was set up in nuclear medicine to transfer images between the various imaging computers. This facility was quite innovative at the time and was developed by Thomas K. Lewellen using twisted pair to communicate data between Apple II computers at 2 Mbitps (Mbit/s) using Corvus OMNINET.

In 1983 John W. Loop and Alan H. Rowberg began a series of meetings with Joseph N. Gitlin and others at the Center for Devices and Radiological Health. These meetings explored the development of a description of a generic PACS, to be authored by representatives of radiology departments, rather than by the marketing managers of medical imaging companies. In 1984 this effort was formally funded, and representatives from about ten universities began meeting on a periodic basis. This led to the publication of a document on the functional requirements for a hospital-based digital imaging network in April of 1985 (MITRE Technical Report, 1985). This report began with a description of the organizations that participated in the development of these functional requirements, and the functional requirements analysis process. It went on to give the profile of a typical radiology department, and then discussed the DIN/PACS concept and how it might work in that department. The final introductory section gave the characterization of the workload in a typical radiology department. The functional descriptions sections of the document covered the areas of workstations, networking, and storage systems, and were followed by a section on training and maintenance.

A follow-up effort explored the system design that would be required to meet these functional requirements and was published in January of 1986 (MITRE Technical Report, 1986). The draft of this document was used as the basis for two procurements initiated in August of 1985, sponsored by a group of federal agencies, primarily the Department of Army. This project was called digital image network/picture archiving and communication system (DIN/PACS). The first of these procurements was to provide for two universities to conduct clinical and basic science evaluations of potential prototype systems. The second procurement was to purchase the two systems that would be installed and operated at the two universities.

Following the conclusion of this evaluation in 1989, an interdisciplinary group of faculty from the School of Medicine and the College of Engineering developed a proposal to pursue the development of a next generation medical image information system (MIIS), built upon new technologies in the context of the experience already gained by the earlier effort. The group was formalized in a Center for Imaging Systems Optimization (CISO) in April of 1990, which was initially funded by the W.M. Keck Foundation and the IBM Corporation. This chapter will present the experience of the PACS group, the current situation at the University of Washington, and will conclude with a description of our current conceptual design of the next generation PACS system.

2. PACS 1980 – 1990

The first move toward automating radiology was a Medical Center commitment to purchase a radiology information system (RIS), and to have it installed and operational by March 1986. A Digital Equipment Corporation (DECrad) system was installed and ready for use by that date. The university developed a PACS prototype evaluation proposal and submitted it in November of 1985.

The review of the PACS prototype evaluation proposals was done and the award was given to the University of Washington (Seattle) in September of 1986, and a similar award was given to Georgetown University (Washington, D.C.), in collaboration with George Washington University. Following the evaluation phase, a request for proposals for installing the prototype PACS themselves was issued; the final due date for proposals was in 1987. Two awards were made: one to AT&T for installation at Georgetown University, and one to Philips Medical Systems for installation at the University of

Washington. Six months later, Philips and AT&T announced a joint venture to produce the CommView® System.

The system proposed by AT&T for Georgetown University went on to become the CommView System. The system proposed by Philips Medical Systems for the University of Washington was also called CommView but was the equipment originally manufactured by Raytel, and being marketed under the CommView name by Philips Medical Systems. Despite the joint venture, the two companies continued their independent efforts to install the two separate systems at the two universities.

Work began at the University of Washington with a detailed baseline analysis, major contributions were by Marty Caudill and Gayle Youngs, including time and cost analyses for each step of the process of completing a radiographic study.

As Philips Medical Systems began staging the system at the factory, they found that there were system integration problems associated with the large size of the network. It involved more computer nodes than had previously been used in any Raytel network. Concurrently with this integration, both the University of Washington and the Department of Army were evaluating the adequacy of the Raytel database and workstation architecture, and found that it would fall short of the requirements. Therefore, discussions were held between the government purchasing authority and Philips Medical Systems, leading to a renegotiating of the equipment list, and the substitution of more modern equipment for the Raytel equipment.

This change in the equipment being delivered, particularly the archive and workstation structure, led to a delay in the installation at the University of Washington, while the installation at Georgetown University proceeded on schedule. The first piece of equipment to be installed at the University of Washington was the Philips Computer Radiography (PCR) device in September of 1988 (Marglin et al., 1990). Initially this was used in stand alone mode, with only a local archive on digital optical disk; eventually, a central computer with its data management system was installed. The major portions of the system were delivered by April of 1989, although the optical disk jukebox, holding 78 platters of 2.2 Mbyte each, was not delivered until October of 1989. The final system delivered included a PCR system with interface to the CommView network. The data management system at the center of the star network included 2 Gbytes on winchester disk storage in addition to the optical disk jukebox. Image viewing was accomplished on 2 four-screen workstations, and 7 single-screen results viewing stations (RVS), which were on Ethernet and connected to CommView through a gateway. Two other two-screen workstations at the Medical Center provided interfaces to the laser film digitizer and video image capture access to computed tomography (CT) and magnetic resonance imaging (MRI) images.

Remote equipment included a CT image acquisition workstation at the VA Medical Center, and a laser film digitizer at Harborview Medical Center, both approximately 5 km from the University of Washington Medical Center. These two remote facilities, in addition to the laser film digitizer located at Madigan Army Medical Center 80 km away, were connected with T-1 telephone lines.

The technical evaluation of the system (Panwar et al., 1990; Saarinen et al., 1990) was conducted by several teams of individuals, with large contributions by Yongmin Kim of the Department of Electrical Engineering. Mitch Goodsitt led the evaluation of the PCR, in addition to assisting with many aspects of the complicated task of site planning (Saarinen et al., 1989a,b).

The clinical evaluation of the system was done by a team led by Dr. Loop and David R. Haynor with major contributions by Suzanne Weghorst of the Department of Industrial Engineering, and many others in the department (Haynor et al., 1988, 1990). The team found and explored many deficiencies in the design and technology of the system. The primary areas of deficiency were the slow speed of image display, the slow speed of network data transfers, and awkward features about the user interface on various workstations. In spite of these deficiencies, the investigators concluded that these problems would be solved in the near future and felt that it was highly likely this technology would be endorsed by the medical community at large.

During the term of the DIN/PACS project, several teleradiology sites were maintained. A site in Sitka, Alaska, was supported by dial-up telephone lines at 2400 baud. For shorter links, the system had three T-1 telephone lines in place, allowing data to be transmitted at 1.5 Mbitps. These lines connected the University of Washington Medical Center with two affiliated hospitals in the Seattle area, and with the Madigan Army Medical Center 50 miles away.

Research conducted at the university was centered around various aspects of evaluation, beginning with baseline studies of the operation of the Radiology Department before PACS was installed, and continuing with evaluation of various aspects of the PACS and its interaction with the department. These included not only evaluations of the workstations and of network capability, but also of an interface to a RIS (Rowberg et al., 1988; Lee et al., 1990), data compression (Wilhelm et al., 1990), image display (Choi et al., 1990), and the possibility of integrating images with printed radiology reports (Loop and Rowberg, 1990).

The interface between the DECrad radiology information system and the CommView PACS system was largely developed by Woobin Lee. This was accomplished on a PC/286 computer running the UNIX operating system. This multi-tasking system uses UNIX pipes to communicate between a variety of tasks, one handling input from the RIS, another handling output to the PACS, while other tasks handle data format translations, operator controls and editing, operator monitoring of system status, and other administrative functions. This software was implemented on a stand-alone PC, so that no changes were required to either the RIS or the PACS. The functionality of the interface was limited, however, because the DECrad system will only send information and the CommView will only receive it, providing only unidirectional data transfer.

The evaluation of usability was led by Judith Ramey, Director of the Laboratory of Usability Testing and Evaluation (LUTE) in the College of Engineering (Ramey, 1989). This included analysis of the user interface, prompts and on-line help functions, and user documentation.

Other activities included an evaluation of how economic analyses could be performed to enable a hospital to predict the benefit, in financial terms, which might be experienced after installation of a PACS. This economic analysis and modelling effort was led by Allan O. Saarinen, assisted by four masters students from the School of Public Health. It led to the development of a modular spreadsheet approach to formalizing the economic model, based on Microsoft Excel (Saarinen et al., 1989a,b).

Related activity in the Department of Electrical Engineering under the direction of Yongmin Kim led to the development of a family of graphic signal processor systems (Fahy and Kim, 1987; Kim et al., 1988; Gee et al., 1989). While the earlier versions of this were based on a PC/AT class machine, the later systems were based on more powerful workstations, such as the NeXT.

The evaluation contract with the University of Washington was extended to November 13, 1989, and final reports were delivered shortly thereafter. The philosophy adopted throughout the evaluation was that for a PACS to be generally clinical acceptable, the internal operation of the system should be as invisible or transparent to the clinical user as possible and meet or exceed the operational capabilities of film-based counterparts. While this is a very demanding requirement, it was felt that a system could be truly successful only when it was fully responsive to the demanding environment of a busy and effective radiology department.

The version of the diagnostic workstation that was tested was not fast enough for routine diagnostic work. Radiologists did not feel that a four-screen workstation was adequate for review of complex studies, although this limitation might be overcome by a more sophisticated user interface and greater speed.

The viewing stations used in the ICU should have two image screens, instead of the one provided. Since space is not easily available in these clinical environments, the separate text monitor is undesirable.

The diagnostic radiologists, most of whom were used to the Apple Macintosh, felt that the user interface for the workstation was unnecessarily complicated on the one hand and not necessarily well-adapted to the reporting task on the other. Functions were sometimes selected by one of three different keys, sometimes by the trackball, and sometimes with a special hardware switch. Many important functions for the diagnostic reporting process were not satisfactorily implemented, even when the hardware could have permitted.

Intelligent image routing over the network could have had a major impact on the perceived utility of the system. This would have allowed routing of selected images automatically to workstations placed in or near the appropriate clinic or nursing station, efficient selecting of comparison studies, and routing of newly performed studies to appropriate reporting stations within the radiology department.

Although there are still many operational deficiencies in the computed radiography technology, it was found to be clinically acceptable in many applications, based on experience, interviews, and surveys.

These findings all combine to point on the importance of continuing end-user involvement in all phases of system design and development. This is particularly important in the case of tasks, such as diagnostic reporting, that are both complex and unfamiliar to vendor systems designers in industrial settings.

3. PACS – present

The PACS at the University of Washington remained in active use after the end of the federally funded contracts. Philips Medical Systems agreed to maintain the equipment for one additional year at their expense, in addition to exchanging several pieces of equipment for new models. By the end of 1990, the university had two of the newer critical care workstations (CCW) installed in the intensive care unit (ICU), replacing the older RVS workstations. Plans are also in place to upgrade one of the diagnostic workstations to the high-speed workstation now offered in the CommView network, called a turbo diagnostic workstation.

Clinical interest in the use of the system remains extremely strong, and requires no encouragement from the radiology department. The clinicians in the ICU actively use their workstations, and are quick to notice and complain when the system is not operational. All of the portable radiographic examinations in the hospital are done using the PCR, and all examinations performed on patients in the ICU are automatically routed to workstations in the ICUs. With this automatic routing, the images may be easily viewed by any of the physicians in the ICU, since all new images are virtually always in local storage, and can be quickly displayed. Since these are two-screen workstations, the next most recent image is automatically displayed whenever a recent image is selected, allowing for easy comparisons.

The acceptance of this clinical facility is impressive. Technical staff in the ICU say that they have never seen a clinical computer system more thoroughly accepted and used by the physicians. Although some users may recognize that there are faster image viewing workstations in existence, and some have more user-friendly interfaces, the only complaints about the system that they will express, even when asked, relate to system downtime.

In October of 1989, a Siemens DRC-80 workstation was installed for evaluation, which included eight screens of $1280 \times 1024 \times 8$ bits and were backed up with 128 Mbytes of video RAM, enabling images to move rapidly from one display to another. This allowed rapid cine loops of images, in addition to rapid paging through large numbers of images, such as through a sequence of 100 CT scans. This was not directly connected to any image sources, but provisions were made for loading a representative test set of images onto the system. These included CT scans and PCR images, both of which were transmitted to the system over the campus Ethernet network. This workstation was used in a series of evaluations, similar to those which were being conducted on the DIN/PACS workstation. These evaluations were designed to test user reactions to features of the workstation, and preferences relating to how these features were accessed and used. The very fast image display on this workstation was a dramatic contrast to the much slower speed of the older CommView workstations, because the newer high-speed CommView workstation had not yet been installed at the University, although one of these workstations was installed at Georgetown University.

More recently, the Department of Radiology has cooperated with the School of Dentistry in an evaluation of dental teleradiology. This particular evaluation is being conducted on advanced video products (AVP) equipment, using a Lumisys scanner on the sending end, and a Megascan monitor on the receiving end. This allowed the small dental radiographs to be scanned and digitized at excellent resolution, and magnified at the receiving end, or many images displayed at the same time.

The purpose of this evaluation is not routine diagnosis, but instead an attempt to accomplish behavior modification using teleradiology. A random sample of films is transmitted from the sending site, which is a remote hospital with staff dentists but without a dental radiologist, to a dental radiologist at the receiving end, the University of Washington Medical Center, who reviews the images which have been transmitted on a daily basis and returns a critique to the site where the images were made. This critique may contain an annotated image, marking an area which requires attention, such as overexposure, missed anatomy, improper film placement, etc.

Another research interest has been quality assurance of images obtained by digitizing the video that comes from a medical imaging device, such as a CT scanner or a magnetic resonance scanner (Rowberg, 1970). We programmed one of the scanners with a variety of test patterns, so that each and every pixel of the image contained a gray scale value which was accurately known. This image may then be displayed at any time using the standard scanner software, and the image may be captured and transmitted to the PACS, where the image is analyzed and the quality of the image is determined by visual verification or by a computer program. For instance, if the displayed image is a gray scale ramp covering all 256 shades of gray from 0 to 255, then the output should cover the same range. The steps should be evenly spaced, and there should be the same number of pixels for each shade of gray. This analysis is easily done on the PACS using a specially developed computer program, so that the analysis proceeds automatically. The computer can then quickly determine what, if anything, is wrong with the current gain and offset settings, or the pixel clock synchronization of the video image digitizer system.

While the presence of PACS at the University of Washington Medical Center started as a purely research-motivated project, these digital imaging devices have now been embraced by both radiologists and referring physicians, and PACS is now part of the routine activities of the department. The system continues to be upgraded and expanded, and additional image management and communication systems are being added at other university-affiliated hospitals.

4. PACS 1990 – 2000 overview

4.1. Conceptual design

As described in the section above, medical imaging is an important aspect of modern medical care. It is a relatively new field and is changing in a number of ways. First, an increasing proportion of imaging is acquired directly in digital form (CT, MRI, and ultrasound (US)). In addition, technologies based on photostimulable phosphors can provide the equivalent of conventional X-rays in digital form. Second, the utilization and complexity of imaging is increasing, resulting in an ever-increasing number of medical images needing to be handled. These must be handled with better efficiency if the cost of medical care is to be kept down. The multiple modalities also provide the opportunities for new techniques (sensor fusion, three-dimensional imaging) for synthesizing and visualizing the information they produce. Finally, these images are not only used for medical diagnosis but also for direct therapy planning in clinical areas such as radiation oncology and surgery.

While certain parts of the system are accepted such as our own experience in the ICU, there is an urgent need for a totally digital system which meets the needs for image viewing and distribution in primary medical care throughout the hospital. This not only requires the archiving and retrieval of images, as supported by an optimal PACS, but also the integration of the full data flow component of medical care. While many prototype systems have been developed, all current systems are plagued by a number of problems. Following is a brief description of some of the more prevalent problems.

4.1.1. Clumsy user interface

The comment has been made that with current systems, radiologists spend more time manipulating the images than viewing them. If these systems are to be competitive with the flexibility offered by conventional film-based radiology, a sophisticated user interface is required. Current displays also do not support enough spatial resolution nor are they consistently bright enough to provide displays that compete with the clarity of film.

4.1.2. Restrictions of the user interface

There is difficulty in simultaneously accessing information and images. A common concern voiced by radiologists about current PACS is the lack of integration with other information sources, such as the hospital information system (HIS) and the RIS. The perceived restrictions on access to data will increase as new systems provide better performance, hold more data per regime study, and more data per patient. The query process needs to be redesigned for the physician to allow the free flow of thoughts and requests for information that is required in clinical diagnosis.

Table 1
Typical image size of medical images.

Modality	Data per image (MBytes)	Image per exam	Data per exam (MBytes)
X-ray	6	1 – 3	6 – 18
CT	0.4	30 – 60	12 – 18
MRI	0.4	64 – 128	25 – 50
US	0.3	20 – 30	6 – 9

Table 2a
Network standard performance.

	Ethernet	Token ring	FDDI
Specified bit rate (Mbitps)	10	16	100
Actual throughput (Mbitps)	1	10	30

Table 2b
Medical image performance based on network technology (transmission times are in seconds).

	Ethernet	Token ring	FDDI
X-ray (best case 6 Mbytes)	48	4.8	1.6
MRI (worst case 50 Mbytes)	400	40	13.3
Average study (20 Mbyteps)	160	16	5.3
Network load (worst case 100 Mbytes)	800	80	26.6

4.1.3. Overall performance

Sets of digitized medical images comprise a large amount of data. Images are acquired by different modalities, such as X-ray, MRI, CT, and US. Most patient exams consist of more than one image. The typical amount of data generated per image for a given modality and a corresponding estimate for a given exam are presented in table 1.

Current networking technology, disc systems and display devices do not have the performance required to provide seemingly instantaneous response to user commands. Typical response times for one patient exam study, based on current network technology, are shown in table 2. (These figures reflect application-to-application communication rates.) A desirable response time requirement for PACS environments is in the range of $1-2$ s. Even the promised performance of FDDI will not meet this requirement.

Another way to predict performance is to estimate that a request for a study (approximately 20 Mbyte of data) might be generated about every 12 s in a 400-bed hospital. This number was based on the following assumptions. In a 400-bed hospital, there are approximately 100 000 studies per year with an average data set size of 20 Mbyte. It is estimated that each study will be looked at six times (including the times it is used for comparison with later studies). If all the image viewing is done between 9 am and 5 pm Monday through Friday, then 600 000 study viewing requests over 2 000 hours per year equals 300 requests per hour, or one request every 12 seconds.

Assuming a peak rate of 5–6 times this, the FDDI network would have marginal performance during regular times and would noticeably slow down during peak times (as shown in table 2).

4.1.4. Scalability and extensibility

The majority of existing prototypes around the country are focused on a minimum set of modalities and functions. These prototype systems typically serve only a single modality or are developed for a small subset of a total operation. They currently are not capable of supporting the full load in a large hospital of more than 100 beds or so, nor are they designed to be extensible either by scaling up to these large capacities or by easily integrating new technology as it comes on-line, particularly when taking into account the expected growth in complexity of medical images.

Another road block that has been observed is the difficulty in extending functionality. This is due to the required compromises in system design necessary to overcome the lack of performance in the system components. For example, software that is not object oriented, i.e., designed for a proprietary system or has a complex set of rules developed to overcome performance limitations, is very difficult to adapt to new hardware configurations. In addition, new functionality cannot be easily added to the system.

4.1.5. Cost of the total system

Due to the complexity of image handling, each node in the system continues to increase in its requirements resulting in a high-cost sophisticated system at every physician node. There is little sharing of expensive items primarily due to the bottleneck of network performance.

Our approach is to design a system that specifically addresses the major problem areas just outlined and satisfies the requirements developed by an interdisciplinary team within CISO (Kim and Haynor, 1991). This system will be based on new technology which is either currently available or will become available within the next three years. Specifically, there are six targeted technologies:
(1) a common platform of the RS/6000 RISC workstation;
(2) a common operating system environment-AIX, X-windows;
(3) very high speed LANs with Gbitps transmission rates;
(4) high-speed parallel disc arrays to support multiple database server machines;
(5) continuous voice recognition systems as the primary input of the user interface; and
(6) high-resolution, 19-inch displays (2 K × 2 K × 8 bits) with an adequate

hardware interface support to allow fast and accurate multiple image manipulation.

These new technologies will be integrated into a single scalable and extensible system. The software will be designed specifically to be modular, conform to existing standards and be extensible. The extensibility will be in functionality as new software modules are developed that add to the system's capabilities and in allowing easy incorporation of new technologies as they become available. The application layers, including the user interface, will be developed in collaboration with the radiologists as users and professional human interface designers from the College of Engineering.

The underlying concept in designing this multi-faceted system is shown in table 3. The primary elements of the system consist of the user interface, the workstation, and the database server. Each of these system elements can be viewed at different layers: an application layer, a logical layer and a physical layer. At the application layer, the user interface consists of the definition of all input/output information that would be described in the user manual; it can be measured against the requirements document in terms of the number of

Table 3
Medical image information system (MIIS) conceptual design.

	System component		
	User interface	Workstation	Database
Application layer	Definition of all input/output User manual describes Measured against requirements	User application program interface Input requests Output display	Database application program interface Query syntax Reply data format
Logical layer	Work flow Radiological methodologies	Database processing Image processing Display processing	Client/server Symbolic/image Data scheme
Physical layer	Displays Input devices	Workstation Processor Memory Disc	Storage Magnetic Optical Parallel Access Processing CPU(s) Parallel system

functions that it fulfills. For the workstation and the database, at the application layer, there is an application programmer interface (API). This interface for the workstation includes all the input requests and output configurations for the displays. The interface for the database includes the query syntax and the required response data format. These APIs are callable library functions used by the application macros.

At the logical layer, each of the components has a set of functions described. The work flow for the user interface is based on radiological methodologies which are being determined by direct observation in addition to physician input. For the workstation, the processes for database access, image processing and display are defined as separate modules which can be added to and modified. For the database, the client – server relationship, symbolic and image information based queries, and the data schema are defined.

The physical layer describes the specific hardware components, such as displays and input devices for the user interface. For the workstation, processor, memory size, and disk storage are described. For the database system, the type of storage (magnetic or optical), architecture, and processors are described. In the following three sections, we will address each of these layers and their components in more detail.

4.2. Conceptual design – physical layer

A physical layer block diagram of the envisioned system is shown in fig. 1. The key component is a Gbit speed LAN and parallel disc systems which dramatically improve the performance, hencing change the design parameters of the system. The higher speed LAN provides the performance required for adequate response time and allows the design of a true client – server architecture. It also addresses the cost issue by reducing the hardware requirements of the workstations and allows sharing of costly elements across multiple workstations through the server design.

The expected performance of the Gbit network is shown in table 4. The throughput is more than adequate for most cases. The time required for transfer in the worst case of a full MRI study is 0.5 s. The total delay in the worst-case peak loading scenario is still only 1 s, well within the design specifications.

To support this high-speed network, the system must be capable of transferring stored data at an acceptable rate. The envisioned architecture would have studies of 'active' patients up to one-week-old on parallel discs, selected studies up to 2-months-old on regular disc, and older studies archived on an optical disc system. Archived studies for comparison purposes would be prefetched before a new exam was performed or when a related study was requested. The

Table 4a
Network standard performance.

	Ethernet	Token ring	FDDI	Gbit
Specified bit rate (Mbitps)	10	16	100	1000
Actual throughput (Mbitps)	1	10	30	800^1 (400^2)

[1] Network

[2] Memory to memory

Table 4b
Medical image performance based on network technology (transmission times are in seconds).

	Ethernet	Token ring	FDDI	Gigabit
X-ray (best case 6 Mbytes)	48	4.8	1.6	0.06 (0.12)
MRI (worst case 50 Mbytes)	400	40	13.3	0.5 (1.0)
Average study (20 Mbyteps)	160	16	5.3	0.2 (0.4)
Average study peak rate (100 Mbyteps)	800	80	26.6	1.0 (2.0)

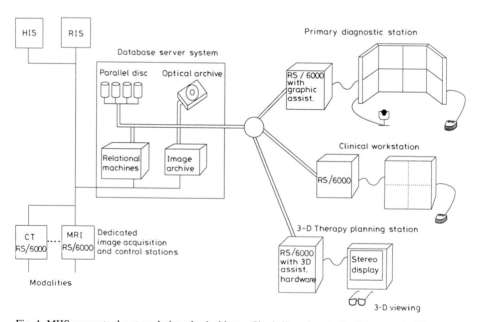

Fig. 1. MIIS conceptual system design physical layer. Single lines denote the Ethernet, double lines the Fibernet (Gbitps LAN).

selected studies would be those most likely to be required for the purpose of comparison and correlation, e.g., a patient under regular therapy treatment. Following our earlier assumptions of 100 000 studies per year, at 20 Mbyte of data per study on the average for a 400-bed hospital, the size of the storage can be estimated. The total data to be stored each year is 2 Tbytes. The amount for 1 week is 8 Gbytes, which is the envisioned size for the parallel disc. The amount of regular disc storage is more difficult to estimate, but a reasonable guess would be around 100 Gbytes. These parameters can be adjusted depending on patient load. The cost of the disc system will be shared across all network workstations due to the support of the Gbit LAN.

Current technology for parallel disc systems supports transfer rates of between 3 Mbyteps for SCSI interfaces and up to 20 Mbyteps for direct Micro Channel attachment. (Note: SCSI interface is defined for 3, 5, 6 and 10 Mbytes depending on whether it is asynchronous or synchronous transmission and whether it is an 8 bit or 16 bit data path. Also, Micro Channel speeds are expected to be doubled in the future.) Assuming direct transfer from the parallel disc system to the network adapter via the Micro Channel bus, one could expect a throughput close to 20 Mbyteps as a best case. This assumes the disc access delays are negligible (currently access is specified at less than 14 ms). If the throughput of a single request is limited to 20 Mbyte, the response time would be less than 2 s for all situations but the largest MRI case. This constraint is acceptable because of the time required by the reviewing physician to do their initial inspection of the early arriving images.

The Gbit speed network would allow significant reduction, if not complete removal of the workstation DASD. These diskless workstations would share the higher speed parallel disc system, and the overall system cost for DASD then becomes more reasonable. This sharing of resources would also be extended to special purpose machines for use in complex database searches.

Central to the design is a database server system consisting of multiple machines that handle the image from the time it is first acquired through archiving and retrieval. The database also contains additional data, such as text from the diagnosis of the radiologist, annotations directly on the image, and other information retrieved from the RIS or HIS. The database server consists of a relational indexing system, an image storage system with high speed parallel discs, and an optical jukebox archive. These database servers are connected through a Gbit LAN to primary diagnostic, clinical, and three-dimensional therapy planning workstations throughout the radiology department and selected clinical areas. All workstation platforms are based on the RS/6000 system.

The database system will be connected to the HIS and RIS through Ethernet. Data is originally acquired from separate RS/6000 systems specifically designed for the control of each modality. These systems will allow the control, review and optimization of image acquisition from a patient during the procedure. Information from the RIS or HIS will be available through X-windows based applications developed specifically for the station. This X-window application will allow access to multiple databases on different platforms. The required information integration will be supported by a local X-window application on the acquisition station at the time of image capture. Once the exam is acquired, the images required will be transferred to the database server through the accepted ACR/NEMA 3.0 messaging protocol standards.

The ACR/NEMA 3.0 protocol will form the basis for the required attributes in the relations used for indexing. The relational database machine(s) will directly index parallel disc systems that support and store the images. Long-term storage of these images will be performed by an optical archive system.

Once the images are available to the database server, radiologists will view images by a primary diagnostic workstation. This diagnostic workstation will consist of eight high-speed resolution displays (2 K × 2 K pixels), large main memory (64 – 128 Mbyte), Gbit LAN connection, and minimal DASD. The physician will interact with the station through a voice recognition system (for transcription) and a pointing device such as a mouse or trackball. Options available to the physician will range from database queries for the studies to be reviewed to the selection of multiple image manipulations necessary for diagnosis. Basic image and display functions will be supported by the workstation, including window and level adjustments, roam, and zoom.

The clinical workstation will utilize the RS/6000 and one or two displays to allow diagnostic images to be viewed remotely by referring physicians in the hospital. The therapy planning three-dimensional stations will be similar to those described above, but will include three-dimensional hardware assist functions for improved performance.

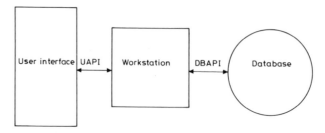

Fig. 2. MIIS conceptual system design application layer. UAPI is the user application program interface. DBAPI the database application program interface, DBAPI the database application program interface.

4.3. Conceptual design – application layer

Both the application layer and logical layer have been developed with the input of radiologist, Dr. David Haynor. The application layer is diagrammed in fig. 2. Basically, the three primary system elements: user interface, workstation, and database are interconnected by APIs. One of these interfaces is between the user interface and workstation, the other interface is between the workstation and the database system. Each of these interfaces consists of a set of specific operations.

4.3.1. Database API

The database API (DBAPI) must allow the formulation of specific requests for input based on any subset of the following: last name, first name, hospital number, exam code, body part, exam modality, start date, end date, text of diagnostic report. The request will return a list of *patients* or *exams*. The interface must also support general SQL query functions, and provide an online copy of the data dictionary for user reference.

A successful query that returns many sets of exams, the most likely being comparison exams, should display these in ranking order. A separate application would set the appropriate rules.

The return of a list of exams will allow retrieval of text of the report only, or the entire exam.

The database can be updated by adding new images, text, annotation, derived images, or other objects to an existing exam. A special request is supported to display a *worklist*. This would be user-specific (i.e., based on the logon). Rules for designing a particular user's worklist would be set by a separate application (this could thus include the concept of a *clinician worklist* as well as the radiologist worklist).

4.3.2. Workstation API

The workstation will maintain a list of active exams. This provides the ability to add or delete exams from the active list. The workstation will also maintain a list of *selected* exams. The interface will allow the definition and alteration of a display configuration. The interface will have the facility to alter the display configuration, maintain a list of visible and invisible (off-screen) images and of selected images, series, and queries concerning these will return information about these lists.

There will be general support for X-window based access to other databases/software. The interface will support an interface-defined overlay (e.g., menus) and user-defined overlays (e.g., annotations) with ability to manipulate each and toggles them off and on.

There will be support for basic operations on images, such as window/level of a selected set of images, zoom/roam, and finally code to support selected image processing operations.

The system will be designed to support multiple user interfaces. The design will also allow incremental improvement and local customization. In general, the system should support extensibility at multiple levels. The system should support multiple user interfaces as described above, allow the inclusion of new functions for image processing, and be transparent to the addition or deletion of workstations on the network.

5. System concept – logical layer

The logical structure of the proposed system is shown in fig. 3. The objective is to develop independent subsystems which are the components of the main system. The links between the system are message strings defined as the user application interface and the database application interface. This software structure will allow independent development of the subsystems and permit interactive refinement of the user interface while minimizing the amount of code that has to be rewritten during the process.

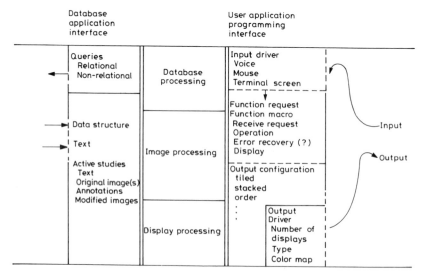

Fig. 3. MIIS conceptual system design logical layer.

The program interfaces are defined as:

(1) The DBAPI will be flexible, but not extensible by applications programmers. It will support general SQL queries and allow modification of the data dictionary. The DBAPI allows the workstation to pass a query to the database for a list of studies (patients, etc.), satisfying certain conditions. The database returns a query answer consisting of the appropriate list. The DBAPI will also accept a request for a fetch-list. The studies or textual information in the fetch-list are retrieved to the workstation and join the list of *active studies* on the workstation (only active studies may be displayed). In the case of a Gbit network with a central server, a study may become active without being actually transmitted (it would, however, be promoted from the optical archive to the parallel disc farm). Although the DBAPI will support these specialized types of queries, it should also be possible to address general SQL queries to the database. The database also stores and sends doctors' comments (addressed to a specific user or associated with a particular study); these comments may consist of both text and annotation. The database has rules for obtaining the *body part* of a study (extracted from the ACR/NEMA implementation of study codes) and can return the set of studies *related* to a given study in descending order of estimated relevance. The DBAPI should require no application-specific modifications, since general queries are supported.

(2) The user application program interface (UAPI) has a workstation part and a human interface part. The workstation section is flexible in that new image processing functions can be added. The input part supports additions to menus and passes messages to workstation and to user-created processes. One or more 'advanced' interface programs will be provided which handle selection functions (point in image, image, histogram, etc.), and display functions. These will be versatile enough to cover needs of new image processing applications. A more detailed description is shown in fig. 3. The UAPI contains a sufficiently rich set of functionalities that two requirements are met: (a) new user views can be easily developed; (b) new functions can be supported with minimal extensions. Several user views may be developed. The UAPI supports the following functions: database queries (various specialized queries which may be clinically useful, and generalized queries); fetch commands; selection commands, image modifying or processing commands; display-configuration requests; and status requests (points to studies, pointers to selected images, etc.).

The workstation API handles requests generated by the human interface part, manages the display, performs image processing computations, and handles transactions with the database. It functions as the *window manager* and maintains the list of windows (each associated with a position on a monitor, a size). Each *acquisition* is linked to a set of windows belonging to it, so that the notion of *scrolling* within an acquisition is well defined. Mapping an image to a window requires specifying an origin for the image within the window, a zoom factor, an LUT. As it becomes better defined, the image presentation information from the ACR/NEMA format will be used for a default display. The following ACR/NEMA classes will be supported: curve (time-activity curve, profile, histogram, ROI, table filter); report; and overlay. Default methods of display for each are provided. Access to the set of curves associated with a study is provided by the UAPI.

Display-configuration requests are used to change the set(s) of windows or the association between acquisitions and windows. They include the ability to generate a single arbitrarily placed window or a set of windows at a defined spacing on the set of monitors. The display of one series may be slaved to another series (to facilitate comparison). The management of slaved series is transparent to the user interface. Displayed series may run horizontally or vertically.

Display requests alter the mapping of the selected images to their windows. All images have a default map associated with them, whether displayed or not. Originally it is the image itself that is displayed in the corresponding window. If the image is modified in some way, the modified image is displayed but the original image is retained (so that a 'Revert to original' command may be supported).

Every image processing operation produces a new image. In many cases these images are best thought of as modifications of one of the existing images (e.g., filter, or adaptive histogram equalization), in which case they become the *displayed* image. In a few cases (e.g., the MAX of a series of images), the image processing operation creates a new image. Methods are provided to save modified images if specifically requested by the user, in which case they become part of the study. The original images are always saved unchanged in the database and exist in unchanged form at all times on the workstation. Image selection operations allow the user to select one or more images from a series on which a particular operation is to be performed. Image selection may be performed either on visible images (by selecting them from the monitor) or on non-displayed images (selecting them from a gallery view or from a list of image descriptors). Image processing operations are performed on all selected images. If it is desired to perform different but similar image processing operations to a series of images, this must be implemented by the application.

Only images from *active studies* may be selected, displayed or modified. The UAPI provides methods to delete from or add to the set of active studies. A reasonable set of image processing operations and the basic display operations (flip, rotate, zoom, roam, change window/level) are provided. The ability to do a *cine* display of a series is provided (this is the analogue of scrolling, but in a conceptual direction perpendicular to the plane of the display). The WS configuration can be saved for resumption later. Functions for turning selected annotation layers on or off are provided.

An earlier CISO document described the requirements for a realistic solution to the medical imaging information system (Zick and Haynor, 1991). The primary needs were: performance, system independence, flexible user interface, and multiple image manipulation. The system described in the conceptual design document addresses each of these four areas through the integration of new technology. A summary of the new technologies and their impact is given below.

Technologies	Impact
Common RS/6000 platform	Compatibility, software migration, future speed improvements
Software standards	(AIX, OSF/motif, TCP/IP, ACR/NEMA 3.0)- open systems, common tool set, distributed system capability.
Gbit networks	Provide required response time, allow true client server architecture, allow reduced workstation requirements, allow increased sophistication.
Parallel disc drives	Use capacity of Gbit LANs, ensure acceptable response time.
Voice recognition system	Overcome primary physician resistance to PACS interface.
High resolution display	Compare favorably to film and light box.

This, combined with the modular software approach to support scalability and extensibility, will produce a system that can be built upon as better technology is available and as we continue to evaluate and improve the software.

6. Conclusion

The development of a PACS that can be effectively used in the clinic is a complex task. A task that must draw on the experience and expertise of an interdisciplinary group of developers. In this chapter we have reported on the history of the University of Washington experience in PACS. This was followed by a brief description of the current status. Finally, we have attempted to give a broad picture of our current concept of what the design of the next generation medical image system will be. This concept is based on six new technologies which significantly impact the design. First are a common RISC-based platform and operating system environment which contributes to scalability and extensibility. Next are Gbit speed networks and parallel disc systems which contribute to overall performance and cost reduction. Finally, the continuous voice recognition system and very bright high-resolution displays allow the development of flexible and acceptable human interface.

References

Choi, H.S., H.W. Park, D.R. Haynor and Y. Kim (1990) Development of a prototype electronic alternator for DIN/PACS environment and its evaluation. In: Dwyer III, S.J., and R.G. Jost (Eds.), Medical Imaging IV: PACS System Design and Evaluation, *Proc. SPIE* 1234, 532 – 540.

Fahy, J.B., and Y. Kim (1987) A UNIX-based prototype biomedical virtual image processor. In: Schneider, R.H., and S.J. Dwyer III (Eds.), Medical Imaging, *Proc. SPIE* 767, 479 – 485.

Gee, J.C., L.A. DeSoto, Y. Kim and J.W. Loop (1989) User interface design for a radiological imaging workstation. In: Schneider, R.H., S.J. Dwyer III and R.G. Jost (Eds.), Medical Imaging III, *Proc. SPIE* 1093, 122 – 132.

Haynor, D.R., A.H. Rowberg and J.W. Loop (1988) Clinical evaluation of a prototype digital imaging network. In: Schneider, R.H., and S.J. Dwyer III (Eds.), Medical Imaging II, *Proc. SPIE* 914, 1431 – 1443.

Haynor, D., S. Weghorst, A. Saarinen, J. DeSoto and U. Schmiedl (1990) Clinical evaluation of PACS workstation – methodology and results. In: Dwyer III, S.J., and R.G. Jost (Eds.), Medical Imaging IV: PACS System Design and Evaluation, *Proc. SPIE* 1234, 408 – 417.

Kim, Y., and D. Haynor (1991) Radiology Requirements Document. *CISO Technical Report,* 91-001.

Kim, Y., J.B. Fahy, L.A. DeSoto, D.R. Haynor and J.W. Loop (1988) Development of a PC-based radiological imaging workstation. In: Schneider, R.H., and S.J. Dwyer III (Eds.), Medical Imaging II, *Proc. SPIE* 914, 1257 – 1264.

Lee, W., A.H. Rowberg, Y.M. O'Leary and Y. Kim (1990) Integrating a radiology information system with a picture archiving and communications system. In: Dwyer III, S.J., and R.G. Jost (Eds.), Medical Imaging IV: PACS System Design and Evaluation, *Proc. SPIE* 1234, 661 – 669.

Loop, J.W., and A.B. Drui (1971) A mechanized film viewing system, *Hospitals* 45(23), 111 – 116.

Loop, J.W., and A.H. Rowberg (1990) Augmenting text with images in radiographic reporting: a pilot evaluation study. *Proc. Symposium for Computer Assisted Radiology, Proc. S/CAR 90,* 132 – 135.

Marglin, S.I., A.H. Rowberg and D.J. Godwin (1990) Preliminary experience with portable digital imaging for intensive care, *J. Thorac. Imag.* 5(1), 49 – 54.

MITRE Technical Report (April 1985) The DIN Report: Functional Requirements for a Hospital-Based Digital Imaging Network and Picture Archiving and Communication Prototype System, The Center for Devices and Radiological Health. The MITRE Corporation, McLean, VA.

MITRE Technical Report (January 1986) Technical Specifications for a Hospital Based Digital Imaging Network. The MITRE Corporation, McLean, VA.

Panwar, R.K., C.S. Wang, L.A. DeSoto, H.W. Park and Y. Kim (1990) University of Washington

PACS prototype performance measurements, computer model, and simulation. In: Dwyer III, S.J., and R.G. Jost (Eds.), Medical Imaging IV: PACS System Design and Evaluation, *Proc. SPIE* 1234, 869–880.

Ramey, J. (Oct 1989) Working with users to design online documentation. *Proc. IEEE International Professional Communications Conference,* 17–20.

Rowberg, A.H. (1970) Objective analysis of image quality of video image capture systems. In: Medical Imaging IV, *Proc. SPIE* 1232, 61–70.

Rowberg, A.H., Y.M. O'Leary and J.W. Loop (June 1988) Interfacing a radiology information system to an image database system. Computer Applications in Radiology, RISC/ACR, Harrisburg, PA.

Saarinen, A.O., M.M. Goodsitt and J.W. Loop (1989a) Logistics of installing PACS in an existing medical center. In: Schneider, R.H., S.J. Dwyer III and R.G. Jost (Eds.), Medical Imaging III: PACS System Design and Evaluation, *Proc. SPIE* 1093, 159–170.

Saarinen, A.O., D.R. Haynor, J.W. Loop, L. Johnson, J. Russel, K. Mitchell and M. Nemerever (1989b) Modeling the DeSoto of PACS: What is important? In: Schneider, R.H., S.J. Dwyer III and R.G. Jost (Eds.), Medical Imaging III, *Proc. SPIE* 1093, 62–73.

Saarinen, A.O., G. Youngs, D.R. Haynor and J.W. Loop (1990) Clinical determinants of PACS acceptance. In: Dwyer III, S.J., and R.G. Jost (Eds.), Medical Imaging IV: PACS System Design and Evaluation, *Proc. SPIE* 1234, 817–822.

Wilhelm, P., D.R. Haynor, Y. Kim, A.C. Nelson and E.A. Riskin (1990) Lossy image compression for digital medical imaging systems. In: Medical Imaging IV, *Proc. SPIE* 1232, 348–358.

Zick, G., and D. Haynor (1991) Conceptual Design Document. *CISO Technical Report,* 91-002.

PACS in Europe

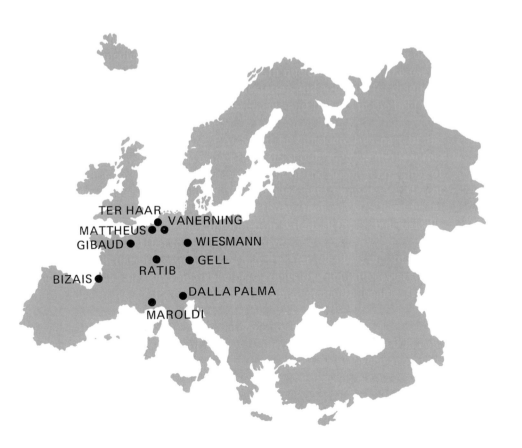

Integrated Diagnostic Imaging
Editor: J.P.J. De Valk
© *Elsevier Science Publishers B.V., 1992*

Chapter 6

Digital PACS in medicine 1980 – 2000

G. Gell and M. Wiltgen

1. Introduction

The concept of a picture archiving and communication system (PACS) and an image management, archiving and communication system (IMACS) is the result of a long development. Starting with nuclear medicine more and more imaging methods have been either digitized or, like computed tomography (CT) and magnetic resonance (MR), have started as digital methods from the beginning. On the other hand, radiology has always been a pioneer in the use of computer methods in medicine: since 1950 computer calculation of radiation doses for radiotherapy, signal and image processing in nuclear medicine, the use of computers for report generation and documentation and as an aid for diagnosis are examples of early developments, achievements and failures in the field that is now called medical informatics.

From a general point of view, a PACS can be considered as part of the hospital information system (HIS) concept. A HIS should manage all the information needed for patient care and the operation of the hospital and this, of course, includes images. The volume of the image data requires a different technical approach but it is well understood, today, that a PACS must be integrated into a HIS (or a radiology information system (RIS) – but logically that is also a part of a HIS) to be fully effective.

PACS means digital processing, archiving, transfer, display, etc. of image data and this should, in principle, make hard copies on film unnecessary. The hoped-for advantages of PACS over conventional methods include several points:

- *Financial.* Reduced costs for films, archive space and personnel.
- *Archiving.* Better availability of images. Experience has shown that in conventional film archives 25 – 35% of films are not available when requested (because they have been lent to somebody, are misplaced, etc.).

– *Communication.* Faster image transfer and simultaneous access from multiple points.
– *Interpretation.* The image processing capabilities of a PACS workstation, like windowing, filtering, three-dimensional visualisation, quantification, etc. might be an aid to diagnosis because all the information in the images can be exploited.

In conventional radiology the X-ray film serves as a detector medium for the radiation, as the viewing or display medium for the interpretation of the images and as a medium for image transport and image archival.

Even where the film has been replaced as a detector (CT, MR, etc.) hard copies on film are made for interpretation, communication and archival. As will be discussed later it seems to be relatively easy to introduce digital means for the 'technical' functions like communication and archiving. The crucial point for the introduction of a complete PACS will be the acceptance of digital display consoles as the medium or tool for primary diagnosis and image interpretation.

2. PACS 1980 – 1990

It is not our intention to try to give a comprehensive history of PACS and we will only mention those developments that have been in some relation to our own work.

2.1. History

In 1985, when we entered the PACS field, the European PACS-scenery consisted of very few active centers: two big European manufacturers of X-ray equipment, Siemens (Greinacher et al., 1984) and Philips (Tiemann et al., 1985) were developing PACS strategies and most of the research in radiology departments was more or less connected with them. The high price of networks, the dependency on interfaces to the image equipment, etc. made it almost impossible to pursue a completely independent development. From our point of view the most striking difference in the approach of the two manufacturers was in the design of the PACS network. There was no doubt, that the transmission speeds of the available local area networks (LANs) were not sufficient for a real PACS. The solution adopted by Philips was to develop a proprietary high-speed star-like network for image transmission, while Siemens opted for the use of commercially available standards (Ethernet), hoping that the standards would evolve fast enough to provide the necessary transmission capacities when PACS would reach a marketable level.

At the Free University in Brussels (VUB) a diagnostic console was installed in december 1987 by Siemens, Erlangen. In 1988, the PACS configuration included two CT-scanners, an MR-scanner, a Philips DSA and a Dupont film scanner. An archive with optical disks was added later (Mattheus, 1990).

In the Netherlands, the Dutch PACS-project has been started in 1986. This project was a cooperative effort of Utrecht University Hospital, University of Leiden, BAZIS and Philips Netherlands until 1989. The group has done preliminary research in PACS-HIS coupling, modelling and simulation of PACS, clinical evaluation and cost analysis (Stut et al., 1989; Barneveld Binkhuysen et al., 1989).

Since 1984, annual meetings, the so called EuroPACS meetings, are organised as a common platform for the exchange of information, ideas and experiences.

In 1985, the American college of radiologists – national electrical manufacturers association (ACR-NEMA) standard publication 300 appeared that specified a hardware interface, software commands and data formats for communication between imaging devices. To avoid limitations of the ACR-NEMA standard, Siemens and Philips developed in a joint project the standard product interconnect (SPI). The SPI added to ACR-NEMA the concept of an image management system (IMS) including a set of commands to manage data in an image database.

The early PACS projects were directed to gather experience in realistic but restricted subfields of PACS.

As an example, the Dutch PACS, installed in Utrecht, tried to incorporate all kinds of imaging modalities (digital ones and conventional X-rays, where the films where to be scanned for entry into the system) – and was, in that sense, a model of complete PACS – but for a small percentage of the patients, namely patients from one ward with a few beds.

The Graz-PACS (Gell et al., 1989) on the other hand included only one type of modality (CT-scanners), but here all the CT-examinations of all the patients of the hospital were to be processed by the PACS; another aspect of a complete PACS.

Brussels, to cite yet another possibility, set out to cover a specific function (emergency diagnosis) with PACS.

In the years between 1985 and 1990 the number of PACS installations (or should we say the number of PACS projects) has increased considerably, in part stimulated by the beginning availability of commercial products – usually 'mini-PACS' systems, providing a digital archive on optical disc for one or a few modalities and a PACS-workstation – and in part triggered by the advanced informatics in medicine (AIM) program of the EC.

The progress made is best summarized in the proceedings of the specific conferences: EuroPACS, computer assisted radiology (CAR)-Berlin (Lemke et al.,

1987, 1989, 1991) Grazer Radiologisches Symposium (Schneider et al., 1990), Medical Imaging (Schneider et al., 1989), ISPRAD-Florence (Planning Considerations in Diagnostic Imaging and Radiation Therapy) (Chiesa et al., 1988), Digitale Radiographie in Bad Nauheim (Riemann et al., 1988), or books like the monograph about PACS and HIS by Rienhoff and Greinacher (1988), etc.

2.2. Present state of PACS (in Europe)

If we divide the development stages of a technical system into:
- basic research (research without direct relation to an application);
- feasibility studies (implementation of certain features of the planned system
  - to see if it is technically possible at all);
- pilot projects (implementation of a real system for a subdomain of the problem);
- site-specific systems (full systems, but developped in an ad hoc manner for specific needs and environments; usually not transferable); and
- marketable products,

then most PACS installations today are more or less pilot projects.

Only mini-PACS have yet reached the status of a product (a mini-PACS is a PACS for the service of one imaging subspeciality without much communication to the outer world, e.g., a MR with an archive on optical disc and a workstation, all of them linked together in a LAN). Today (1991) to our knowledge there exists nowhere a full PACS, serving all the image management, communication and archiving needs of a hospital. Furthermore, there seems to be no proof that for primary diagnosis the X-ray film may be replaced by workstations with electronic screens. In other words – up to now there is no place where the PACS-workstations are used for routine diagnosis of all cases in one of the typical digital routine examinations like CT. However, there are a few instances where image display is routinely used in ICU-units by non-radiologists (Mun et al., 1989)*.

On the other hand, concerning PACS components, much progress has been made. Digital networks are used in routine to transmit images and the same holds true for digital archives. There exists a full range of image display workstations and many specific PACS-related problems have been solved. Last, but not least, there exists a widely accepted standard for image formats and image transfer: ACR-NEMA. (This is only true for the higher levels of the standard. The physical interface design with its 50-pin connector of ACR-NEMA seems to be a dead born child.)

---

* Addendum in proof. Since April, 1992, a PACS in the Vienna Danuble Hospital runs in 'preliminary' routine including diagnosis on diagnostic consoles

3. PACS 1990 – 2000

3.1. Patterns for the introduction of new technologies in medicine

In the past the introduction of new technologies into medicine has followed two different patterns which might be exemplified by two computer-based methods: CT and HIS.

- *CT.* CT has been established as a valuable routine method all over the world in a few years, surpassing all expectations and forecasts. Other examples of similar penetration are the introduction of diagnostic X-rays a hundred years ago, magnetic resonance imaging (MRI), laser applications in ophthalmology and many more.
- *HIS.* Quite a different pattern is shown by the extremely slow evolution of HIS for real patient care (not billing). More than twenty years ago much has been written about the benefits of computerized HIS, which should not only give the physician all the necessary information about the patient from different sources but also give advice and help for diagnosis and treatment. And yet, progress has been painstakingly slow and today even very advanced institutions do not have a really complete system, one which fulfills all of those early promises.

There are many reasons for this divergence, but, in our opinion, the main difference lies in the fact that CT has a primary effect on patient care, providing the physician with new, previously unavailable information about the patient leading directly to better treatment and care (neurosurgery, radiation therapy, etc.). If there is a definitive advantage for diagnosis or treatment, the introduction of a new method is not obstructed by a poor user interface, complicated operations, old habits, high prices, etc.

On the other hand, the benefits of a HIS for patient care are much more indirect and of secondary order. No really new information is created, but already available information is collected, made easily accessible, etc.

If we try to classify PACS in that sense, there is no doubt that PACS belongs to the HIS category, i.e., the effects of PACS on patient care are of secondary order only. This does not mean that the introduction of PACS must be as slow as the introduction of HIS, but every step has to be justified with respect to ease of use, cost, functionality, etc.

3.2. Future developments, 1990 – 2000

Research in PACS is likely to continue on a broader scale and on all aspects. The forthcoming EC program for informatics in medicine (AIM mainphase) will also sustain projects in the PACS-field. Besides that a growing number of non-research oriented hospitals is launching PACS-projects; a particularly spectacular one is the PACS project of the US military hospitals, where actually the proposals of the industry have been delivered (Goeringer et al., 1989). Decision is planned for the first half of 1991 and implementation over the following years. Another example − on a much smaller scale − is the plan of the SMZ-Hospital in Vienna, a new hospital under construction that should be operational in 1992, to have a comprehensive PACS and an almost filmless operation from the beginning (Mosser et al., 1989, 1991).

The further penetration of PACS into hospitals will largely depend on the success of those early full-scale projects. We are sceptical that comprehensive PACS will rapidly spread out − too many questions are still open and too many problems remain to be solved. We would rather expect a relatively rapid introduction of PAC subsystems with limited aims and functionality that serve a specific (local) purpose: fast availability of images at different locations, image transfer over greater distances (depending on local circumstances a distance of a few hundred meters may already justify electronic transmission to speed up operation), storage systems when archival space is scarce, teleradiology, special purpose image processing (discussed below under special function workstations), etc. These subsystems will eventually merge into a really integrated PACS.

3.3. Problems to be solved

3.3.1. Communication and data transfer
Standard networks like Ethernet have proved to be reliable and successful in small-scale pilot projects, especially if the image transfer is organized as a background process. It is, however, clear that the high data rates generated by a modern film scanner or a computed radiography (CR) device cannot be sustained by Ethernet and probably not even by an FDDI token ring in the usual one ring (backbone) configuration.

If, therefore, CR and film scanners are to be integrated today in a PACS, special solutions must be found. Besides the speed of transmission lines all components of the system, e.g., storage devices and internal bus systems must be capable to deal with these high data rates.

3.3.2. Storage capacity
Here again present day technology (juke-boxes, disk arrays) provides storage capacities sufficient for on-line storage of the traditional digital modalities (CT, nuclear medicine, MR) for one or a few years. If we add conventional radiology (either by scanning films or generating digital CR images), the optimum will be to keep the images in direct access during the stay of the patient in the hospital.

In addition to the optical disk juke-box a large and fast 'cache memory' on magnetic disk is necessary, to buffer the slow juke-box.

3.3.3. Compression

Problems with transmission speed and storage capacity can be eased by compression techniques. Error-free compression (which means that the decompressed image is identical to the original) can only be guaranteed with low compression rates (ca. 1 : 2). It is an open question, if non-errorfree compression with factors like 1 : 10 – 1 : 20 can be used without degrading diagnostic quality. Finally there are experiments with completely new methods like compression with fractals.

3.3.4. Image workstation

A whole gamut of different workstations with different functionality will be necessary, to exploit the possibilities of a PACS. We will discuss three types of such stations in detail, although their functions may be combined in one or spread over even more stations.

3.3.4.1. Primary diagnosis. This is the workstation for the radiologists, which must compete with the traditional light box or alternator.

The basic functionality of this workstation must be better or at least equal to that of the traditional film. The basic parameters include: ease and speed in calling and arranging the images on the screen, strain on the eyes (flicker free, nonglaring surfaces, brightness, etc.), spatial resolution, simultaneous display of all the images of actual and previous examinations, etc. The functional equivalence must be verified by controlled studies concerning the diagnostic quality, speed, fatigue, etc., but this will not suffice if radiologists do not feel subjectively at ease with the station. Despite a few preliminary results, the equality (or superiority or inferiority) of display stations to films for primary diagnosis has not yet been established on a broad and incontestable empirical basis. Necessary additional functions (ordered with decreasing importance) include windowing (grey level windows) to exploit the greater dynamic range of digital methods, a few measurements (pixel values, distance and angle, etc.), zooming and the capability to add annotations to the image. Advanced features like filtering, edge enhancements, three-dimensional reconstructions, etc. are optional for primary diagnosis, since their diagnostic value has not been established so far. The workstation for primary diagnosis should be linked to the RIS or HIS to allow for the retrieval of additional patient information (see also the discussion below about PACS-HIS integration).

Future features may include the use of the diagnostic station for the preparation of the diagnostic report via voice recognition and/or editing capabilities for preformatted reports, etc. which may be sent directly to the HIS.

However, all those additional features cannot substitute for a failure in one of the basic parameters.

3.3.4.2. Special function workstation. It is likely that the easy availability of digital medical images through standardized interfaces (see discussion below) will trigger the development of many new algorithms and methods to solve special problems (examples may be: all kinds of three-dimensional visualisations for therapy planning, dynamic studies, color coding of different parameters, overlay synthesis or comparison of images from different modalities or different times, planning and preview for plastic or constructive surgery, teaching, etc.). At least some of these methods will also require special hardware.

3.3.4.3. Simple image display. There is a great need for access to images from different places of the hospital outside of radiology for different purposes of patient care. In essence the functional need is a display of an image with reasonable speed and resolution with a predefined window setting. Preferably the diagnosis of the radiologist (possibly with annotations on the image) should be available together with the image. In most cases, the necessity to retrieve and review images will only arise occasionally between many other communications- and computer-related tasks. It is, therefore, difficult to see separate display stations or terminals for PACS and HIS in the usually already overcrowded space in a ward or consultation room. In the long run, there will be one multifunctional medical workstation, probably with a (X-) window like user surface, capable of displaying (and to some degree manipulating) laboratory data, medical charts, schedules, images, orders etc. Currently several such multifunctional workstations are under development (e.g., in the EC's AIM program, or (Ratib et al. (1991)).

3.3.5. PACS logistics (PACS-HIS integration)
The management of the image flow in a comprehensive PACS is a non-trivial problem, but the main question is the relation between PACS and HIS. Since a HIS shall per definition control and manage the whole information flow in a hospital, the PACS is logically a part of the HIS. Since many hospitals do not have a HIS or a RIS (as a subsystem of the HIS) capable to support a PACS, manufacturers and developers will be constrained to produce stand-alone PACS with their own database, duplicating many functions and features of a HIS. However, this can only be an intermediate step and those systems should be implemented in such a way that standardized interfaces exist to a HIS

(or RIS) which allow the HIS to keep track of the image information, to link it with other patient data and to request retrieval and display of images (if necessary in advance). Eventually it should be possible to remove non-image-related data to the HIS (avoiding duplication and ensuring data consistency) and to treat PACS as a HIS subsystem like laboratory systems, etc. Ideally, the HIS (RIS) should be able to display, for example, the list of patients waiting for an examination at the operating console of the imaging modality, and the demographic data should be directly copied for image identification, etc.

3.4. Open PACS (expectations and recommendations)

The development of comprehensive HIS which go beyond administrative tasks and encompass medical information and medical procedures has been slow, but there exist many examples of very successful solutions for subsystems on a smaller scale, e.g., for the clinical laboratory, for departmental systems like radiology, oncology, intensive care, etc. The top-down approach has failed, because too many problems must be solved at once. To remedy this situation, there is now a strong trend towards standards and open systems (Miller, 1990). Communication standards like health level seven (HL7) (McDonald, 1990) should allow for the integration and communication of successful subsystems, Syntax standards like the Arden syntax (Hripcsak et al., 1990) should enable the sharing of knowledge bases between different institutions.

PACS seems to be in a similar situation. The top-down planning of an integrated PACS for a whole hospital represents a huge investment with many unknown parameters concerning acceptance and cost – benefit relations. This risk can only be accepted if the system is planned as a modular open system, relying as much as possible on standards (e.g., for the communication network, for data formats and messages, etc.) and well-defined interfaces. Otherwise the hospital may soon be in a position to be wholly dependent from one manufacturer only and unable to incorporate newer technologies from other sources or to integrate the PACS in the HIS. We think that the development of standards and interfaces for open PACS is necessary before the introduction of PACS in hospitals on a wider scale can be justified.

4. PACS – Graz: 1985 – 1990

The Department of Radiology of the University Hospital Graz (a general hospital with 3000 beds) has a long tradition in advanced computer applications. The use of computers for documentation and outpatient management in radiotherapy dates back to the sixties. The development of a documentation system for radiology started in the early seventies. This system which eventually became a full RIS is called AURA and includes today 120 terminals covering almost all aspects of patient management, reporting, retrieval and scientific evaluations (Gell, 1982). AURA has been extended to include pathology and neurosurgery, allowing the sharing of data for patient care, scientific studies, feedback and quality control (Gell, 1983). Other developments include radiologic image processing (Gell and Fotter, 1984), computer-assisted diagnosis, etc.

In 1985, the department of radiology in Graz and Siemens Medical Systems in Erlangen decided to begin a common PACS pilot project. This project should implement a PACS for the CT division of the department and evaluate all aspects of the operation in clinical routine. The necessary hardware and software has been installed and implemented step by step:

1986 Installation of the Ethernet-based 'CT net' linking together three CT-scanners (Siemens, Somatom) and an old Siemens evaluation console (EVA). Installation of a diagnostic console (PDM) with two displays and a special non-standard keyboard. The console was not linked to the net; the images had to be transferred via magnetic tapes.

1987 The diagnostic console is connected to the network and the special keyboard is replaced by a mouse as the standard user interface. The diagnostic console is enhanced with a third monitor. A short-term image database (Microvax with magnetic disks) is linked to the network.

1988 Two optical disk drives are added to the image database computer and, throughout the year, more and more images are stored on optical disks. The PACS is linked to the hospital wide network (Ethernet) and logically integrated into the RIS (AURA).

1989 The MR-scanner (Philips) is linked to the net and software for image transfer is developed. A fourth CT-scanner from radiotherapy with a distance of about 1 km is integrated into the system via the hospital network. All CT-images are routinely archived on optical disk and the use of magnetic tapes is terminated. The old diagnostic console is replaced by a new one with three high-resolution monitors.

1990 Begin of a project to give workstations (PC) in the hospital network access to PACS images. Installation of an 'intelligent' supervisor process to watch PACS operation.

In a first phase (1985 – 1987), the main efforts were concerned with the establishment of the basic structure, network communication and the user interface and use of the diagnostic console. In a second phase (1988 – 1990) emphasis has been shifted to the problems of routine operation, archival and the PACS-RIS integration.

5. PACS-Graz. The actual state

5.1. PACS configuration

The general configuration is shown in Fig. 1. PACS includes four CT-scanners (one of them in a distance of 1 km), an evaluation console, a diagnostic console and an archive with two optical disk drives. Within the hospital network (KH-net), many more computers exist, one of them supporting the RIS (AURA).

5.1.1. Network and communication

Hardware and low-level protocols of our networks are based on Ethernet. CT-net is a Siemens proprietary protocol (a subset of Decnet) for linking Siemens modalities via Ethernet. The hospital network (KH-net) is based on Decnet, a proprietary protocol of digital equipment corporation which should eventually evolve into a ISO/OSI network. Fiber optic cables link the different buildings of the hospital; within the buildings thick or thin wire Ethernet is used. The hospital net and the PACS net are linked via a VAX (see Fig. 1) which serves as a bridge. CT-net and Decnet coexist – the CT-scanner in radiotherapy is linked via the hospital network using the CT-net protocol.

Different tasks in the PACS are achieved by software processes which permanently reside in the different computers (they are initialized once at system start-up) and are triggered into action by events like a user command or a message from another process. A process on the archive, for example, receives the images from a modality (CT) and stores them into a file. The process then sends a message to another process responsible for converting the images into

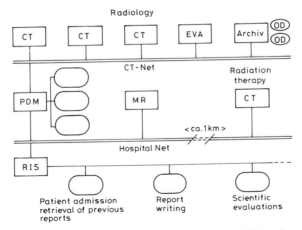

Fig. 1. The PACS at the Department of Radiology of the University of Graz.

ACR-NEMA format. This process in turn submits the images with the corresponding messages to another process for archiving on optical disk and to another process on the diagnostic console to arrange the images for reporting. In a similar way, the RIS sends a message to request rearchiving of old images of a patient. The whole structure realises the high levels of ACR-NEMA as specified by system product interconnect (SPI), an agreement between Siemens and Philips. The pipeline of processes operates automatically in the background while the user continues with other work. Most of this software is proprietary by Siemens. The company provides (sells) software tools to link other equipment to these structures.

5.1.2. Imaging

CT scanner: Siemens Somatom DRH, DR3, DR3, DR2, based on PDP11 computers. There is little flexibility for communication (with RIS, for example). They deliver images with 256 × 256 or 512 × 512 pixels in a non-ACR-NEMA format via the Decnet protocol. Two bytes per pixel are transferred although only 12 bit contain image information.

MR-scanner: Philips Gyroscan, 256 × 256, 12 bit (two bytes transferred), based on a VAX 750. The VAX supports Decnet and can transfer ACR-NEMA formats, although the ACR-NEMA protocol is not yet supported. Image transfer is via DEC utility programs (copy).

5.1.3. Archive

Microvax II with two optical drives (LD 1200 WORM). One drive is used for archiving and short-time retrieval and the other for reading disks from the 'manual' archive. Two magnetic disks with 450 Mbytes each are used for temporary storage and as a fast buffer to the slow optical drives (The LD1200 has a net transfer rate of 1.5 Mbytes/s and the average access (seek) time is 150 ms). The optical disks (12 inch) have a total capacity of 2 Gbytes (1 Gbyte on each side).

If an optical disk is full, a corresponding message is displayed on the archive console and also on the monitors of the CT-scanners. Then a new disk must be inserted into the disk drive. The disks are identified by sequential numbers which are automatically assigned at the initialisation of the disk.

5.1.4. Diagnostic console

The diagnostic console includes 3 monitors (20 inch) with a resolution of 1050 × 1280 pixels and a refresh rate of 60 Hz. The computer of the diagnostic console is a MicroVAX II. Special processors are used for image processing and mouse handling. The console has a local Winchester disk store of 500 Mbyte.

After the log-in on the keyboard every function on the console is called by clicking a mouse. First a list of all the available examinations is displayed. After the selection of an examination an overview with all the images of this examination is displayed. The overview consists of so called token images (128 × 128). Up to 64 token images can be displayed on one monitor.

The images are selected from the overview by clicking with the mouse and displayed on the two other monitors. It is possible to show up to 16 images with 256 × 256 pixels or 4 images with 512 × 512 pixels simultaneously on each screen. The images are displayed with a preset gray-scale window which depends on the kind of examination. The radiologist can also chose windows from a table of preset values or he may freely change center and width with the mouse. The console enables image processing functions like zooming, mirroring, rotating, etc. With the pixel lens the radiologist can determine the Hounsfield value of every single pixel in the image. It is also possible to make line and area histograms.

If an examination is transferred to the diagnostic console, the RIS is checked for previous examinations. If previous examinations exist, the report texts are copied automatically to the diagnostic console where they can be displayed on the overview screen.

5.1.5. Data structures

Before the archiving and after the retrieving patient-, examination- and image-data are organized in so called folders (in analogy to the conventional folders with the images used in the routine of every radiology department). Folders are collections (pointers to) images which belong to one examination, one patient or one problem. There exists an actual examination folder (AEF), which contains the unreported examinations and a final examination folder (FEF), which contains the reported examinations. The access to the folders is performed via patient ID-data. The folders are managed by the image database IMS. In addition all examinations of a patient are collected into a patient folder and images may be grouped into a special folder according to special criteria (e.g., diagnosis).

5.1.6. PACS – RIS-interface

As explained earlier, we consider PACS to be logically a part of a RIS (or a HIS). Although our PACS and RIS have been developed independently and may operate independently, we tried to avoid too much duplicity of data and to give the RIS the control over the entire long-term database, consisting of free text reports, coded data and pictorial data. The RIS sends patient data about previous examinations to the PACS and requests the rearchiving of old patient folders from the optical archive thus enabling the PACS to display all relevant information about a patient (reports and images from previous examinations) on the physician's console. We would like to have an even tighter coupling with a display of patient's lists on the monitor of the modality – but this proved to be impossible with our 'pre-PACS modalities'. On the other hand, the PACS sends the information about new examinations and their (physical) location on optical disks to the RIS for incorporation in the database. The coupling with the RIS makes it easy to select images with an arbitrary logical combination of parameters (sex, age, diagnosis, clinical question, findings, etc.).

The structure of the PACS – RIS interaction follows the message process pattern outlined above.

5.2. PACS operation – the users view

At the admission desk, the operator enters the patient's ID-data into the RIS which automatically performs a search in the full radiology database for previous encounters. A list is displayed and the operator selects those examinations, which might be relevant for the present problem. As explained above, this triggers background processes to rearchive images and to transfer images and reports to the diagnostic console (prefetching).

At the examination the radiographer has to enter again the patient's name, birthdate and an examination identification at the console of the CT. We hope that future modalities will be able to accept those data directly from the HIS/RIS. After the examination the radiographer sends the images to the archive – in fact, he/she initializes the transfer which then runs in the background, inserting images in the database, routing them (selected examinations) to the diagnostic console and archiving them on optical disks.

If the radiologist starts the reviewing process at the diagnostic console the necessary data are preloaded and immediately available: the images of the actual examination, the reports of previous examinations and the digital images of previous examinations. After reporting, the images are deleted from the local store.

The send command allows also to copy images from one modality to another one (e.g., to make hard copies, if the local hard copy unit is not working).

5.3. PACS operation – quantitative data

5.3.1. Network and communication

Image transfer: In the department of radiology CT examinations are made 24 hours a day. Up to 60 examinations are made during the day shift (between 7 in the morning and 3 in the afternoon) and 5 – 10 examinations during the night shift. On weekends we have an average of 10 examinations per day. 8 – 12 examinations per day are transferred to the archive from the remote scanner in radiotherapy.

The copying from the CT-scanner to the archive needs 4 s for images with 256 × 256 pixels and 16 s for images with 512 × 512 pixels. To convert an image into ACR-NEMA needs 4 s for images with 256 × 256 pixels and 8 s for images with 512 × 512 pixels. Submitting into the image database takes 1.5 s per image. Because the different processes are running simultaneously the time needed to transfer and archive a whole examination is less than the sum of the single steps.

If an examination with 30 images is transferred to the archive, it takes 5 min until the whole examination is submitted into the image database and another 5 min to copy the examination on optical disk. An examination with 30 images is available at the diagnostic console about 7 min after the retrieval request from the RIS.

5.3.2. Archive

Storing all images in a reduced 256 × 256 format and with lossless compression about 26 000 images, roughly corresponding to 1 000 CT-examinations or the production of one week, can be stored on one side of an optical disk. Using both sides we need about 25 disks for the image production of one year (four CTs).

5.4. Experiences and discussion

5.4.1. Acceptance by radiographers (communication and archiving)

Those features of PACS that effect radiographers, are well accepted and established in clinical routine: sending images over the network, archiving on optical disks, etc. Radiographers generally feel PACS made their work easier in most places; there are still complaints concerning some duplication of work because of insufficient integration of modalities (cf., the discussion on PACS-logistics).

5.4.2. Acceptance by radiologists (primary diagnosis)

Our somewhat disappointing experience is: radiologists do not like to use the diagnostic console for primary diagnosis! To give another disappointing fact: we (in Graz) do not really know the reason why radiologists do not use the console. The reasons put forward are: not all the relevant images of one case (actual examination, previous examinations, images from other modalities) can be seen 'simultaneously'; operation is slightly more inconvenient, than that of the traditional lightbox; the difference in brightness makes it difficult to have a lightbox besides the monitor (for viewing, e.g., a chest X-ray of the same patient), etc.

In the early phases we tried very hard to get radiologists to work with the console; we were told over and over again to just add another feature and then it would be accepted. When that feature was implemented, the console was used for some time in routine and then use stopped again.

5.4.3. General operation

Usually radiographers are able to do all the necessary operating for running the entire PACS. Sometimes, however, as a consequence of hard- or software failure or of some other unusual situation, the intervention of a software specialist becomes necessary. Those events tend to cluster − the mean time between such clusters is about two weeks.

Outgoing from our experiences in routine work we perceive that for a smooth and reliable operation the PACS should conform to a set of requirements like autonomous supervision, automatic elimination of malfunctions, automatic catch of wrong manipulations, communication with the user, etc.

The system must inform the user about successful completion of procedures as well as about malfunctions which occur during the routine work and check automatically if all the necessary functions are executed. The system should supervise autonomously the single processes and be intelligent enough to recognize, localize and eliminate faults automatically.

For a detailed discussion of our experiences and of what we perceive as necessary software requirements of a successful PACS see Wiltgen and Gell (1991).

5.4.4. Discussion

From a functional point of view, the system benefits are higher than the costs (in terms of human efforts and running costs) except for the use for primary diagnosis where our experience does not allow to make a well-founded statement.

Finally we do not know: do we just need a little bit more user friendliness on the side of the console or a little bit of change in user attitude to get full acceptance or is there some much more fundamental problem to solve?

It seems, however, from many visits at other PACS-sites and discussions with other PACS-developers and users that our experience is not a singular one (although the fact is not always stated clearly in published papers)!

Due to the easy handling and the high storage capacity of the optical disks, there exists an economization of labor and time for the radiographers. The price for optical disks is at the moment 0.02 US$ per image and therefore lower than for magnetic tapes (0.03 US$ per image).

We are not able to make a complete cost−benefit analysis because the original hardware for the pilot project was given by Siemens and still has no definite price tag.

6. PACS-Graz. Developments since 1990

The PACS project in Graz currently (1991) has very limited resources. We therefore plan to position our development efforts in such a way as to achieve maximum benefit (in terms of improved patient care and scientific output) with the available means.

The most urgent clinical interest in PACS seems not to be in primary diagnosis in radiology, where only a small additional benefit is to be expected by the replacement of films, but in the wards, where images are presently not available or only with delays and incomplete. To achieve this we want to capitalize on the ubiquitous presence of PCs in the hospital and we have developed software to turn every PC (with an Ethernet card and VGA) into a cheap PACS terminal for viewing images without much functionality (just windowing). This will not be a competition for the PACS terminals of the industry, but a cheap access to PACS that will create a need, first for the introduction of PACS and then for more sophisticated workstations and monitors.

A necessary prerequisite will be a much larger on-line storage and we consider the installation of an optical jukebox.

Large image databases will create completely new possibilities for using images in medical education and for integrating images into computer-aided medical decision systems. We want to explore those possibilities and have a project to improve our existing system for the computer-aided diagnosis of bone tumors (Gell and Fotter, 1984) by the integration of images.

Another development is a software process (PACS-monitor) to handle and survey image communication and archiving. This process monitors the background activities of the PACS and allow the user to get information about the status of the system at any time. The PACS-monitor is used for the supervising of the PACS.

There is an increasing need for software which allows the user to easily localize and eliminate malfunctions during the routine work. So a smooth operation of the PACS should be possible, independently from the permanent presence of an EDP-expert in the radiological department. This software (OPERAS: operating assistent) is based on a rule based system. OPERAS is started via the PACS-monitor and gains information about the state of PACS, analyses the situation via condition – action rules and gives then either advices to the user or eliminates the problem automatically.

A DSA and a Siemens DRC 101 workstation have been added. We plan to activate the MR connection and study the integration of nuclear medicine.

A new section for pediatric radiology is under construction. Given our experiences, we do not plan for a filmless operation, but we shall install the infrastructure to allow for easy communication of pediatric radiology with the rest of the department, again using the RIS as the common database to access images in different locations.

References

Barneveld Binkhuysen, F.H., F.P. Ottes, B.M. Ter Haar Romeny, P.L.M. Klessens, C.G. Vos, L.H.L. Winter, P.T. Calkoen and J.H.T.H. Andriessen (1989) First results of the diagnostic evaluation studies and the clinical efficacy in the Dutch PACS project. In: Schneider, R.H., S.J. Dwyer III and R.G. Jost (Eds.), Medical Imaging III: PACS System Design and Evaluation, *Proc. SPIE* 1093, 13–19.

Chiesa, A., Gasparotti and R. Maroldi (Eds.) (1988) Planning Considerations in Diagnostic Imaging and Radiation Therapy, *Proc. ISPRAD V Florence*, 20–23 April 1988. Clas Int., Brescia.

Gell, G. (1982) AURA: a clinical data bank based on free text. In: Moore, R.R.O., B. Barber, P.L. Reichertz and F. Roger (Eds.), Lecture Notes in Medical Informatics, 16, 850–856 (Springer, Berlin).

Gell, G. (1983) AURA: routine documentation of medical texts, *Meth. Inform. Med.* 22, 63–68.

Gell, G. and R. Fotter (1984) Experiences with the use of a foreign system for computer assisted diagnosis. In: Roger, F.H., J.L. Willems, R.O. Moore and B. Barber (Eds.), Medical Informatics Europe 84, Lecture Notes in Medical Informatics, 24, 337–340 (Springer, Berlin).

Gell, G., G.H. Schneider and M. Wiltgen (1989) Klinische Erfahrungen mit einem PACS. In: Riemann, H., J. Kollath and O. Rienhoff (Eds.), 3. Frankfurter Gespräch über Digitale Radiographie in Bad Nauheim, pp. 196–201 (Schnetztor-Verlag, Konstanz).

Goeringer, F., S.K. Mun and B.D. Kerlin (1989) Digital medical imaging: implementation strategy for the defense medical establishment. In: Schneider R.H., S.J. Dwyer III and R.G. Jost (Eds.), Medical Imaging III: PACS System Design and Evaluation, *Proc. SPIE* 1093, 429–437.

Greinacher, C.F.C., K. Müller and D. Fuchs (1984) Digitale Bildinformationssysteme in der Radiologie Stand und Entwicklungstendenzen, *Digitale Bilddiagnostik* 4, 87–104.

Hripcsak, G., P.D. Clayton, T.A. Pryor, P. Haug, O.B. Wigertz and J. Van Der Lei (1990) The Arden syntax for medical logic modules. In: Miller, R.A., (Ed.), SCAMC Symposium on Computer Applications in Medical Care, *Proc. 14, IEEE Comp. Soc. Press,* Los Alamitos, California, 200–204.

Lemke, H.U., M.L. Rhodes, C.C. Jaffe and R. Felix (Eds.) (1987) Computer-Assisted Radiology. *Proc. 2nd International Symposium Computer-Assisted Radiology,* Car 87 (Springer, Berlin).

Lemke, H.U., M.L. Rhodes, C.C. Jaffe and R. Felix (Eds.) (1989) Computer-Assisted Radiology. *Proc. 3rd International Symposium Computer-Assisted Radiology,* Car 89 (Springer, Berlin).

Lemke, H.U., M.L. Rhodes, C.C. Jaffe and R. Felix (Eds.) (1991) Computer-Assisted Radiology. *Proc. International Symposium Computer-Assisted Radiology,* Car 91 (Springer, Berlin).

Mattheus, R. (1990) PACS and PACS-related research in Belgium. In: Huang, H.K., O. Ratib, A.R. Bakker and G. Witte (Eds.), Picture Archiving and Communication Systems (PACS) in Medicine, *NATO ASI Series F* 74, 251–258 (Springer, Berlin).

McDonald, C.J. (1990) Standards for the electronic transfer of clinical data: progress, promises and the conductor's wand. In: Miller, R.A., (Ed.), SCAMC Symposium on Computer Applications in Medical Care, *Proc. 14, IEEE Comp. Soc. Press,* Los Alamitos, California, 9–14.

Miller, R.A. (Ed.) (1990) SCAMC Symposium on Computer Application in Medical Care – Standards in Medical Informatics, *IEEE Comp. Soc. Press,* Los Alamitos, California.

Mosser, H., A. Mandl, M. Urban, H. Hradil and W. Hruby (1989) The Vienna SMZO project. In: Huang, H.K., O. Ratib, A.R. Bakker and G. Witte (Eds.), Picture Archiving and Communication Systems (PACS) in Medicine, *NATO ASI Series F* 74, 247–250.

Mosser, H., W. Rütger, M. Urban and W. Hruby (1991) Planning a large scale PACS: the Vienna SM70-project. In: Adlassnig, K.-P., G. Grabner, S. Bengtsson and R. Hansen (Eds.), Medical Informatics Europe 1991. Lecture Notes in Medical Informatics 45, 187 – 192 (Springer, Berlin).

Mun, K., H. Benson, S. Horri, L.P. Elliot, B. Shih-Chung, B. Levine, R. Braudes, G. Plumlee, B. Garra, D. Schellinger, B. Majors, F. Goeringer, B. Kerlin, J. Cerva, M.-L. Ingeholm and T. Gore (1989) Completion of a hospital-wide comprehensive image managment and communication system. In: Schneider, R.H., S.J. Dwyer III and R.G. Jost (Eds.), Medical Imaging III: PACS System Design and Evaluation, *Proc. SPIE* 1093, 204 – 213.

Ratib, O., Y. Ligier, M. Funk, D. Hochstrasser and J.-R. Scherrer (1991) Modular development of a hospital wide picture archiving and communication system (PACS). In: Adlassnig, K.-P., G. Grabner, S. Bengtsson and R. Hansen (Eds.), Medical Informatics Europe 1991, Lecture Notes in Medical Informatics 45, 182 – 186 (Springer, Berlin).

Riemann, H., J. Kollath and O. Rienhoff (Eds.) (1988) Digitale Radiographie, 3. Frankfurter Gespräch über Digitale Radiographie (Schnetztor-Verlag Konstanz).

Rienhoff, O, and C.F.C. Greinacher (Eds.) (1988) A General PACS – RIS Interface. Lecture Notes in Medical Informatics 37 (Springer, Berlin).

Schneider, R.H., S.J. Dwyer III and R.G. Jost (Eds.) (1989) Medical Imaging III: PACS System Design and Evaluation, *Proc. SPIE* 1093.

Schneider, G.H., E. Vogler and K. Kocever (Eds.) (1990) Digitale Bildgebung, Interventionelle Radiologie, Integrierte digitale Radiologie, 6. Grazer Radiologisches Symposium (Blackwell Ueberreuter Wissenschaft, Berlin).

Stut, W.J.J., M.R. Van Steen, L.P.J. Groenewegen, A.R. Bakker and B.M. Ter Haar Romeny (1989) PACS design issues: modelling and simulation. In: Schneider, R.H., S.J. Dwyer III and R.G. Jost (Eds.), Medical Imaging III: PACS System Design and Evaluation, *Proc. SPIE* 1093, 523 – 536.

Tiemann, J., R. Heu and G. Tesche (1985) Digitale Bildarchiving und Kommunikation. In: Schneider, G.H., and E. Vogler (Eds.), Digitale bildgebende Verfahren Integrierte digitale Radiologie, 4. Grazer Radiologisches Symposium, 908 – 912 (Schering, Berlin).

Wiltgen, M., and G. Gell (1991) An intelligent software process for the survey management and error detetection in a PACS. In: Lemke, H.U., M.L. Rhodes, C.C. Jaffe and R. Felix (Eds.), Computer-Assisted Radiology. *Proc. International Symposium Computer-Assisted Radiology.* CAR 91, 863 (Springer, Berlin).

Wiltgen, M., G. Gell and G.H. Schneider (1991) Some software requirements for a PACS: lessons from experiences in clinical routine, *Int. J. Bio-Med. Comput.* 28, 61 – 70.

Integrated Diagnostic Imaging
Editor: J.P.J. De Valk
© *Elsevier Science Publishers B.V., 1992*

Chapter 7

Communication services: a key issue in the PACS of the year 2000

R. Mattheus

1. Introduction

In the past decade, the emphasis in medical equipment has shifted from the application of microelectronics to system-level solutions. This includes the incorporation of computers and associated software in existing products. The integration of these products through local area networks (LANs) and dedicated software into medical information systems is on its way. Attempts to combine the existing isolated departmental medical information systems into a hospital information system (HIS) have proven the importance of integration. The management of the vast amount of medical images and information generated by today's clinical services is a growing problem. For the management of this enormous amount of images, the concept of picture archiving and communications systems (PACS) was defined in the early eighties.

The introduction of PACS shows problems similar to the ones experienced in other application areas, as office or plant automation. In 1982, PACS was first introduced as a concept. Different solutions where proposed, but the medical community has not yet been satisfied. In a clinical environment, a large-scale host computer system seems not to be effective for PACS. A distributed system is more flexible and makes it possible to maintain and expand the system in relation to the organization and needs of the imaging department.

The role of advanced technology needs continuous reevaluation. Introduction of new technologies has raised a number of issues. Changes in patient flow were brought about by the new imaging technologies. It became important to review the hospital organization in order to accommodate the changes in decision making processes and patient care, driven by the new technology.

The transmission of the medical information, including images, has to be carefully coordinated, with appropriate users at various locations serving specialized purposes. PACS will change the way that diagnostic information is presented and decisions are made. The PACS concept as first defined is changing and will increase focus on the communication service aspects, allowing to add different other functions as image processing, image phone, teleradiology. The benefits will not be found in cost saving in film in the next decade. The same problems hold here that held for the paperless office: more paper is generated than before the introduction of the computer. The benefits will be in the area of image management, image processing, remote consultation, shorter stay in hospital, better coordination between different departments and more accurate selection of the diagnostic procedure.

Modular network architectures, capable of reacting to growth and changes in traffic patterns are essential. Partitioning the network into subnets will reduce bandwidth requirements and increase response time by distributing network traffic. A hierarchical system structure will make it easier to use existing transmission techniques with an optimum choice on each level. As an additional benefit, this design strategy offers the possibility to start introduction of PACS into a given environment by establishing the local subsystem first. In subsequent steps, the integration of subsystems into a complete PACS could be performed, accompanied by a step-by-step training of personnel and a gradual change of work routines. Using building blocks from the information technology and telecommunications (IT & T) market is essential. Moreover, standardization work going on in medical informatics and IT & T will stimulate the PACS activities. In the year 2000 PACS will be no science fiction any more, but a useful tool. Like a telephone for voice communication, we will have a medical image (maybe multi-media) 'phone'.

2. Health care and PACS

2.1. Components of health care

If we look at it from the medical informatics point of view, medicine can be divided in four main components.

- *Preventive medicine.* Averting or protecting persons from the occurrence of a particular condition or disorder, and forecasting and/or identifying the individuals at risk of acquiring a particular illness at some time in the future. This class is starting to grow, e.g., mammography screening. To allow expansion, the necessary communication services need to be available and PACS can play an important role in this area by providing image communication.
- *Diagnosis.* Determining the nature and circumstances of a disease condition

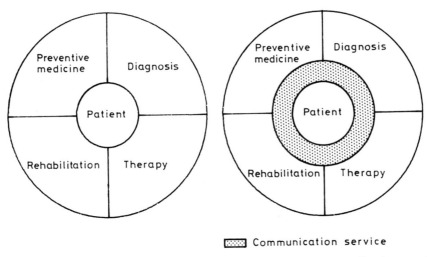

Fig. 1. The health care glasses, focusing on communication. The information flow between the health care components. Left figure before introduction of communication services, right after introduction.

through examination, tests, evaluation of information and monitoring. Remote consultation and advice will be one of the applications of a PACS.

– *Therapy.* Deciding on how to treat the patient for the diagnosed disease condition with a combination of curative, supportive and/or interventional processes, and the treatment itself. The integration of the diagnostic information, as images, with the therapy systems will allow more accurate procedures; e.g., use of CT (computed tomography) images for the calculation of isodosis for oncology and the use of CT/MRI (magnetic resonance imaging) images for prosthesis developments. PACS will be acting as a service allowing these and other image processing applications.

– *Rehabilitation.* Restoring or reestablishing a condition of good health, the ability to work, or integration into society, ideally at the level that existed before the illness. Due to the existence of a good communication infrastructure more adequate rehabilitation can be performed and feedback to therapy easier.

The different components of health care will be more integrated by means of the communication services which will be developed during this decade (fig. 1). Information will be digital available through the components so that processing becomes possible on each level. Information can be shared between the different components. It can be patient specific but also general statistical information, needed for preventive medicine.

2.2. Advanced medical equipment and systems

Science and technology are evolving rapidly. This creates the potential for applying its innovations to health care products too. Improved and/or cheaper older technologies and products, and sometimes even new ones, will continue to emerge as a consequence of this. On the basis of medical, economic and technical assessments, the users should decide which old technologies should be replaced and which new ones put into use. New materials and computer technology are the driving forces behind advances in medical equipment. Indication must be made that hardware is becoming better performing and cheaper, but that on the other side software and services are becoming more complex and much more expensive. For example, the maintenance of software must not be underestimated. By combining means of networking and system integration, new systems will be created.

- Patient-monitoring equipment, comprising sophisticated transducers, such as transcutaneous oxygen transducers, together with microelectronics, microprocessors and software for processing the measured signals.
- Information systems for patient-data management and for decision support integrating various sources of patient data and incorporating, e.g., knowledge-based techniques (artificial intelligence, expert systems) for the interpretation of the compiled data. Such systems are used and developed for intensive care, clinical laboratories, etc.
- Imaging of the anatomy and functions of the human body, a rapidly expanding area where many imaging modalities are currently available. The technology for obtaining and storing the images is changing from film to digital. Integration of the various image sources with PACS and image processing stations is the present trend.
- Automated laboratory equipment for the processing of patient samples (blood, urine, etc.), an area that has been highly cost-effective. It incorporates many technologies necessary in the handling, dispensing, incubation and analysis of the samples. Information systems are extensively used to manage the process, for quality control and for producing laboratory reports to wards and treating physicians. The ease with which these analysis can be performed led at one point to undue proliferation of this technology.
- Technical aids for the handicapped (and for the elderly), comprising both simple and complex tools. Lately developments in IT and in robotics have yielded up new possibilities in environmental control and communication both at home and at work.

Multi-disciplinary initiatives are the main thread in this new development. Integration of information is the key stream, and PACS is one of these. Medically relevant information will be communicated through the hospital and even further; but the integration and display of the most relevant information will be the most demanding and will need a knowledge base for the handling of these difficult tasks.

2.3. *Digital medical imaging*

Digital medical imaging is an interdisciplinary field which bridges mathematics, engineering, computer sciences, physics and medicine. PACS development is very dependent on the evolution in these fields. It responds to the need for a non-invasive technique to view the interior of the body. The current practice involves trade-offs in computing requirements and matching of different techniques.

Medical imaging is a global discipline that mainly evolved from radiology. Conventional radiology, skeleton, chest X-ray, is a discipline that originated at the beginning of the century, and that is based on films, lightboxes, and classical (paper)files. New methods were, however, introduced more recently. High-performance acquisition techniques and advanced medical knowledge gave rise to the development of computed tomography, digital angiography, single positron emission tomography, and more recently magnetic resonance imaging. Note that images are also generated and manipulated in disciplines like nuclear medicine, macroscopy, endoscopy, pathology, cytology, orthopedics and radio-therapy.

The major problem is the handling of all the image and image-related infor-

Data	Text and other patient data, administrative and medical
Two-dimensional	Techniques for displaying CR images and CT or MRI slices
Three-dimensional	Techniques for more realistically displaying anatomical objects reconstructed from CT, MRI, US data
Four-dimensional	Digital processing and manipulation for visualisation of dynamic images
Five-dimensional	An additional dimension used for parameters like wavelength or energy, necessary to obtain lists of images; e.g., spectroscopic sequences in MRI
Multi-modality	Mapping of different types of information, for example, functional information, PET and CT anatomical information.
Multi-media	Text, images, graphs, signals, voices, documents

Fig. 2. Medical information type. The evolution of the type of information, from the imaging point of view, having an impact on the range of acquisition units to display devices.

mation like patient name, acquisition parameters, regions of interest and other even more complex data. Handling can be visualizing, processing, transmitting, storing, manipulating and managing this multi-media information. The research in the scope of computer applications in medical care has entailed great benefits in terms of patient care, but it has also raised a variety of concerns regarding the implications of uncoordinated use of this new technology. Since the discovery of X-ray, mostly two-dimensional imaging was done, a projection of the view of interest (fig. 2). The introduction of the computer allowed the computing power, with which reconstructions could be calculated, necessary for CT and MRI and allowing three-dimensional imaging. Imaging with the time component is referred to as four-dimensional and is well known in the US (ultrasound) and DSA (digital subtraction angiography) environments. Lists of images can be generated based on the variation of a parameter like the wavelength or energy. Next steps will be the mapping and correlation of different types of images. Multi-media information will be a combination of the relevant information on a patient, the total digital medical record, including voice reports, ECG measurements, and video communication. Advances in the direct digital imaging techniques will stimulate the need for PACS. Computed radiography (CR) based on phosphor plate or similar techniques will soon be implemented world wide, not because PACS demands them, but because a lot of other benefits are gained using this technology: lower doses, image processing, less miss exposures, less personnel and, of course, they are digital. The major current problems are the prices, but they will drop in time (WHO, 1990).

2.4. PACS-IMACS: a definition

A lot of different definitions and acronyms were given in the past, probably in this book too, and one might expect not for the last time either. The definitions of PACS and IMACS given below are in this chapter not used in the restricted context, but more as synonyms.

PACS

After a digital radiological image is acquired (compressed or uncompressed), it has to be transmitted to a storage device for archiving and to be available for later retrieval, display, manipulation and review. This procedure and the associated computer system, both hardware and software, are called a PACS.

IMACS

Image management and communication systems (IMACS) describes an advanced, image based, medical information system. The system can manage varieties of medical images and is capable of retrieving and displaying alphanumeric information from the conventional medical information system, or facilitates information transfer by sound. The IMAC system could be one of many configurations ranging from a single module capable of supporting a small medical operation, to a network of modules shared among major medical centres. IMACS covers the total hospital and PACS is more or less restricted to the radiology department.

3. PACS characteristics and technology impact

3.1. PACS-topology

Two main reasons can be given why the setting up of a PACS environment takes place in different phases. The first reason is that the cost price of a PACS environment in a hospital is rather high. The other reason is that there is still very little experience in setting up such an environment. Mostly, a PACS is built with new equipment and later on extended with the already existing equipment. It is dubious if activities in a hospital could be shut down in order to perform a few PACS experiments.

Because there are different phases, PACS-environments of different hospitals can hardly be compared, unless one knows exactly in which phase they are. Standard modelling methodologies and terminology need to be defined before comparison is really possible (Mattheus et al., 1990; Nosil et al., 1990)

Closed line architecture
Closed line architecture (fig. 3) is the first phase from which one starts for the development of a PACS environment. This one is specifically oriented towards a specific type of acquisition station. This type of PACS environments is in

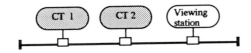

Fig. 3. A closed line architecture with two CTs and a viewing station.

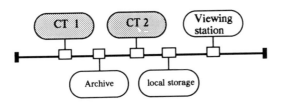

Fig. 4. A central line architecture.

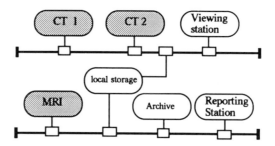

Fig. 5. A distributed network architecture. A computer is used for the integration of two networks or more.

general supplied by the manufacturer of the machine. Two or three acquisition stations of the same type are linked to a viewing station. It is possible to store the images temporarily, but no form of archiving is offered yet.

Central line architecture
In a central line architecture (fig. 4), a central computer is linked to a local storage medium, a local database and archiving possibilities. This approach is commonly the first real step towards a PACS environment.

Distributed network
In a distributed network (fig. 5) two central line networks are linked. This creates the possibility to have a network in which different types of acquisition stations occur. There is still one archive, and the network manager still is in the hands of a single computer.

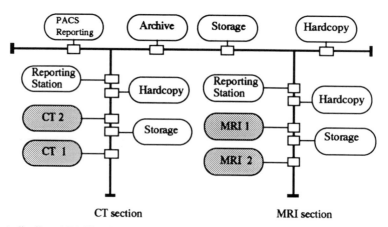

Fig. 6. A distributed PACS subnetwork. The two departments on the figure are interconnected through the PACS-backbone, resulting in two PACS clusters.

Distributed subnetworks

In a distributed subnetwork (fig. 6) each subsegment cluster has a local storage unit, reporting consoles and hard copy equipment. The archive is distributed over the subsegments. Each segment is linked with another segment via a gateway: this enables both linked segments to transport images undisturbedly. Small PACS-islands are created, communicating trough a higher level structure controlled by a network manager. The network manager is a kind of traffic policeman that lets images through if the segment or one linked to it needs them. It is an addition to pre-fetching techniques. A distributed database handles and distributes the data, while the images are stored in hierarchical local storage (Huang et al., 1990).

3.2. The requirements of a PACS/IMACS architecture

These requirements are:
- Continuous access by many users to large amounts of distributed data. The underlying technology must provide high system availability, the ability to repair the system while it is on-line, high performance to handle unpredictable peakloads in utilization, large storage capacity to accommodate the massive corporate database, and high-speed communication for rapid response.
- The ability to accommodate rapid and unpredictable growth in the size and use of the application. The underlying technology must support system expansion without lengthy software conversions. Many PACS applications generate high growth and require the ability to increase capacity without significant system outrages.
- The ability to manage large networks of heterogeneous computers. Most acquisition vendors have a heterogeneous computer environment, with many different types of equipment purchased from multiple computer vendors. One of the biggest challenges of the 1990s will be the management of this resource.

3.3. PACS revolutions

PACS is a complex item, it is a trade-off between technical, medical, economic and organisational issues. As mentioned before, PACS combines efforts of different disciplines. It is therefore not evident to describe the phases in its evolution: they are set by one or more events in the various disciplines. Characteristic for this evolution is the IT & T and hospital integration (HI) involvement. HI covers different items, e.g., integration with the HIS, interaction with the clinic environment and adaptation of medical knowledge. As we are moving towards a film-independent system, the realization of this technology needs to be map-

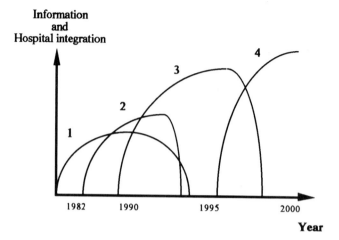

Fig. 7. The four PACS revolution phases. Evolution in PACS concepts and the driving forces behind it. Phase 1: experimental phase; phase 2: technical driven approach; phase 3: medical user approach; phase 4: open system phase.

ped to the information technologies, and this in close relation to the open system approach. The four phases of PACS revolution are shown in fig. 7.

3.3.1. Phase 1: experimental phase
Since 1982, when the 'PACS' acronym and concept was defined, research has been done in different domains, but the major approach for some of the installations in hospitals had a lot of technical problems which needed to be solved before the real introduction in hospitals could occur.

Large projects where set up in the experimental phase. Characteristic for this phase is that most of the components where developed from scratch. Fast networks were under development, display stations were implemented and archiving was a concern. A lot of manpower and money was put into these systems, with not always the expected results. The focus was on the radiology department and less attention was given to other departments, where most of the users kept waiting.

3.3.2. Phase 2: technology driven approach
The first generation of PACS implementations, as they were developed in the last decade, were mostly technologically driven. Most proved to be technically quite successful, and were important in order to acquire experience. It is however generally accepted that they failed to demonstrate a real utility in the clinical environment and were just not effective. As a consequence, PACS is

not yet universally recognized as a useful medical system by all the actors of the health care community.

This failure is partially due to the lack of maturity of the technical tools (e.g., storage, network, digital radiology), the absence of recognized standards and some misconceptions in the system itself. After 1986, a further development was performed in different directions and several tentative implementations were performed. These implementations were immediately challenged by serious technical problems.

Large archiving possibilities were needed. Storage possibilities became available with the introduction of the write-once-read-many (WORM) optical disk technology and became more resulting with the erasable optical disk or magnetic optical disk (MOD). New technologies are available allowing fast access to Gigabytes. The bottle-neck was moved to the networking environment and faster communication became available, but interfacing remained difficult. Moreover, other more drastic technology appeared while struggling with the large amount of information (Inamura et al., 1990; Huang et al., 1991)

3.3.3. Phase 3: medical user driven approach

In addition to the new hardware which became available, or as solution to some of the problems we still have, medical knowledge is added to the architectural structure of the IMAC's environment.

First generation PACS was rather technology driven, although the diagnostic benefits were stressed from the beginning. PACS design started in the mid-eighties with a technology push: the introduction of new optical mass storage technology offered the potential of cost-effective picture archiving, replacing the photographic film as an information carrier. The perspective of a fully digital communication system including appropriate facilities for image transport and viewing was added later on.

The technology of communication components, however, had developed much slower. It is still not mature enough to be used in fully digital imaging systems. In first generation PACS environments, inappropriate equipment was nevertheless installed.

The proposed bottom-up procedure to set up the model description of the user's situation — the organization and work routines in a hospital department — requires, first of all, rules for a decomposition into less complex segments.

A natural breakdown would be patients, medical professionals, and technical devices (imaging machines). Patients propagate through the diagnostic department following distinct temporal and geographical rules. Physicians and assisting personnel perform activities requiring cooperation, or at least communication. Imaging machines and support devices add another dimension because they also communicate with each other. Thus, three separate 'virtual networks' can be defined (Mattheus et al., 1988).

Common nodes can be recognized when the networks are superimposed. These common nodes represent functions in the user sense. Analyzing user functions leads to defining technical functions of the devices installed at the individual nodes. Analyzing the connections between the nodes leads to defining the communication structure of the network of devices – the PACS. To the user, the PACS appears to be geographically decomposed systems defined in terms of user functions (nodes) and communication tasks. Some characteristics can be summarized:

- medically driven to suit the needs of the different clusters of users;
- options for modular architecture (specialized small systems, integrated as a logical whole with a distributed network);
- 'open' architecture multi-vendor environment, making use of recognized standards and a maximum use of digital interfaces;
- architecture allowing progressive and phased approach;
- upgradability;
- distributed database and/or multiple local temporary storages with pre-fetching and preloading capability;
- integration with radiological and/or hospital information system, inclusive provision for pre-fetching and preloading strategies;
- knowledge-based networking allowing an intelligent distribution of the image within a distributed network; and
- adaptive user interface.

3.3.4. Phase 4: open system phase

As mentioned in the third PACS phase, a lot of medical knowledge is added to the technical realisations. The medical knowledge is based on the medical professionals education and habits. The first problem for the next phase, is that this 'medical knowledge' will in the future change the function of the result of the installation. A way to trigger this in time, is the organisation of education in applied medical informatics. The technical tendency will be towards standards and open systems.

The techniques can be divided in two major components: hard- and software. The total cost will remain constant here. One must, however, not underestimate the maintenance cost for software. It is not realistic to assume a lot of dedicated hardware will be developed for this small market segment. This is specially true for the big investments, e.g., network and storage. Instead, the technical innovations will come from the office automation market and electronic data interchange programmes. The realisation will certainly be a multi-vendor environment, where the key issue will be integration. Moving to phase 4 will be more easy.

For the medical technical world, the push comes from the digital environment. One does not buy a MRI or CR because one can connect it to a network, but one probably will buy a network if one has a MRI or CR, because it will give one more processing and management possibilities and is less expensive if resources are shared! The broad-scale introduction of CR will be a real stimulation for PACS. This approach serves as a model for final system specification, procurement, and implementation. The architecture has been designed modularly to facilitate the assessment of new technologies and algorithms that come into being prior to the time of procurement.

Distributed systems are particularly attractive to users whose tasks are diverse, interactive, and require significant processing capacity. The manager of a distributed system is able to extend the system as the demand for service grows without replacing any of the existing components. High reliability and rapid access to stored information can be achieved by maintaining several copies of data in different server stores.

When one of the components in a distributed system fails, most of the work in progress need not be interrupted. Only the work that was using the failing component must be moved to another unit, if the one it was using breaks down. Such an open architecture is attractive to system developers, but software security measures are needed to protect the services against intentional or accidental violation of access control and privacy. PACS will be seen as a service based on services like communication and supporting dedicated applications.

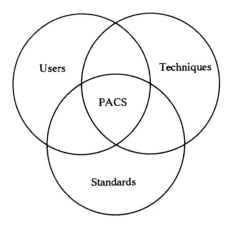

Fig. 8. Main ingredients of a PACS/IMACS world.

4. *Components of an IMACS environment.*

PACS is closely linked with the development of digital modalities in today's hospitals and the concept of a filmless hospital. The current hybrid PACS uses both digital and film techniques, and we have to keep in mind that the majority of images are still recorded in an analog form today. The emergence of totally filmless hospitals will depend on the development of digital radiography equipment to replace X-ray radiology. The term image processing includes a broad range of different applications. The most simple ones are changes of the grey scale or contrast enhancement in an image. They are already very useful to the physician. One of the most spectacular applications is the three-dimensional reconstruction of, e.g., CT or MRI slices, which needs very sophisticated algorithms to run on very powerful workstations.

The future in digital image processing may be the use of artificial intelligence for diagnosis or therapy support or automatic image interpretation.

Three main ingredients (fig. 8) are needed for the realization of a PACS environment. Users coming from different medical disciplines need to be provided with the necessary information including images and functions to manipulate and process this information.

Technology, the second ingredient consists of three components:
- the medical imaging equipment, which has its own evolution;
- the IT component, which needs to be used where possible as basic building block; and at last
- the special developments that are done mostly on the application level.
  These three components makes it difficult to integrate.
  The remaining ingredient is standardization.

5. *Introducing PACS*

One of the most difficult and risky tasks is the introduction phase of a PACS. Good background education for the users is necessary, but the key issue is the reliability of the system, which means that it must perform the functions expected by the users. If the system fails in the introduction phase, it will be hard to convince the user to use it later. This issue is very hard to deal with and calls for a decentralized approach in upgradable phases. When installing new medical equipment, it is important to keep in mind that PACS will come and that some preparations that will save costs later, can already be done. The most critical issue is of course the integration within the HIS. PACS without HIS is impossible. A logical way for combination of patient data with digital images is needed.

Images need to be distributed to the different locations, departments, private doctors, etc. Setting up an installation at all departments at once is dangerous if one cannot provide these with images. In this direction more clusters need to be defined (sub-networks). Such a cluster might, depending on local situations and needs, also be implemented partly outside the hospital, e.g., for remote consultation.

On-screen presentation of the image is another critical issue. In the evaluation of the project, different classes of image display stations need to be defined.

An innovative idea is the introduction of three-step viewing modes: overview, full resolution and zoom mode. These functions can be implemented on one screen system and on a three screen unit.

Legal issues will change too. The main problem here is that they will change rather slow. One of the questions at stake is: Which medium is allowed for archiving and how long? Education and standardization are needed to stimulate these aspects and come to a consensus on legal issues worldwide and for continents. Maintenance contracts need to be studied and discussed carefully: in a multi-vendor environment, companies will blame each other if anything goes wrong due to, e.g., problems with the network connections (Irie et al., 1990).

6. Important evolutions

The IT market is preparing the grounds for medical informatics. It can be expected that the efficient use of computer technology (both hardware and software) will result in several significant changes, providing faster diagnosis with greater specifics, using less invasive techniques (like MRI).

6.1. Trends that influence the PACS/IMACS architecture

There are five major trends directly affecting PACS/IMACS architecture. The first is growth in processor performance. Processor performance advances generally signal forthcoming developments in other areas. Processor performance is a major determinant of a system's ability to provide a fast response to a request or an adequate response to a very complex request. For example, image compression will be available on each system without special hardware.

The second trend consists of the need for continuously available systems.

The third trend is the cross-domain endeavour of distributed database technology.

The fourth is the evolution toward distributed on-line enterprise networks.

The fifth is the user's need to control these technologies in a network, using network and systems management. All these trends will determine the pace at which PACS will progress.

Availability is one of the four attributes that all future PACS will possess; the others are reliability, expandability and maintainability. Reliability is a measure of the likelihood that a component in the computer will fail and/or require service. Expandability means that the system can grow easily, transparently, and cost-effectively to handle a greater workload. Maintainability covers important issues like maintenance, soft-hardware upgrades and service resources.

Availability is a measure of the degree to which a user experiences uninterrupted service from his computing system. In case of 100% availability, a component or software failure means the system continues to operate, and an online service call can be completed before another failure occurs. Availability requires fault tolerance, which means the system's ability to operate in spite of component failures and a service that is both timely and performed without having to interrupt use of the system. Availability will take on new meaning as a result of distributed computer networks and the application models they will make possible.

6.2. Trends in graphics display technology

Character-based terminals, the common computer display in the 1970s, have been replaced by bit-map graphic workstations for personal or scientific use during the 1980s. Bit-map technology allows manipulation of individual picture elements (pixels) on a screen. Products suitable for displaying two- and three-dimensional medical images have been appearing at an increasing rate in the last years and each succeeding generation has more capabilities than the preceding ones.

A first progress was the achievement of resolutions of 1280 × 1024 pixels. Monochrome systems are now available with resolutions greater than 2048 × 2048, and limits as high as 4 K × 4 K may be achieved in future years. Spatial and contrast resolution will be no problem stricto sensu anymore at the level of the report or viewing station. Spatial resolution of 2 K × 2 K seems to be adequate for most of the applications. Only a few functions are generally needed. Centre/windowing, panning and zooming are key functions. Flicker free 14 × 17 inch and good luminance screens would do a good job, unfortunately do only a few companies have such screens available. Most of the manufacturers concentrate on image resolution, processing capabilities and forget about the major functions.

6.3. User interface

The successful introduction of PACS in hospitals will decisively depend on the user interfaces, i.e., image stations. Several user acceptance problems must be solved if the clinical work procedures of medical-image interpretation and consultation are to be based on electronic display systems instead of using the traditional photographic films and lightboxes. Image workstations will be the principal and critical interaction devices for radiologists to access, process and communicate information. The design of image workstations has to focus on solutions for man – machine interfaces that protect the users from involvement in the technical details and that fit into the organization of the radiology departments and adapt to the various clinical tasks and to the users.

The user interface plays an important role in the success of the PACS application; it is a common feature to all applications targeted at professionals. It is therefore essential that a close interaction should exist between the designers and users, and that development be based on prototyping involving the users.

While alphanumeric keyboards are still very important in computer applications, additional devices are predominantly used to interact with imaging applications. They are mice, or better, trackballs to point at selected areas of the images or to operate 'iconic' commands. Resistor matrixes or digitising tablets offer more accurate guidance for selecting a region of interest in the display. Rotating knobs and function keys can be designed to enhance ergonomy. For manipulation of the centre and window function, rotation knobs seem to be the favourites of most radiologists.

6.4. Standardization

Standards cannot be used unless they are really available in the market place, which means that the active early involvement of the suppliers is essential. For suppliers, open system standards, allowing the flexibility to interface with and accommodate local requirements, provide the opportunity to compete in a world-wide multi-vendor environment. Health care communication standards should build on existing open systems standards including OSI, taking full advantage of the investments which have already been made by the computing industry.

It is necessary for the support of the standards by the manufactures of systems platforms, that these standards for health care communications be international. This standardization effort will bring together different market segments and also influence the products (specifications, cost, . . .). To be cost-effective, a large market segment is necessary and standards are needed to fulfill this. Standardisation is not limited to communication issues but terminology, coding, privacy, safety are important topics too.

The American College of Radiology and the National Electrical Manufacturers Association (ACR/NEMA) joint committee is working on version 3.0

of their standard. Here, more emphasis is given to open system interconnection, where in previous versions the focus was more on point to point communication.

ACR/NEMA and other standardisation activities are clearly going in the good direction and we must try to support them. It is not realistic to reinvent the wheel over and over again. We need a standardisation soon, with migration and harmonisation paths world-wide. Moreover, this will decrease the prices of the systems, and ensure the medical effectiveness.

CEN, the European Standardization Institute has set up a committee dealing with medical informatics. TC 251 has seven working groups in this area covering the domain. Working group 4 is the responsible for 'imaging and multimedia', a strict workscheme is defined and performed, which will result in European standards in 1992. Of course in this world-wide field, international coordination and cooperation is needed (Mattheus, 1992).

ANSI, the American National Standardization Institute has formed a Health Care panel which will coordinate this issue in the U.S.A. and work close together with CEN TC 251 where needed.

ANSI and CEN already have coordination efforts going on in this field, and we hope that others will join this initiative. This will on short-time basis hopefully result in standards for the world market. Standards are needed to stimulate this market and to decrease prices.

7. Conclusion

The introduction of high-technology medical equipment into health care requires changes to be made in the training of the staff and in the ways of operation, in order to utilize and maintain the equipment efficiently.

High-technology infrastructure normally requires more skills from the user although it at the same time relieves them of trivial routine tasks. To control the correct functioning of the system, one has to understand its basic operation principles and be able to apply some relevant quality (performance) assurance tests. The physicians utilizing the results produced with this equipment need to understand the limitations of the technology, e.g., as concerns its sensitivity and specificity. The efficient use of a technology also requires motivation from the users. An important step towards achieving this is adequate training.

The effective utilization of high-technology equipment and systems necessitates the technical expertise of clinical engineers, hospital physicists and/or computer scientists. The efficient and cost-effective utilization of a new technology also requires careful planning in organization and ways of operation. This includes consideration of what are the appropriate hierarchical levels in health care for a new technology, and whether it should be centralized or decentralized.

High-technology equipment requires regular servicing. This servicing can be done either by an institution hiring its own personnel or by an outside contractor.

The introduction of computer radiography will stimulate the need for the PACS.

For the development of the PACS components it will be crucial to use existing building blocks. The use of standard modular systems is important. Backward compatibility is an important issue. The cost versus benefit issue will be difficult to handle at the start phase. Imaging technology is rapidly moving towards total dependence on computers. Early in the next millennium, 90% or more of medical images will be digital. Computers will help us to analyze and think, and they will be doing a few simple intelligent tasks independently. Sophisticated communications will remove spatial constraints that we now take for granted. Increasingly 'realistic' images will converge what end users see in fact and what they see in their mind's eye. These last two developments will substantially alter the current relationships in medical specialty practice. It is likely that the imaging revolution supported by other advances in medical informatics will constitute the bridge to some new paradigm of health delivery.

The seeds of the foregoing exist. A dozen years will dramatically develop these functions. We can predict fairly well by extrapolation, as Jules Verne so able demonstrated. But the unexpected must also be accommodated. For both,

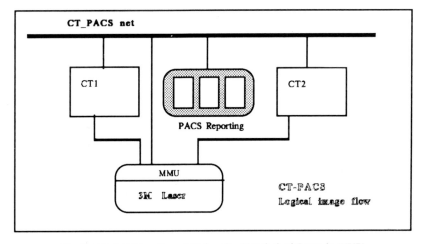

Fig. 9. CT-PACS section at University Hospital of Brussels (VUB).

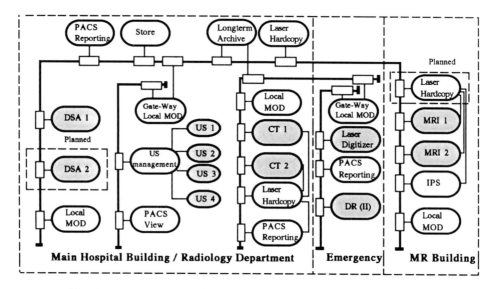

Fig. 10. PACS architecture at the University Hospital of Brussels (VUB) 1991.

we must build open, flexible systems to accommodate both variety in the expected alternatives and the complete surprise.

PACS/IMACS will come soon. The trade-off between partial and full implementation is not always clear. A full-scale infrastructure is expensive, and though technically this seems not possible to realize now, it will be possible within the next five years. The trade-off will be that the best benefits can be optimal in a full scale PACS.

A possible way to solve this problem, will be to set up the image services infrastructure and applications on particular departments.

A full integration from consultation to diagnosis and to therapy, for example, is an example of the total health care glasses concept. The concept of a filmless radiology (or hospital) is confronted with the same problems as that of the paperless office. Still more paper is produced than before, but the means to access information, processing and handling are extended. PACS will allow faster treatment and optimize use of the health care infrastructure.

PACS and IMACS will be implemented soon, but not with as main objective to replace film or archives as the acronym was supposed to say (PACS; A = Archive). What we need is IMACS to manage and communicate multimedia information (IMACS; M = Management, C = Communication).

8. Case study University Hospital Brussels (VUB).

The VUB-PACS/IMACS project is executed in distributed upgradable phases. In a first step in 1985, a limited scale PACS system was installed: a local network with two CTs as acquisition units, a two 512 × 512 screens reporting console, and storage possibilities. This was a typical example of a closed line architecture.

In early 1989 we decided to shift towards a totally distributed approach resulting in small PACS islands for medical subsections: the distributed subnetworking approach (fig. 10).

The CT-PACS consists of two CT units (Siemens), a prototype three 1 K × 1 K screens reporting station (Siemens), local storage and archiving possibilities (2 Gbyte). A hardcopy unit (3M) is shared by the two CTs and the reporting console.

The installation of the 3M laser hardcopy unit at the CT-PACS is an example of a full usable image management environment with low down time (fig. 9). The MMU (multi-modality unit) is used for the connection of the two CTs and the PACS network (server of the reporting console).

Operation: CT1, CT2 – – – > Laser Hard Copy
PACS reporting console – – – > Laser Hard Copy

A component may break down without having problems making hard copies. On the PACS reporting console, instead of using the keypad (3M) to produce hard copies, selection on the screen can be done by mouse. Options like 'format' and 'print' have been implemented. A unique item is the possibility to place images of different examinations of one patient on one film, which can be useful during operation in the operation room. A patient history film is a combination of the important images of that patient. These documents are easier to handle.

The MR-PACS section consists of two MR units (Siemens), two powerful image-processing stations with array processors, local storage, shared hard copy (3M) and archiving possibilities (3.2 Gbyte).

At the emergency department the PACS section consists of a laser-digitizer (Kodak), a two 1 K × 1 K screens reporting console (Kodak) and a prototype DR (II) (CGR-GE) system based on image capture on the image intensifier tube. Evaluation studies are being carried out for the emergency-PACS, with promising medical results. Currently technical problems at the level of the integration of the patient identification on the laser scanner and at the throughput of a set of images are being dealt with.

The digital subtraction angiography (DSA) (Philips) system is integrated in our network and for next year a logical step will be the connection of the DSA (Siemens) which was installed early 1991. This will result in the creation of our DSA-PACS section, with local storage, reporting and hard copy units.

The ultrasound management application (Medicom Technologies Europe) allows the user to archive, retrieve and manipulate echo images. Examinations can be compared locally. The system allows the retrieval of the echo images together with the report. This US unit is based on standard Macintosh hardware and allows the connection of up to four ultrasound units, and integration of the hard copy unit.

In 1992, a test at the orthopedics department with a 1 K $\times$ 1 K viewing station (Imlogix) will be set up with a personal computer based image server (Macintosh). These subsystems are linked to an acquisition backbone network in the radiology department via Ethernet. This backbone network consists of a buffer storage (MOD), optical archiving, a multi-modality reporting console and a hard copy unit (3M). The currently used network (connecting MR, emergency and radiology departments) has a length of 300 metres. An optical fibre network with a length of 1.5 km was completed at the end of 1990. This network, consisting of 20 parallel fibres will not only serve the PACS, but also a number of other hospital informatics projects. It will allow for further extension of the PACS system towards the nursing units. Ethernet, TCP/IP and DECnet will be used on this fibres until other protocols and interfaces become more cost effective (FDDI). Experiments are also being considered which could extend outside the hospital premises (e.g., towards a radiologist on duty, who may then, during the weekends, give advice based on images sent to his house to less experienced radiologists on duty inside the hospital). A project for interhospital communication based on ISDN and B-ISDN is under study.

ISDN is offered by the Belgian PTT, as a 2 Mbit service for multi-media data communication between two or more users. Broadband ISDN (experiments will allow more users in Belgium) a throughput to 160 Mbit/s and will take place in 1995. Terminals are integrated within the different acquisition modalities containing the control functions to request image transfer. At each modality the radiologist can select various functions: archive, report, special study and temporary storage. The messages on the control layer are sent to the network management process. The image-manipulation and reporting console communicates at image-transfer, control and security level. The communication with the optical-disk image database takes place in time-sharing mode via message structure, at the control level and by batch processes created by the control layer on image-transfer level (making use of statistical information). Images are converted to the SPI (ACR/NEMA) format.

SPI (Special Product International) is an extension of ACR/NEMA defined by the two manufacturers Siemens and Philips. The major difference with

ACR/NEMA V2.0 is the folder concept (grouping of images) and the introduction of groups (examinations) operations, where ACR/NEMA id dealing with single images.

The PACS at the CT and MRI departments are in real clinical use, and provide the following advantages:
– less missing films;
– multiple copies and mixed films;
– feedback for assistant radiologists;
– more images for research;
– sharing hardcopy units;
– fully redundant system.

Network manager

Network management and control is one of the research topics going on at our university. Based on five years of experience a network is implemented managing the PACS architecture. The network manager shell insures that traffic on the network is optimal. Buffering, decentralization and pre-fetching are techniques used to allow faster access of examinations (possible delays are due to image transport).

During the night, a link between the radiology information system (RIS) and PACS allows the search in the archives of all images of patients scheduled for control or new examinations the following day. A program database in KEE is used to maintain, change and further develop these programs. KEE is a commercially available knowledge representation system embedded in Lisp. The installation has a hierarchical architecture introducing several levels for image transport, control, security and management. The system is distributed according to the image, data, hardcopy and control level.

Terminals are integrated with the different acquisition modalities containing the control functions to request image transfer. At each modality the radiologist can select different functions: archive, report, special study and temporary storage. The messages on the control layer are stored on queues managed with different priorities. The image-manipulation and reporting console communicates on image-transfer, control and security level. The communication with the optical disk image database takes place via a message structure, in time-sharing mode on the control level and by batch processes created by the control layer on image-transfer level (making use of statistical information). The network management and security level is recursively defined for each sub-network. The management level performs the logical handling of the stored images and takes care of all supervisory and administrative tasks. In addition it performs the logical link of images to related non-image information such as patient data. The security level forms the top layer, which supervises the different tasks, notes the history of events and controls login and password information. This hierarchical structure of the network allows the workload of the network to be optimized and enables us to handle image transport 24 hours a day. The network shell uses different input parameters, correlations between the workload and report and image generating functions at the radiology and emergency departments (amount of images per hour or day). By processing this information and other statistical data (appointments, priorities, etc.) we have a constant continuous throughput function instead of a highly variable discontinuous function, and we can use our PACS environment in clinical practice.

The layered approach to the design of computer networks has been well developed in the contexts of distributed data processing and office automation. By studying the first three layers, several design equations appropriate to PACS can be obtained. These equations, combined with estimates of the flow of digital images, provide a methodology for the prediction of the performance of various PACS designs. The rapid response requirements of a department of radiology, coupled with the quantity of data, suggest architectures that differ markedly from the popular store and forward approach to computer networks.

The PACS will eventually serve all of the imaging modalities provided by the department and will be linked to the RIS already in place and which is also in-house developed and based on the most recent evolutions in technology. Decentralized, unix based, X-terminal as user and integrated in a FDDI clinical-server architecture.

The performance of the PACS in terms of speed and reliability of communication, is determined by the individual modalities. Inefficiency of communication can limit even the most successful of digital modalities on render valuable diagnostic information virtually useless. In the absence of film and paper records, the PACS must be planned such that, at least, the users (radiologists and referring physicians) experience the same level of service that they currently enjoy using the film-based system. That the information presentation to the user via PACS must mimic the current patient-film folder system of image communication, has been widely acknowledged.

Reflection of the profile of a medical imaging department on the architecture of PACS environment

The introduction of PACS in a clinically useful way is only possible if the PACS-architecture reflects the profile of a medical imaging department. With a background of four years clinical experience with PACS at our hospital, a PACS architecture has been established that closes in on the needs of a clinical use.

The PACS configuration and architecture will be different for each hospital, and even each department. A profile of the department can be described in different layers: geographical, patient-flow, radiologist-flow, image data-flow and related data. Each item has its own related information, e.g., radiology-flow: localisation, work description, and specialty. All this information is used in our approach to define the organisation and the topology of the PACS environment. This reflection can be summarized as different small PACS islands for each medical subsection. In this way a hierarchical PACS-world will emerge. Introduction of PACS in this way results in a phase upgradable, decentralized and cost realistic PACS at the department level. It furthermore results in easier education of the users and faster availability of examinations on the display screens.

Clinical experience

The introduction phase of a PACS cluster is one of the most critical points. If the user is unhappy with the system due to technical failure, it is hard to convince him to reuse the system. Careful introduction, good education and in-house support are the messages.

A push from the responsible clinicians is needed to set the new technology to move. For clusters where there is a direct personal benefit this is more easy. For example, MRI where additional image handling (reconstructions) tools can be offered this the acceptance is rapid.

More procedures need to be avoided. An experiment at the emergency department shows that the interaction is very critical, the way image are digitized, patient identification is added. All this may not delay the normal process.

Clinicians are more motivated if they have direct benefit, technical problems need to be avoided after introduction and education is needed.

References

Huang, H.K, S.L. Lou, P.S. Cho, D.J. Valentino, A.W.K. Wong, K.K. Chan and B.K. Stewart (1990) Radiologic image communication methods, *Am. J. Roentgenol.* 155, 183–186.

Huang, H., H. Kangarlooh and R. Tecotzky (1991) Multi-channel fiber optic broadband video communication systems for monitoring CT/MR examinations. In: Medical Imaging V: PACS Design and Evaluation, *Proc. SPIE* 1446.

Inamura, K., T. Umeda, A. Takigawa, K. Inamoto, T. Kozuka and N. Ohyama (1990) Trial of PACS employing magneto-optical disks. In: Dwyer III, S.J., and R.G. Jost (Eds.), Medical Imaging IV: PACS System Design and Evaluation, *Proc. SPIE* 1234, 50–59.

Irie, G., K. Miyasaka, K. Miyamoto, T. Kojina and L. Yamamoto (1990) PACS experience at the University of Hokkaido Medical School. In: Dwyer III, S.J., and R.G. Jost (Eds.), Medical Imaging IV: PACS System Design and Evaluation, *Proc. SPIE* 1234, 26–33.

Mattheus, R. (1992) The European Community and their standardization efforts in medical informatics. In: Medical Imaging VI, *Proc. SPIE,* in press.

Mattheus, R., R. Luypaert and M. Osteaux (1988) Hierarchical layers in a clinical PACS environment, *Med. Imag. Technol.* 6, 157.

Mattheus, R., F. Moyson, Y. Temmerman and M. Osteaux (1990) Hospital integrated picture archiving and communication systems: a European project, SCAR 90 Computer Applications to Assisted Radiology, Symposium Foundation, 396 – 404.

Nosil, J., L. Scobic, C. Justic, B. Clark, W. Ritchie, W. Weigl, H. Gnoyke and P. Fisher (1990) Performance of a partial PACS and its applications to the development of a fully integrated digital medical imaging department in a community hospital. In: Dwyer III, S.J., and R.G. Jost (Eds.), Medical Imaging IV: PACS System Design and Evaluation, *Proc. SPIE* 1234, 186 – 204.

WHO (1990) Effective choices for diagnostic imaging in clinical practice, *WHO TRS 795*, World Health Organization Geneva.

Integrated Diagnostic Imaging
Editor: J.P.J. De Valk
© *Elsevier Science Publishers B.V., 1992*

Chapter 8

Management and processing of medical image information

Yves Bizais and Pascale Chiron

1. Introduction

Half way between 1981 (birth date of picture archiving and communication systems – PACS) and 2001 (expected date of clinical acceptance of PACS), the year 1991 seems to be the right time to review where we come from, and where we go to in this field.

To begin with, it is most important to define the concept of PACS (Marceau, 1982). The technological objective of PACS is to provide digital means to store and remotely retrieve image data (Duerinckx and Pisa, 1982). Because the technological components were (are?) not available, technological aspects of PACS were focused on, and medical aspects were neglected during the infancy of PACS. When PACS prototypes started to be built, medical aspects were naturally introduced. Unfortunately, a specific medical objective was defined for each prototype, depending on local constraints (builders' will and wishes), and no global and formal medical objective was ever clearly defined. Retrospectively two main types of medical objectives were considered in prototypes:

(1) *Departmental PACS* or PACS for radiology departments, which is seen as *extensions of the radiological information systems* (RIS). In this case, the medical objective consists in managing all the information used in a radiology department (patient, appointment, procedure, report and images), with the hope to make such departments more efficient.

(2) *Hospital-wide PACS*, which is seen as *extensions of the hospital information systems* (HIS) (Bakker, 1986). In this case, the medical objective consists in managing all the information used during the diagnostic and therapeutic processes, and images are just considered as a piece of information used in addition to clinical records or biological data. This type of PACS can be easily extended to metropolitan or regional PACS.

The two above approaches are quite different because of the technology involved, and because of the requirements induced. For instance, response times and image processing functionalities may be quite different for departmental PACS and hospital-wide PACS.

We can reformulate what has been said in the previous paragraph as follows. The acronym of PACS defines a technological objective in the medical imaging field. Because of technological difficulties, the issue 'How can we build PACS?' was addressed first. As a first approximation, we can say that this question is answered, at least partially. Then when first PACS prototypes were built, a second question 'What can we do with PACS?' was asked, and this one is not fully resolved.

Consequently this chapter is organized in the following way. In the second section (PACS 1980 – 1990), PACS research efforts in the past are summarized: Why is PACS a difficult issue from a technological standpoint? What kind of components are needed? How can these components be integrated? What kind of standards are needed? In the third section (PACS 1990 – 2000), the medical usefulness of PACS is addressed: Do physicians need departmental or hospital-wide PACS? Must PACS only replace film-based archives and communications or does it have to provide additional services? In our opinion, there exists no definitive answer in this field, and in the last section (here and now) we focus on research efforts carried out in our institution, as a contribution to define such an answer.

2. PACS 1980 – 1990

2.1. Data requirements in medical imaging

It is extremely easy to understand why PACS is a difficult issue: from a technological standpoint the *volume of manipulated data* is considerably larger than in most other application fields (e.g., office automation). Images are usually represented by two dimensional arrays, the size of which varies from 64×64 to 2048×2048, i.e., from 8 Kbyte to 8 Mbyte for 16-bit deep pixels, with a median value of 0.5 Mbyte. An appropriate unit to express the volume of a piece of information in medical imaging is therefore the Mbyte (it is the Kbyte in office automation).

Moreover, imaging devices (such as the ones used in cardiac angiography) may generate up to 50 images per second. It means that the required *digital throughput* may be as high as 12 Mbyte/s, which corresponds to a very large bandwidth.

Finally, despite the large differences between medical imaging practices throughout the world, the *amount of digital image data* produced per day is estimated to be the same (1 Gbyte/day/100 bed) in several studies (Dwyer III et al., 1982). It corresponds to a 7500 Gbyte archive for a 600 bed hospital with 250 working days every year, if images are kept for five years. If all films were to be digitized, this figure should be multiplied by ten.

In summary, it is enough to remember that an image corresponds to 1 Mbyte, the bandwidth in medical imaging is in the range of 10 Mbyte/s, and the size of an image archive is about 10 Tbyte (Terabyte, i.e., 10 000 000 Mbyte). These figures explain why technological solutions suitable for other archiving and communication applications cannot be used for PACS. It follows that the feasibility of PACS is not fully certain yet, and it explains why a lot of research efforts have addressed technological issues until now.

2.2. User requirements

As the volume of manipulated data is large, the *system response time* (Lodwick, 1986; Toshimitsu et al., 1990) is seen as the most important requirement by users. This is especially true in a departmental PACS, because radiologists want to access many images very quickly. From a practical standpoint, they want to have an image displayed on a monitor as quickly as they can pull out a film from a folder and hang it up in front of a lightbox. Moreover, as several images can be displayed simultaneously on a lightbox, they want to switch from one image to the next even more quickly to simulate simultaneity. In a hospital-wide PACS, requirements for response time are not as stringent: physicians understand that images are 'far away' and that it takes time to carry images from the archive to the display. However, two aspects must be mentioned.

(1) The response time is the combination of the response time of the archive to locate an image after a request and the one needed to transfer the image. Usually the former is longer that the latter. Acceptance of PACS by the user depends on the global response time, and not on its components.

(2) Today, for those who do not use PACS (prePACS environment), the total time spent to access an image is shared between employees who physically carry patient folders, and physicians who look at images. In a PACS environment the total time spent to access an image is likely to be less than the total time spent in the prePACS environment, but it is spent by a physician only. In this case, hospital managers may be satisfied with PACS because image access costs (related to total time) decrease. However, physicians are not satisfied because they spend more time waiting for images using PACS than in the prePACS environment.

The second requirement made by physicians about PACS is *user-friendliness*. In a radiology department, and even more in clinical wards, especially in university hospitals, physicians' turnover is very high. For this reason, physicians must be able to use PACS workstations very quickly, in an efficient and safe manner. Again user-friendliness of PACS workstations is evaluated by comparing it to the prePACS situation: 'Is it as easy to display a digital image, as to pull a film out of the folder and to hang it onto a lightbox?' Obviously this is a requirement difficult to meet.

Finally, if the two previous requirements are met and if fully digital operation is expected, physicians want a *100% reliable PACS*. As a PACS is a highly complex computer and communication system, it is extremely difficult to build such a reliable system: redundancy must be systematically implemented, and degraded modes of operation must be built into such systems. This can be achieved only at very high cost.

A final constraint on PACS is *cost* (Dwyer III et al., 1982; Ottes et al., 1990). Imagine for the moment that a completely satisfactory PACS from a physician's standpoint is available. If this system only replaces film-based solutions for archiving and distributing images by digital means, and if its cost (investment and operation) is higher than the cost of film solutions (which is the case

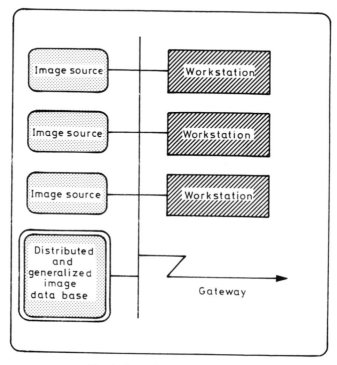

Fig. 1. General PACS architecture.

today), whatever the quantitative (not qualitative) improvements provided by such a PACS are, is there only one hospital manager throughout the world ready to buy it? For this simple reason, PACS is a rapidly progressing field of research, not a reality at the present time. And the added value is extremely important.

2.3. A general diagram for PACS

In the same way as in any information system, data must be created, updated, deleted, moved around and stored. Such functionalities are provided by a PACS system as shown in fig. 1:

(1) *images are created by image sources* which must be interfaced to a network;
(2) *images are manipulated in workstations* which must provide appropriate image processing functionalities;
(3) *images are stored in an image database* which may be centralized or distributed;
(4) *images are moved around using a network;*
(5) as *images* must be associated to other data, a PACS *must be connected to a RIS and a HIS.*

Conceptually, a PACS has a very simple structure. It is worth mentioning some important features of it. Each component has a well-defined and unique functionality. For example, data production is provided by image sources. Data management is realized by the image database. In this regard, the PACS structure describes medical imaging in a better way than today solutions, in which production, processing and management of image data are mixed together. For instance, today CT (computed tomography) scanners ensure acquisition of slices, processing and display, and local storage, within the same system. It is difficult to clearly separate these functionalities, and to understand how they interact. However, *the simple structure described above does not solve all PACS issues.* For example, it is clear that image data may be produced by image processing in image workstations. In this case, the latter can also be seen as image production devices, able to update the image database. Another example is even more important: all image sources can process images to some extent, and it is likely that all images produced by acquisition and processing within an image source are not needed to be stored in the image archive. The above structure does not tell us which fraction of image information has to be stored in the image archive (and this is an important issue as we will discuss later). In other words, the above described PACS structure clearly defines the functionalities required to handle images, and identifies the devices realizing such functionalities. But it does not precisely tell us how such functionalities fulfill medical requirements, and thus does not specify global PACS functionalities with enough details. Moreover, each of the above functionalities is difficult to implement in a satisfactory manner. In the following sections, we address each of these issues.

2.4. Interfacing image sources

The first and main difference between PACS and other data management systems comes from data acquisition. Images exhibit three major characteristics, as far as data acquisition is concerned.

(1) They do not own an internal meaning such as an ASCII string. Their meaning is provided by image characteristics (number of rows and columns, pixel depth, etc.) which are a separate piece of information.

(2) Until a recent time, there was no standard to describe image characteristics. Rather each manufacturer had its own standard, making exchange of images difficult.

(3) Images are usually acquired as analog signals, which are digitized in a second step, even though analog signals are not available such as for CT scanners. It turns out that image digitization may be a technologically difficult process.

It follows that interfacing image sources to a PACS is a major task for essentially two reasons:

(1) most digital image sources still make use of proprietary *image formats*, such that images must be reformatted before they are introduced into a PACS;

(2) today image sources are not provided with *standard network interfaces*, making interfacing to PACS extremely difficult.

The *ACR-NEMA standard* (ACR-NEMA, 1985; Alzner and Murphy, 1986; Lehr, 1986; Oosterwijk et al., 1986; Horii, 1990) provided an answer to the first point: it can be considered as a major breakthrough in the PACS field. Among other issues to be discussed later, it specifies how to describe an image. The corresponding *data dictionary* defines semantically related groups of items which uniquely specify an image. Consequently, an ACR-NEMA compatible image source is straightforwardly able to formally exchange meaningful image data with other PACS components. The ACR-NEMA standard also tried to answer the second point by defining a *hardware interface and a 5-layer communication protocol* dedicated to medical imaging. It turned out that the corresponding interfaces were difficult and costly to build because of stringent requirements and of a limited market. A *new version* of the standard to be published in the coming months (Dicom V3.0 1993) makes use of standard protocols such as TCP/IP, such that the second bottleneck in interfacing image sources should be solved. Consequently, image sources able to communicate with other PACS components, using standard network protocols and a common data dictionary, should be available in the very near future. Moreover, extensions of the ACR-NEMA standard allowing one to handle higher level image data (e.g., patient folders) such as SPI or Champollion (Appel et al., 1990) are being proposed. It is our opinion that a world-wide adoption of the standard is a major advance which must not be underestimated. It solves the problem of interfacing digital image sources (CT, MRI, nuclear medicine).

Another important issue in this field is the *digitization of X-rays* (known as digital radiology or DR), necessary to integrate radiograms into PACS. It is important because X-rays are still (and for a long time) the main source of medical images and because they turn out to be difficult to digitize. Two main solutions (Huang, 1986) have been investigated.

(1) The first one consists in digitizing films, using a *laser scanner*. Today, 1 K × 1 K or even 2 K × 2 K digital X-ray images can be produced in such a way. Even with such arrays, digital resolution is less than analog resolution and it may decrease the diagnostic ability of an observer. Moreover, the noise introduced by digitization turns out to be important, again decreasing image quality. Finally, such a solution is hardly justified from an economical standpoint since films are still used.

(2) The second solution consists in using *phosphor plates* instead of films. They are read by a laser beam, the output of which is digitized. It has mainly been investigated by Fuji. It has the same drawbacks as the previous solution, in terms of resolution and noise. However, it suppresses films (except if digital images are output to film for interpretation) and X-ray equipments can be easily upgraded to handle phosphor plates.

It follows that there is no satisfactory solution to digitize X-rays today. This is an important limiting factor to total digital imaging.

Before ending this section, it is worth mentioning our work in this field as a case example. When we started our PACS project (the DIMI project) (Bizais et al., 1986b), there was no ACR-NEMA compatible image sources. For this reason, a part of the project consisted in developing compatible image sources for nuclear medicine and DSA (digital subtraction angiography), by using the same computer system (modified VICOM image processor), the same operating system (Unix), and the same data structure. It allowed us to easily access images at least for research purposes. It demonstrated the necessity of defining a common image format more generally accepted than our own standard, such as the ACR-NEMA standard.

2.5. *Image workstations*

If an image workstation is connected to an image source, it results into a rudimentary PACS. Many industrial PACS prototypes are not more than that. The initial version of the ACR-NEMA standard only defines a point-to-point communication protocol, and many interesting issues can be studied with such a two node system.

The first one is to define the functionalities which are to be available in image workstations. During the eighties, applied research and testing demonstrated the necessity of *three types of workstations*, corresponding to various physicians' needs. The first class is known as the *upper-end image workstation*. It is characterized by its ability to display high-resolution (1 K $\times$ 1 K, or even 2 K $\times$ 2 K) images, to process such images using complex algorithms (three-dimensional representation (Herman, 1986), image analysis), and to communicate with other PACS components. It is clear that such workstations provide image processing functionalities not permitted by film, but are extremely costly. If they were not as costly, they would be the only needed type of workstations. Because only a limited number of them can be bought, they are seen as a shared resource, essentially used by radiologists. The second type corresponds to *middle-line workstations* (Johnston et al., 1986), able to display 1 K $\times$ 1 K images, with limited processing capabilities. By using several monitors, alternators can be emulated. Their cost is rapidly decreasing such that several of them can be available in an imaging department, and be used to interpret the bulk of produced images. Finally, there exist *lower-end workstations* (Ho et al., 1990). They are low-cost systems, able to display 512^2 images, with very limited processing capabilities. They can be used in clinical wards, by referring physicians inside and outside hospitals to display images supporting a diagnosis. The definition of the above three classes of workstations is important because it shows that various image users exist, and that an appropriate (in terms of functionalities and cost) solution is available for each of them. However, there are other important and less clear issues about workstations.

The main issue is probably the possibility of *reading images directly from monitors* (Carterette et al., 1986; Horii et al., 1986; Pizer, 1986; Arenson et al., 1990; Britton et al., 1990; Dwyer III et al., 1990; Good et al., 1990; Slasky et al., 1990; Taira et al., 1990). As we already suggested, one of the objectives of PACS is to suppress (or at least reduce) the consumption of films. Several experiments were carried out to assess the diagnostic capabilities of physicians, reading images from monitors. In terms of *resolution*, today monitors are appropriate for digital images (CT, MRI and nuclear medicine). *Contrast* is usually acceptable even though it is less than that of lightboxes. It follows that lighting environment must be more strictly controlled with monitors than with lightboxes. 50 Hz *refresh rate* causes fatigue and thus a decrease in diagnostic capabilities of the reading physician. Most authors agree that a newly available standard (75 Hz) should suppress this problem. Up to day, there is no long-term study demonstrating the possibility to read medical images from monitors. Moreover, moving from film to monitors would correspond to a drastic psychological change for physicians. Finally, the contrast available with 2 K $\times$ 2 K monitors does not seem acceptable for image reading, such that the possibility of reading digital X-ray images is questionable. This is a second reason why the feasibility of integrating X-rays into PACS is not demonstrated.

Another interesting question concerns the *management of image processing in workstations*. As we already mentioned, image reading requires a lot of image processing even if it is simple. In this regard, an image workstation can be seen as an image production system. Some of the results produced by processing must be stored in the image archive. This is difficult to achieve because the ACR-NEMA standard is very poor in describing processed image data. Which results are to be kept? How to describe the relationships between acquired and processed data? Who is authorized to update the database with processed data? Until which step of the image procedure life is updating allowed? All these questions are unsolved yet, and in most prototypes management of processed data is very limited. We come back to this issue in Section 3.

One more point which has to be solved is the *location of reading*. More precisely, the above described general PACS architecture specifies that images are processed and read in workstations. It means that, at the same workstation, a physician may either read a specified image procedure (e.g., a CT scan) using specific tools, or he processes several image procedures at the same time (e.g., several CT scans performed in the same patient at various times, or several procedures performed in the same patient at almost the same time). In the first case, he is doing '*monomodality*' reading, in the second case, '*multimodality*' reading. But in both cases, he acts as a radiologist, and he is likely not able to clearly distinguish between these two activities, even though they are different from a computer standpoint. In today PACS prototypes, 'monomodality' reading usually involves an *image source* rather than a *workstation*. Such an approach facilitates the management of processed images during the active period of a procedure (until reporting), data are acquired and processed within an image source; only image data supporting the report are sent to the image archive; workstations are only used to consult the latter, and to perform post-processing (e.g., three-dimensional), the results of which are not kept. However, for the radiologist, this is not a good solution, because he must move from the image source to a workstation back and forth, each time he switches from 'monomodality' to 'multimodality' reading. The exact role of workstations is thus not fully clear, and we will come back to this issue in Section 3. In some way, it relates to what we want to do with PACS.

In our PACS project, the above issues were tackled in the following way. At each terminal of the image processors, the two modes of operation were possible. During the active period of an image procedure (until reporting), monomodality processing was allowed and data could be accessed only inside the node where data had been acquired. After reporting, image data were made public, and could be accessed by any authorized user. Consequently, at the same terminal, multimodality processing could be performed by accessing data produced in other nodes. To manage the data produced by multimodality processing (i.e., processing performed after reporting), the concept of virtual procedure was introduced: processing, reading and reporting associated with multimodality images were considered as forming a new image procedure. For example, if the same patient underwent two different procedures (e.g., a cardiac DSA and a myocardial scintigram), the comparison of the two studies and the corresponding findings formed a third study. Some cases are more ambiguous. For instance, ventilation/perfusion lung scintigrams can be seen as three distinct entities: a ventilation scan, a perfusion lung scan, and the comparison of ventilation to perfusion defects. However, it can also be seen as a single entity, mostly aiming at diagnosing pulmonary embolism.

2.6. Archiving

Two main aspects must be presented concerning image archiving. Quantitative aspects refer to the way used to handle huge amounts of data (see Section 2.1). Qualitative aspects deal with the way to access a particular image.

Specifying *quantitative aspects* is fairly simple: 'How to handle Terabytes of data?' A satisfactory answer to this question was not available ten years ago, but PACS research and technological advances have provided appropriate devices and concepts. Today optical *jukeboxes* which can store about 800 Gbyte are available, i.e., ten such devices are enough to archive all digital images produced in an hospital. They are likely to be cost effective in the very near future. However, there is no standard format available concerning 8 inch digital optical record (DOR), contrary to 5^1_4 inch DOR. Moreover, images may be *compressed* (Haskell and Hang, 1986; Noh and Jenkins, 1986) by a factor of ten, without noticeable degradations using standard techniques (e.g., discrete cosine transform − DCT), even though the latter are still to be carefully evaluated. Consequently, it is our opinion that the technology exists to build large medical image databases. Because the response time of optical devices is long, magnetic disk caches and local stores attached to image sources and workstations are necessary to ensure response times acceptable for users. A *multi-layer archiving strategy* (Meyer-Ebrecht, 1986) is commonly accepted today. Finally, a complementary device consists in storing the most meaningful images of a patient into an '*image credit card*' including an optical tape strip: it contains some Mbytes.

Qualitative aspects are as important as quantitative aspects, even though they have been neglected by PACS researchers. In most prototypes a simple but restrictive solution was adopted: patients and image procedures are registered in a *relational database* (Assman et al., 1986; Liu Sheng et al., 1990; Seshadri et al., 1990; Stewart and Taira, 1990), which also includes pointers to images stored outside. Therefore, images are accessed by issuing requests to the database which returns image pointers; pointed images are then read from the image archive using standard file system routines. If only patient and image procedure oriented requests are provided, digital images are essentially accessed as film images. If more advanced requests are defined, other access modes are specified, providing PACS with functionalities not available with film-based solutions. For example, if image procedures can be retrieved on the basis of image findings, then a physician may be shown similar cases when he is reading a difficult case (computer-assisted diagnosis). Using a relational database to access images which are located outside it does not guarantee *data security*, and usually results into (too) long *response time*. Partial responses to these problems are provided by the Copernique multimedia database machine experimented in the Sirene project (Renoulin et al., 1987) (see Chapter 9, this volume), and by *prefetching strategies* (Levin and Fielding, 1990). None of the existing PACS prototypes does provide a satisfactory solution for the management of processed data. This is an extremely important point to which we come back in Section 3.

In our project, we implemented some of the above concepts. Each node, acting as a modality-specific system and as a multimodality station, could store data locally, while a central image archive centralized all public image data. Image access was patient or image procedure oriented, and was based on a relational DBMS (empress 32). Unfortunately, image archiving used magnetic tapes because DOR were not available, making the archiving process very cumbersome.

2.7. Networking

In the same way as for archiving, quantitative and qualitative aspects of networking must be discussed. At the very beginning of PACS, it was clear that *high throughput* was necessary, because of the size of medical images and of acquisition rate (see Section 2.1). High throughput means large bandwidth of the network medium, high throughput of network interfaces and minimal overhead of software protocols, because a high transfer rate is expected from memory to memory between a *small number of nodes*. These characteristics are quite different from office automation applications, and explain why most standard networks are not suitable for PACS.

During the last ten years, various solutions have been experimented. Most of them made use of *Ethernet* and *TCP/IP*. Such standard solutions turned out to be too slow for an actual use in hospitals, but proved the feasibility of PACS in this field, and the necessity to base PACS networks on standard solutions. Several other experiments used *locally developed solutions* (broadband network, optical fiber, etc.). They showed that an effective throughput of several Mbyte/s was necessary to make PACS accepted by physicians, but turned out not to be viable solutions, especially because user-friendly interfaces were difficult to develop and because maintenance and upgrade were too costly. These drawbacks are also true for *ACR-NEMA solutions*: the standard defines a ISO-OSI like protocol, with a maximum throughput of 8 Mbyte/s, such that interfaces must be based on high-tech, expensive components. The definition of the *FDDI standard* and the recent availability of FDDI products can be considered as a milestone in the feasibility of acceptable PACS networks. Recent experiments show that an effective throughput of 1 Mbyte/s is achievable using FDDI, and this figure is likely to increase with the development of improved interfaces. For these reasons, the new version of the ACR-NEMA provides an alternative to the original proposal: medical image communication may be based on standard networks and interfaces (such as FDDI products), the aspects specific to medical imaging and high-level protocols being located at the application layer (Stewart, 1990). It seems to us as being a good solution. PACS may benefit from network developments realized for a large market, while the ACR-NEMA standard essentially takes care of medical image communication applications. To speed up data transmission, one fact may be taken into account: each type of medical images is likely to be moved through a well-defined path within the PACS, corresponding to a subset of the network. For this reason, the network is sometimes organized into subnetworks, thus minimizing the traffic.

Concerning the distribution of images to *remote sites* (teleradiology, shipping of images to referring physicians), a solution based on *ISDN* (Blaine et al., 1990) is being available in most European countries, and in the U.S.A. The current ISDN standard provides one or several 64 Kbit/s channels, such that medical images can be transmitted in a minute or two at low cost. This is quite acceptable in most clinical situations.

Finally, it is worth mentioning that *image compression* (Cho et al., 1990) is important in image transmission as well as in image archiving. Reducing the amount of data to be transmitted by a factor of three (reversible or lossless compression) to ten (irreversible or lossy compression) decreases the transmission time in the same proportion. Using fast CPUs and efficient compression software, or videorate compression boards, compression becomes effective.

The actual content of transmitted information and connection to HIS (Heu et al., 1986; Parrish et al., 1986; Bakker, 1990; Levine et al., 1990) can be included into the *qualitative aspects* of PACS communication. Who are the receivers of data transmitted through a PACS network? What kind of information do they need? How does this information relate to HIS data? These are the basic questions to be answered. The ACR-NEMA standard provides partial solutions in this regard. More precisely, it specifies the type of data (essentially images and graphics) to be transmitted, and the commands which are used to transmit the data. As such it defines the scope of PACS, and implicitly how a PACS relates to other information systems. However, it is our opinion that the ACR-NEMA is incomplete in this regard, because the data types are too restricted (especially processed data are poorly described), and the available set of commands is too limited to encompass the various types of medical activity. We have to go back to users' requirements (Who needs images? For which purpose? Do they simultaneously need other information such as HIS data?) in order to precisely specify functionalities: the *tools for transmitting images* are available, the *medical use of image transmission* is not fully specified at the present time. We come back to this issue in Section 3.

In our project, we took part in the development of a high speed, dedicated network (Imopnet) able to transmit data through DMA (direct memory access) interfaces 1 km away, using optic fiber. Five years ago, the throughput was about 20 Mbit/s with minimal software overhead. Consequently, a 512^2, 16 bit deep image was transferred in about 3 seconds. Moreover, each imaging division was organized around an image processor concentrating several image sources. In this way images were acquired and processed essentially within a subsystem, such that traffic was minimized. Unfortunately, network breakdowns were quite frequent and maintenance turned out to be extremely difficult and costly. For this reason, we decided to stop our work in PACS networks, waiting for FDDI to come.

2.8. User-interface

The computer processes involved in PACS are numerous and complex. They have to be hidden to the final user who is usually not a computer specialist and must concentrate on medical problems. For this reason, user-interfaces (Nievergelt, 1986; Wendler et al., 1986) are key components of PACS. This was an unsolved problem until recent times. Thanks to the wide acceptance of windows, menus and mouse interaction in the medical community, and the availability of such an interface generator in a network environment (*X-window*) (Ratib et al., 1990), the user-interface issue seems to be solved. It will take time to develop PACS interfaces, but the appropriate tools are available now.

2.9. Integration

After reviewing the various components of a PACS, we may conclude that, after ten years of PACS developments and of parallel technological advances, most components are becoming available (ACR-NEMA compatible image sources, high-quality workstations, large archives and relational DBMS, high-speed networks and ISDN). It is one thing to buy such items, it is another one to integrate them. For this reason, PACS integration is a PACS research field by itself, focusing on hardware and software *compatibility* of components, uniformity of user interfaces, *reliability* and degraded modes of operation.

Feasibility of integration can only be tested by building prototypes (Bizais et al., 1986a; Hegde et al., 1986; Hemminger et al., 1986; Preston et al., 1986; Stockbridge and Ravin, 1986; Irie et al., 1990; Minato et al., 1990; Ravin, 1990). Some of them (essentially the UCLA project and the Georgetown University project in the U.S.A., the Hokkaido project in Japan, the AZ-VUB project in Belgium and the Sirene project in France) are being evaluated. All of them can be considered as pre-industrial projects, providing key results in assessing the feasibility and the medical acceptance of PACS.

2.10. Social and economic aspects of PACS

It is not our purpose to discuss these points in too much details, because we think that PACS is still an applied research issue, rather than an available product. A lot of work has still to be done to come up with satisfactory solutions and by this time the cost of PACS is likely to significantly decrease.

However, a crucial point of PACS is its *acceptance by physicians* and especially radiologists. By providing an efficient means to access data which are now confined inside imaging departments, clinicians and surgeons daily exposed to medical images will become more and more able to read them correctly. Consequently, the role of radiologists will be modified. Actually, the situation is quite different in the U.S.A., in Europe and in Japan, for legal reasons. It is our opinion that radiologists should not fear PACS for several reasons:

(1) their experience cannot be replaced for difficult cases; they will have more time to focus on them by having simple cases read by referring physicians;

(2) they have to develop an experience in multimodality imaging which is quite immature at the present time;

(3) because of HIS to PACS links, they will be able to access clinical and biological data, which are necessary to properly read images, and are nevertheless not available at the present time.

3. PACS 1990 – 2000

Before jumping from past to future, let us spend some time in the present to summarize where we stand as far as PACS is concerned. *Several issues are clear today*, which were not clear ten years ago:

(1) a formal architecture is agreed upon, defining each required functionality and the corresponding component;

(2) most of the technological components are available, and PACS integration is being tested;

(3) communication between PACS and the other medical information systems is being specified, providing a synthetic view of the information useful to be managed in health care;

(4) the specificity of PACS, due to image features is demonstrated.

However, *several issues are still to be solved*:

(1) Is it possible to include DR into PACS in the near future?

(2) Do we need departmental PACS (i.e., RIS extensions) or hospital-wide PACS (i.e., HIS extensions)?

(3) How to include image processing and management, depending on the answer to the previous question?

(4) Are PACS to be a simple replacement of film by digital means, or are PACS to provide additional functionalities (added values of PACS)?

All the above questions can be summarized as follows. *Why do we need PACS from a medical standpoint?* There is no definite answer to it, and it is our belief that PACS research is about to move from technological to medical issues. We explain how it is likely to happen in this section.

3.1. Digital radiology

A major technological issue has not been cleared up until now. The possibility of producing and displaying digital radiographs, allowing the same diagnostic performances as films, is not demonstrated. *Laser-scanning* of films is not satisfactory because it still makes use of film. *Phosphor plate* technology can still be improved and is likely to be the most appropriate solution in the near future, because it involves slight modification of X-ray equipments. A third alternative does exist: the *flying spot* or *linear detector technology* with which radiograms are digitized in real time during acquisition. Moreover, irradiation is substantially reduced. Theoretically such a solution provides images comparable to film radiographs (even better because of scatter reduction). However, today X-ray equipments cannot be upgraded, such that this solution will not be widely used in the near future. For this reason, we do not forecast filmless medical imaging before the second half of this decade.

On the other hand, the *fraction of digital images increases rapidly*, such that

X-ray systems will progressively represent a smaller and smaller market. This statement can be understood in two ways. It is less and less important to digitize radiograms for physicians, or for manufacturers. In the first case, it means that PACS without DR is satisfactory for physicians. In the second case, it means that the development of DR and thus of filmless medical imaging will be slowed down.

3.2. Hospital-wide PACS

From a technological standpoint, it is easier to build a hospital-wide PACS than a departmental PACS, because the functionalities of the latter are more numerous. Consequently, it is useful to precisely define a hospital-wide PACS from a medical standpoint. To improve the efficiency of the diagnostic and therapeutic processes, it is crucial to be able to access medical information. For clinicians and surgeons, clinical data are readily available, and biological data can be accessed through a HIS. However, images represent a main piece of information for most pathologies, and are not included into a HIS. *A hospital-wide PACS can be defined as an image extension of a HIS.*

Such a solution implies *several modifications in the formal structure of a PACS.*

(1) Image sources are still used to acquire, process and display images. The radiologist exclusively makes use of them to read image procedures and to report.

(2) After reporting, image data are selected by him, are archived into the PACS database, while the report is archived into the RIS. Because HIS, RIS and PACS databases are interconnected, it becomes possible for a physician to access images and reports remotely.

(3) Images selected in the PACS database can be displayed on image workstations in wards and operating theaters. Depending on processing functionalities, clinicians and surgeons may post-process image data according to their needs.

(4) There is no major legal reason to store post-processed data (the latter are seldom used to support a diagnosis or a treatment). Consequently, the PACS database is highly static updated after reporting in one transaction by radiologists, only consulted by physicians afterwards.

Such a viewpoint corresponds to the *replacement of film-based solutions by digital means.* The latter has several advantages over the former:

(1) images can be accessed easily, quickly and simultaneously by all physicians needing them, even if they are located far away;

(2) a second reading can be asked to a remotely located expert, or primary reading can be performed remotely (teleradiology);

(3) images are available as soon as possible, such that patients may be hospitalized for a shorter time;

(4) images cannot be lost anymore because only copies are transmitted;

(5) because a large database is progressively built, it is possible to define strategies in order to perform cheap and safe image procedures first;

(6) high-end workstations may be shared by several occasional users, even though results are displayed on low-cost personal workstations.

However, *such a solution has several drawbacks*:

(1) the cost of a PACS is extremely high (several million dollars) and savings (decrease in film consumption, strategies) is not likely to compensate PACS investments, at least at present;

(2) time responses do not compare favorably to those of film-based solutions for physicians;

(3) user-friendliness of PACS is not as good as that of film;

(4) film is an easy-to-carry hard copy, while digital images are soft copies which must be displayed on a static device, and medical practice takes place in many different rooms;

(5) reliability of film is incomparable when it is available (i.e., when it is not lost).

It is our opinion that in the coming years, several manufacturers will come up with such hospital-wide PACS, because technological advances will provide cost-effective and reliable components, because physicians are gradually accepting computers, and because the medical objectives of such PACS are clearly defined. For them to be fully accepted, one key point must be solved. In most cases *images supporting the report are processed images* (windowing, smoothing, edge enhancement, etc.). Today processing conditions are known by the reading physician because he is located close to the image source. In a PACS situation, this is not the case anymore, and the PACS database must be able to provide this type of information to remotely located physicians. For this reason, the ACR-NEMA standard must be extended in order to provide appropriate means to describe processed images. If this was not the case, the meaning of images would be considerably reduced, proper post-processing might be hazardous, such that the report might contain all the relevant information: 'If the report is enough to understand the information provided by an image procedure, why would we need PACS?' In other words, we advocate for a description of processed data: because of medical practice reasons it is necessary to know how an image was produced (acquisition and processing) to read it properly.

3.3. Departmental PACS

A second class of medical objectives which can be achieved with a PACS corresponds to departmental PACS. To improve the efficiency of an imaging department and the diagnostic performances of radiologists, it is desirable to disconnect the various functions to be performed (acquisition, processing, reading, reporting) and to provide radiologists with as much additional information as they want (previous image procedures, biological data, clinical records). This is theoretically achieved with a PACS as the one we formally described in Section 2. Obviously, it is *more difficult to build than a hospital-wide PACS*, because functionalities are more numerous. However, we favor such a solution because it provides a comprehensive view of medical imaging (including management and processing).

It is worth mentioning some *important features of departmental PACS, as compared to hospital-wide PACS* because our definition of departmental PACS is not standard.

(1) Image sources are in charge of image acquisition only.

(2) Acquired images are at least temporarily archived in the PACS database.

(3) *Radiologists process, read and report image procedures using workstations having the same image access functionalities as clinicians' workstations.* Consequently, they can access previous image procedures and HIS data during the interpretation process. Monomodality and multimodality processing tasks are performed at the same workstations, eventually simultaneously.

(4) Processed image data supporting the report may be included into the PACS database. Therefore, the same data as in the case of an hospital-wide PACS are accessible to clinicians and surgeons.

(5) *Post-processing* is considered exactly in the same way as *processing before reporting*, such that the data resulting from it may be included into the database, and later used by another physician. The only important point is that the producer of data must be identified for legal purposes.

(6) If the database used to access image data is organized properly, *additional functionalities* may be provided such as access to similar cases to help reading of difficult cases, building of teaching files, statistical processing of image data.

It turns out that *departmental PACS provide all the functionalities provided by hospital-wide PACS*. They do not artificially separate processing performed before and after reporting. Every image user may include his own knowledge into the database. Radiologists and clinicians mutually take advantage of their complementary expertise. *The formal superiority of such an approach is thus clear*. However, *from a practical standpoint, it suffers a major drawback*: a mechanism must be developed to describe the image processing process and the resulting data. In other words, the PACS database must include the semantic description of the items it includes. This is a formidable task which requires

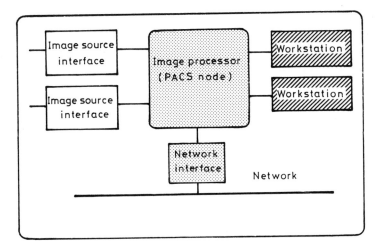

Fig. 2. DIMI project, structure of a node.

years of research. For this reason, we do not expect departmental PACS to be available before the end of this decade.

3.4. Summary

During the coming years, PACS research should move from technological to medical issues, we should know whether a totally filmless hospital is possible or not; and the management of digital images (not of image processing) by hospital-wide PACS should be commercially available. By the end of the century, image processing should be included (departmental PACS) and PACS cost should be low enough to be attractive for potential buyers.

4. Here and now

To illustrate the above points, we describe three PACS related projects carried out in our institution, in collaboration with other centers.

4.1. The DIMI PACS project

We already mentioned several aspects of our PACS project (Bizais et al., 1986a,b) which was carried out from 1984 to 1988 in Nantes. The objective was to develope an *integrated medical imaging department* in a new hospital. For this purpose, we developed compatible image sources (nuclear medicine and DSA) and connection to other image sources (CT). Each imaging division (fig.

2) was organized around an image processor able to acquire, process, store and transmit – receive images. Image processors were linked together and to a VAX computer acting as the database through high-speed optic fiber links (fig. 3). The database was based on a relational DBMS pointing to image files.

The project was stopped in 1988 essentially because of the unreliability of the network. However, image sources are still in use, and a lot of practical experience was gained in the field of PACS, even though PACS technology has evolved significantly in the last three years.

4.2. The medical image database project

Four years ago, three French PACS teams joined into the NRV (Nantes, Rennes, Villejuif) PACS group, in order to carry out PACS projects. We all had a previous experience with PACS databases using relational DBMS. We decided to tackle the database problem from a medical standpoint (Aubry et al., 1991; Bizais et al., 1991). We selected a set of *30 image procedures*, routinely performed in our institutions, and we defined a *form* listing the items describing a procedure throughout its life time. Then we *interviewed* radiologists, referring physicians, clinicians and surgeons in order to fill out the forms for each procedure. This *inventory of image data* allowed us to specify all the image objects used in medical imaging. They turn out to be more numerous and more complex than those proposed by the ACR-NEMA standard. Moreover, the relationships between image objects are quite complex. They define the meaning of image objects and their role in the diagnostic process. In a second step we used this inventory to build a *data model*. Several attempts were made to

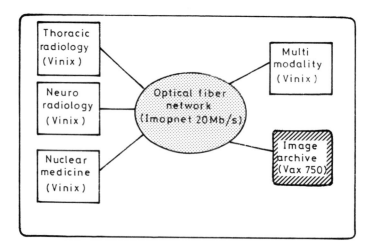

Fig. 3. DIMI project, general architecture.

use a relational model, but we ended with an *object-oriented* model which describes image data in a very clean and concise way. We are in the process of *implementing* this model. It is not clear yet whether the object-oriented model can be implemented using a relational DBMS or not; using a relational DBMS would make the process easier due to the lack of reliable object-oriented databases at the present time. *This work can be seen as a contribution to the PACS database issue as a whole.* A reduced version might be used to build hospital-wide PACS databases, allowing to provide end-users with the meaning of images they look at. An advanced version might be used to build departmental PACS databases; it would include a full description of image processing.

4.3. Intelligent analysis of medical images

Locally, we started a project two years ago about intelligent analysis of medical images (Forte and Bizais, 1991). The basic concept of this project consists in assuming that processing of medical images is too complex a process to be formalized by a simple (mechanized) algorithm. Consequently, we model the *image processing process* by an *intelligent system able to activate image processing procedures*. More precisely, the intelligent subsystem is an expert system including an inference engine, *generic* (application independent) knowledge bases (scene, image source, image processing), and *specific* (application-dependent) knowledge bases. When a specific knowledge base is consulted, its own rules or the rules of the generic knowledge base may activate various image processing procedures (algorithmic component of the system), until the goal of the consultation is reached (image data, which can be straightforwardly used to interpret the image procedure, are generated). A *database* is able to store intermediate and final results, and an *advanced user-interface* is used to make the system user-friendly. After consultation the system is able to tell which rules and which procedures were used to obtain the results.

This project is consistent with the MIDB project since an object-oriented data model similar to the one presented in the previous section is used. This project can be seen as an attempt to *manage medical image processing*, and thus as a research work in the field of *departmental PACS*. The workstation with which the project is developed should be connected to image sources, and the database located in an independent server for this purpose.

5. Conclusions

Medical imaging has become a major investigation tool during the last 40 years, thanks to the availability of several complementary imaging modalities. It is clear that the information provided by medical imaging is so large that it is difficult to utilize it completely. For this purpose, processing tools are being developed especially in the field of *multimodality medical imaging* (data integration or fusion, etc.). Moreover, image data must be managed by appropriate information systems. This is the field of PACS. At first, the results of PACS research during the last ten years may seem disappointing. No PACS prototype is actually used routinely. However, it has led to a general agreement on the formal architecture of PACS as well as on its appropriate components. Moreover, several prototypes are being experimented. It is therefore possible and necessary to focus on medical aspects of PACS from now on. Further PACS research should result in image extensions of HIS (hospital-wide PACS restricted to image management) in the near future. By the end of the century, image extensions of RIS (departmental PACS able to manage image processing) should be available. *Generalized handling of medical imaging* is likely to be a formidable tool allowing physicians and researchers to better use medical image data.

References

ACR-NEMA Publication 300-1985 (1985) Digital Imaging and Communication (NEMA, Washington D.C.).

Alzner, E., and L. Murphy (1986) The ACR-NEMA digital imaging and communications standard evolution, overview and implementation considerations. In: Schneider, R.H., and S.J. Dwyer III (Eds.), Medicine XIV/PACS IV, *Proc. SPIE* 626, 506–510.

Appel, R.D., O. Ratib and J.R. Scherrer (1990) CHAMPOLLION: an image file format translator. In: Huang, H.K. (Ed.), Picture Archiving and Communication Systems (PACS) in Medicine, *NATO ASI Series* (preprint), 252–254.

Arenson, R.L., D.P. Chakraborty, S.B. Seshadri and H.L. Kundel (1990) The digital imaging workstation, *Radiology* 176, 303–315.

Assman, K., R. Venema and K.H. Hohne (1986) Software tools for the development of pictorial information systems in medicine: the ISQL experience. In: Hohne, K.H. (Ed.), Pictorial Information Systems in Medicine, *NATO ASI Series F* 19, 333–356.

Aubry, F., Y. Bizais, B. Gibaud, A.M. Forte, V. Chameroy, R. DiPaola and J.M. Scarabin (1991) Object-oriented model for medical image data base. IN: Jost, R.G. (Ed.), Medical Imaging V: PACS Design and Evaluation, *Proc. SPIE* 1446, 168–176.

Bakker, A.R. (1986) Integrated hospital information systems. In: Hohne, K.H. (Ed.), Pictorial Information Systems in Medicine, *NATO ASI Series F* 19, 105–150.

Bakker, A.R. (1990) HIS and RIS and PACS. In: Dwyer III, S.J., and R.G. Jost (Eds.), Medical Imaging IV: PACS System Design and Evaluation, *Proc. SPIE* 1234, 8–13.

Bizais, Y., M. Baba-Ami, E. Boissinot and S. Roy (1986a) The DIMI system philosophy and state of development. In: Hohne, K.H. (Ed.), Pictorial Information Systems in Medicine, *NATO ASI Series F* 19, 433–444.

Bizais, Y., M. Baba-Ami, M. Roy, E. Martin and S. Roy (1986b) The DIMI project, an image processing and management computer facility for an imaging department. In: Schneider, G.H., and

S.J. Dwyer III (Eds.), Medicine XIV/PACS IV, *Proc. SPIE* 626, 656 – 663.

Bizais, Y., B. Gibaud, A.M. Forte, F. Aubry, R. Di Paola and J.M. Scarabin (1991) A qualitative approach to medical image databases. In: Jost, R.G. (Ed.), Medical Imaging V: PACS Design and Evaluation, *Proc. SPIE* 1446, 156 – 167.

Blaine, G.J., R.C. Ferguson, J.W. Studt and R.A. Whitman (1990) ISDN early experiments as a wide area extension to LAN-based PACS. In: Dwyer III, S.J., and R.G. Jost (Eds.), Medical Imaging IV: PACS System Design and Evaluation, *Proc. SPIE* 1234, 140 – 146.

Britton C.A., J.H. Sumkin, H.D. Curtin, R.J. Hoy, E.K. Tabor, S.A. Yousem, M.A. Costa-Greco, R.C. Gennari and E.A. Eelkema (1990) Subjective perceptions of and attitudes toward primary interpretation of X-ray images in a PACS environment. In: Dwyer III, S.J., and R.G. Jost (Eds.), Medical Imaging IV: PACS System Design and Evaluation, *Proc. SPIE* 1234, 94 – 97.

Carterette, E.C., R.A. Fiske and H.K. Huang (1986) Receiver operating characteristic (ROC) evaluation of a digital viewing station for radiologists. In: Schneider, R.H., and S.J. Dwyer III (Eds.), Medicine XIV/PACS IV, *Proc. SPIE* 626, 441 – 446.

Cho, P., K.K. Chan and B.K.T. Ho (1990) Data storage and compression. In: Dwyer III, S.J., and R.G. Jost (Eds.), Medical Imaging IV: PACS System Design and Evaluation, *Proc. SPIE* 1234, 35 – 46.

Duerinckx, A.J., and E.J. Pisa (1982) Filmless picture archiving and communication in diagnostic radiology. In: Duerinckx, A.J. (Ed.), Picture Archiving and Communication Systems (PACS) for Medical Applications, First International Conference and Workshop, *Proc. SPIE* 318, 9 – 18.

Dwyer III, S.J., A.W. Templeton, N.L. Martin, L.T. Cook, K.R. Lee, E. Levine, S. Batnitzky, D.P. Preston, S.J. Rosenthal, H.I. Price, W.H. Anderson, M.A. Tarlton and S. Faszold (1982) Cost of managing digital diagnostic images for a 614 bed hospital. In: Duerinckx, A.J. (Ed.), Picture Arciving and Communication Systems (PACS) for Medical Applications, First International Conference and Workshop, *Proc. SPIE* 318, 3 – 8.

Dwyer III, S.J., G.G. Cox, L.T. Cook, J.H. Macmillan and A.W. Templeton (1990) Experience with high resolution digital gray scale display systems. In: Dwyer III, S.J., and R.G. Jost (Eds.), Medical Imaging IV: PACS System Design and Evaluation, *Proc. SPIE* 1234, 132 – 138.

Forte, A.M., and Y. Bizais (1991) Analyzing and interpreting pulmonary tomoscintigraphy sequences realization and perspectives. In: Loew, M.H. (Ed.), Medical Imaging V, Image Processing, *Proc. SPIE* 1445, 409 – 420.

Good, W.F., J.M. Herron, G.S. Maitz, D. Gur, S.L. Miller, W.H. Straub and C.R. Fuhrman (1990) Implementation of high resolution workstation for primary diagnosis of projection radiography images. In: Dwyer III, S.J., and R.G. Jost (Eds.), Medical Imaging IV: PACS System Design and Evaluation, *Proc. SPIE* 1234, 105 – 110.

Haskell, B.G., and H.M. Hang (1986) Comparison of discrete cosine transform and vector quantization of medical imagery. In: Schneider, R.H., and S.J. Dwyer III (Eds.), Medicine XIV/PACS IV, *Proc. SPIE* 626, 399 – 408.

Hegde, S.S., A.O. Gale and J.A. Giunta (1986) AT&T PACS architecture. In: Schneider, R.H., and S.J. Dwyer III (Eds.), Medicine XIV/PACS IV, *Proc. SPIE* 626, 618 – 625.

Hemminger, B.M., B.G. Thompson, S.M. Pizer and P. Stancil (1986) The ongoing implementation of a prototype medical communications system at the University of North Carolina. In: Schneider, R.H., and S.J. Dwyer III (Eds.), Medicine XIV/PACS IV, *Proc. SPIE* 626, 574 – 580.

Herman, G.T. (1986) Three dimensional computer graphic display in medicine: the MIPG perspective. In: Höhne, K.H. (Ed.), Pictorial Information Systems in Medicine, *NATO ASI Series F,* 19, 181 – 210 (Springer, Berlin).

Heu, R., R. Hass and B. Scharnberg (1986) Implementation of a data exchange procedure between RIS and a PAC-system. In: Schneider, R.H., and S.J. Dwyer III (Eds.), Medicine XIV/PACS IV, *Proc. SPIE* 626, 594–596.

Ho, B.K., P. Zhu, S. Cho and H.K. Huang (1990) Dedicated radiology viewing station for low cost and high performance. In: Dwyer III, S.J., and R.G. Jost (Eds.), Medical Imaging IV: PACS System Design and Evaluation, *Proc. SPIE* 1234, 418–422

Horii, S.C. (1990) An introduction to ACR/NEMA standards. In. Dwyer III, S.J., and R.G. Jost (Eds.), Medical Imaging IV: PACS System Design and Evaluation, *Proc. SPIE* 1234, 93–113.

Horii, S.C., G. Isles and R.T. Bergeron (1986) Display preferences for viewing CT scans. In: Schneider, R.H., and S.J. Dwyer III (Eds.), Medicine XIV/PACS IV, *Proc. SPIE* 626, 426–430.

Huang, H.K. (1986) Recent developments in digital radiology. In: Höhne, K.H. (Ed.), Pictorial Information Systems in Medicine, *NATO ASI Series F* 19, 369–380.

Irie, G., K. Miyasaka, K. Miyamoto, T. Kojima, I. Yamamoto and T. Kudo (1990) PACS experience at the University of Hokkaido Medical School. In: Dwyer III, S.J., and R.G. Jost (Eds.), Medical Imaging IV: PACS System Design and Evaluation, *Proc. SPIE* 1234, 26–32.

Johnston, R.E., D.C. Rogers, B.M. Hemminger, S.M. Pizer, J.L. Creasy, J.R. Perry, E.V. Staab, J.T. Curnes and L.A. Parker (1986) A multiscreen multiple image display console. In: Schneider, R.H., and S.J. Dwyer III (Eds.), Medicine XIV/PACS IV, *Proc. SPIE* 626, 447–450.

Lehr, J.L. (1986) The ACR-NEMA standard data dictionary: a radiologist's perspective. In: Schneider, R.H., and S.J. Dwyer III (Eds.), Medicine XIV/PACS IV, *Proc. SPIE* 626, 511–514.

Levin, K., and R. Fielding (1990) Method to prefetch comparison images in image management and communication systems. In: Dwyer III, S.J., and R.G. Jost (Eds.), Medical Imaging IV: PACS System Design and Evaluation, *Proc. SPIE* 1234, 270–274.

Levine, B.A., S.K. Mun, H.R. Benson and S.C. Horii (1990) Assessment of the integration of a HIS/RIS with a PACS. In: Dwyer III, S.J., and R.G. Jost (Eds.), Medical Imaging IV: PACS System Design and Evaluation, *Proc. SPIE* 1234, 391–397.

Liu Sheng, O.R., H.C. Garcia, C. Wei, T. Ozeki and P. MacNulty (1990) Distributed database design and modeling for PACS. In: Dwyer III, S.J., and R.G. Jost (Eds.), Medical Imaging IV: PACS System Design and Evaluation, *Proc. SPIE* 1234, 256–269.

Lodwick, G.S. (1986) Pictorial information systems and radiology improving the quality of communications. In: Höhne, K.H. (Ed.), Pictorial Information Systems in Medicine, *NATO ASI Series F* 19, 1–28.

Marceau, C. (1982) What is a picture archiving and communication system (PACS)? In: Duerinckx, A.J. (Ed.), Picture Archiving and Communication Systems (PACS) for Medical Applications, First International Conference and Workshop, *Proc. SPIE* 318, 24–29.

Meyer-Ebrecht, D. (1986) On the architecture of pictorial information systems. In: Höhne, K.H. (Ed.), Pictorial Information Systems in Medicine, *NATO ASI Series F* 19, 151–180.

Minato, K., M. Komori, Y. Nakano, K. Okajima, I. Kimura, T. Takahashi, J. Konishi, M. Abe, Y. Gotoh and K. Sato (1990) Present status of PACS at Kyoto University Hospital: image workstation for clinical education. In: Dwyer III, S.J., and R.G. Jost (Eds.), Medical Imaging IV: PACS System Design and Evaluation, *Proc. SPIE* 1234, 180–185.

Nievergelt, J. (1986) Issues in the design of human-computer interfaces. In: Höhne, K.H. (Ed.), Pictorial Information Systems in Medicine, *NATO ASI Series F* 19, 251–262.

Noh, K.H., and J.M. Jenkins (1986) Comparison of data compression schemes for medical images. In: Schneider, R.H., and S.J. Dwyer III (Eds.), Medicine XIV/PACS IV *Proc. SPIE* 626, 392–398.

Oosterwijk, H., F.W. Gutzwiller and A. Giangrande (1986) Practical and strategic implications of the ACR-NEMA interface standards. In: Schneider, R.H., and S.J. Dwyer III (Eds.), Medicine XIV/PACS IV, *Proc. SPIE* 626, 515 – 521.

Ottes, F.P., E.M. Van Gennip, L. Steenbergen and B.M. Van Poppel (1990) Dedicated software packages to support PACS research. In: Huang, H.K., O. Ratib, A.R. Bakker and G. Witte (Eds.), Picture Archiving and Communication Systems (PACS) in Medicine, *NATO ASI Series F* 74, 399 – 401.

Parrish, D.M., J.L. Creasy, B.G. Thompson, D.C. Rogers, E.R. Johnston, J.R. Perry and E.V. Staab (1986) Functional requirements for interfacing PACS to HIS. In: Schneider, R.H., and S.J. Dwyer III (Eds.), Medicine XIV/PACS IV, *Proc. SPIE* 626, 597 – 602.

Pizer, S.M. (1986) Psychovisual issues in the display of medical images. In: Höhne, K.H. (Ed.), Pictorial Information Systems in Medicine, *NATO ASI Series F* 19, 211 – 234 (Springer, Berlin).

Preston, D.F., S.J. Dwyer III and W.H. Anderson (1986) Experience with a prototype PACS system in a clinical environment. In: Höhne, K.H. (Ed.), Pictorial Information Systems in Medicine, *NATO ASI Series F* 19, 357 – 368.

Ratib, O., Y. Ligier, M. Funk, C. Girard, R. Perrier and D. Hochstrasser (1990) PACS workstation user interface design. In: Dwyer III, S.J., and R.G. Jost (Eds.), Medical Imaging IV: PACS System Design and Evaluation, *Proc. SPIE* 1234, 190 – 194.

Ravin, C.E. (1990) Initial experience with automatic image transmission to an intensive care unit using PACS technology. In: Dwyer III, S.J., and R.G. Jost (Eds.), Medical Imaging IV: PACS System Design and Evaluation, *Proc. SPIE* 1234, 386 – 390.

Renoulin, C., J.M. Scarabin, J.L. Coatrieux, J.C. Launay, G. Babonneau, B. Gibaud, D. Curet, G. Lecerteu, B. Mahieddine, C. Isias-Perez, C. Barillot, M. Launay, F. Heuze, S. Fresne and C. Toumoulin (1987) The Sirene project, CAR (Springer Berlin) 523 – 531.

Seshadri, S.B., S. Kishore, S.S. Khalsa, F.J. Stevens and R.L. Arenson (1990) Software considerations in the design of an image archive. In: Dwyer III, S.J., and R.G. Jost (Eds.), Medical Imaging IV: PACS System Design and Evaluation, *Proc. SPIE* 1234, 2 – 9.

Slasky, B.S., M.S. Rosenthal, C.R. Fuhrman, D. Sashin, F.L. Thaete, J.H. Feist, M.A. Costa-Greco, K.M. Harris, H.D. Curtin and J.H. Sumkin (1990) Primary diagnosis of chest images in a PACS environment. In: Dwyer III, S.J., and R.G. Jost (Eds.), Medical Imaging IV: PACS System Design and Evaluation, *Proc. SPIE* 1234, 120 – 125.

Stewart, B.K. (1990) Three tiered network architecture for PACS clusters. In: Dwyer III, S.J., and R.G. Jost (Eds.), Medical Imaging IV: PACS System Design and Evaluation, *Proc. SPIE* 1234, 203 – 208.

Stewart, B.K., and R.K. Taira (1990) Database architecture and design for PACS. In: Huang, H.K. (Ed.), PACS in Medicine, *NATO ASI Series* (preprint), 209 – 215.

Stockbridge, C., and C.E. Ravin (1986) Phased implementation of AT&T PACS at Duke University Medical Center. In: Schneider, R.H., and S.J. Dwyer III (Eds.), Medicine XIV/PACS IV, *Proc. SPIE* 626, 570 – 573.

Taira, R.K., M.A. Simons, M. Razavi, H. Kangarloo, M.I. Boechat, T. Hall, K. Chuang, K.S. Huang and S. Eldredge, (1990) High resolution workstations for primary and secondary radiology readings. In: Dwyer III, S.J., and R.G. Jost (Eds.), Medical Imaging IV: PACS System Design and Evaluation, *Proc. SPIE* 1234, 18 – 25.

Toshimitsu, A., Y. Fukushima, K. Tawara, M. Osada, T. Ema, T. Ozeki, K. Komatsu and W.J. Dallas (1990) Network data rate requirements analysis for picture archiving and communication systems. In: Dwyer III, S.J., and R.G. Jost (Eds.), Medical Imaging IV: PACS System Design and Evaluation, *Proc. SPIE* 1234, 147 – 158.

Wendler, Th., R. Grewer, K.J. Monnich and H. Svensson (1986) Design considerations for multimodality medical image workstations. In: Höhne, K.H. (Ed.), Pictorial Information Systems in Medicine, *NATO ASI Series F* 19, 401 – 420 (Springer, Berlin).

Integrated Diagnostic Imaging
Editor: J.P.J. De Valk
© *Elsevier Science Publishers B.V., 1992*

Chapter 9

PACS evolution between 1980 and 2000

Bernard Gibaud, Jean-Marie Scarabin and Yves Gandon

1. Introduction

Hospital information systems (HIS) have been intensively studied for more than 20 years and the problem of the integration of its multiple components is of primary concern (Melrose and Ericson, 1981; Bakker, 1991). As with most modern companies, hospitals have to face this problem and it is clear today that information has to be considered as a resource; as a consequence, better information management is one way of increasing productivity. This awareness leads to major transformations, which are especially long and tedious in hospitals as a result of the multiple tasks a hospital must fulfill (patient care, administrative and financial management, research, education, etc.) and the numerous professionals involved in these tasks (doctors, nurses, administrators, researchers, professors, etc.) (Rienhoff, 1989).

Historically, HIS made no distinction between the *various kinds of information* to be dealt with by the system. Consequently, the first attempts to integrate medical imaging information would logically have been carried out in the HIS environment. This, however, has not been the case in practice, as will be shown.

We are going to present first our perception of the beginning of PACS (picture archiving and communication system), through experiments described in the literature and through our own experience. Secondly, we will present several possible developments towards integrated information systems by the year 2000.

2. The 1980–1990 period

Two major periods can be identified during the 1980–1990 decade. Between

1980 and 1985 a lot of PACS experiments were initiated and carried out, but most of them actually failed to provide clinically usable systems. This was really an *exploratory period* since a lot of enthusiasm and energy had been spent in prototyping and most teams suffered from the fact that the technology had not been fully developed, from the lack of standards and from their own methodological and organisational inadequacies.

The second period (between 1985 and 1989) issued *second generation projects* which were much more well-thought-out and diversified. Their objectives were more to assess given aspects of the PACS impact, rather than just prototyping.

2.1. First generation PACS projects

2.1.1. Motivation
Before we give further details of the characteristics and results of these two generations of PACS projects, it seems necessary to review the general motivation for PACS, at the beginning of the 1980s.

Four major categories of motivation arise: medical and organisational issues, potential of a digital management of images, the feeling of new opportunities brought by new technology, and economic issues.

Medical and organisational issues. The rapid evolution of medical imaging at the end of the 1970s and the beginning of the 1980s demonstrated the necessity of a consistent management of images within radiology departments. The rapid increase in volumes of data created by digital image sources resulted in increasing management and storage problems. Radiology information systems (RIS) started to be developed at that time, so the idea of using computer-based procedures to manage, archive and communicate the images within and outside the radiology departments seemed a very natural approach; this explains why most experiments were initiated in radiology departments which became aware of the problems involved.

Potential of digital imaging. This potential is perceived by the whole medical staff, but more or less acutely according to the various specialties which range from the improvement of image reading as a result of digital windowing capabilities (CT (computed tomography) images are a common example), up to multi-modal image comparison or fusion. Researchers have shown a major interest in such new features because they opened-up a very fruitful and unexplored field of research. When one looks back to the 1982 – 1983 literature, it is surprising to notice a certain mixture between *immediate* and *potential* benefits, some of the latter being more or less realistic at that time. Actually, such a mixture did not provide a sound basis for a gradual introduction of

PACS, which would have been able to lead to a good acceptance of the PACS concept, since the benefits that could be anticipated and actually noticed by end users were not made clear. On the other hand, this mixture may explain some disillusions.

Technology opportunities. The beginning of the 1980s was marked by the very rapid expansion of local area networks. Moreover, the decrease in cost of increasingly powerful micro-computers and workstations and the arrival on the market of high-capacity storage media like optical disks have certainly given *the impression* that the technology necessary for building PACS was available. One experienced how wrong this feeling was. The mistake certainly deals with the level of development of technology (which remains a difficult problem that will be further discussed), but also with the dangers brought by this evolution. The difficulty of choosing a computer, especially when it has to be integrated into a complex system, is well-known, now.

Economic issues. Most 1982 – 1983 papers explain that significant savings can be expected as a result of the introduction of PACS. Looking back, one realizes that these expectations were mostly extrapolated from a few economic studies comparing a film-based archiving and a digital one. The distinction is not clearly made between *direct savings* (films, chemicals, personnel managing films, etc.) and *indirect savings* that could result from PACS introduction throughout the chain of image production and utilization (savings of radiologist time, reduction of lost films, etc.). Even more hypothetic are those which could result from the reduction of patient stay or from the optimization of diagnostic and therapeutic procedures.

Industrial challenges. This feeling essentially concerns manufacturers providing PACS components like networks or archiving systems, or storage media like optical disks. These manufacturers felt that a major market could possibly be opened-up and they decided to collaborate with PACS prototype developments. On the other hand, a very cautious approach could be noticed among medical imaging manufacturers who obviously preferred to *follow* this evolution rather than trying to anticipate it.

2.1.2. Main experiments

These various, more or less precise motivations have been catalysed by the enthusiasm of physicists and researchers for this new technology and a lot of teams got involved in PACS prototyping. The major experiments have been carried out by the Department of Radiology of the University of Kansas, in partnership with NCR (Dwyer III et al., 1982; Bulatek and O'Connell, 1983), the Department of Radiology of the New York University Medical Center (Maguire et al., 1982; Cywinski et al., 1983; Horii et al., 1983), the Department of Radiological sciences of UCLA (Huang et al., 1983a,b), the Mallinckrodt Institute of Radiology at St Louis (Cox et al., 1982; Blaine et al., 1983), the University of Pennsylvania in Philadelphia (Arenson et al., 1982, 1983), and the University of North Carolina in Chapel Hill.

2.1.3. Main difficulties

None of these experiments succeeded in providing a clinically useful system in the anticipated time. The difficulties encountered by these pioneer groups enabled researchers to fully understand the PACS 'problem'; the major ones were due to:

(1) Technological reasons, mostly related to the immaturity of available technology (expensive, nonreliable, and globally not very efficient). The lack of standards for the digital sources interfacing also required tremendous efforts to provide only specific and nondurable solutions.

(2) Methodological reasons; these projects aimed at too many goals, without clear milestones. Consequently, a lot of energy was spent with little concrete outcome. Ergonomics and organisational issues were underestimated, leading to systems which could be little used in a clinical context.

These difficulties were more or less acutely perceived. In a paper which remains famous, Maguire gives an almost caricatural description of the disillusions which marked the end of this exploratory period (Maguire, 1986).

2.2. Second generation PACS projects

The 1985 – 1989 period is characterized by a sharp contrast with the former one. A number of new projects were issued, some of them in continuity with a previous experiment, some others completely new.

2.2.1. General characteristics

Two major characteristics can be drawn.

(1) These new projects certainly attest *pragmatism* as far as technology is concerned; whereas former experiments did not hesitate in offering hazardous solutions, people try to rely on proven technology even if it is less efficient. Ethernet-TCP/IP turns out to be the most popular solution for communication. Frame-grabbing is used to make the interfacing of medical image sources easier, as long as no standard is really available.

(2) The objectives are also much better defined than during the previous period; the major difficulties for building PACS had been highlighted by first generation projects so the new experiments can be focused on given

aspects of PACS in order to elucidate and solve them. The example of the Dutch PACS project provides a very good illustration of this new approach. The aspects studied in this project concern mainly the evaluation of the clinical impact of a PACS (reduced to the scale of a 15 bed ward in an internal medicine clinic), the coupling between the PACS and the RIS-HIS, the evaluation of the quality of diagnosis on consoles (compared to film) and the measurement of the cost efficiency ratio in order to derive when PACS costs will be equal to savings (ter Haar Romeny et al., 1987, 1989; Lodder et al., 1988; Barneveld Binkhuysen et al., 1989; Ottes et al., 1989).

2.2.2. General lessons

2.2.2.1. General aspects. Such well-focused studies have been very numerous all over the world and have brought significant contributions to the understanding of PACS problems, especially on the organization of radiology departments, like those carried out at the University of North Carolina (Parrish et al., 1986; Rogers et al., 1986), on the evaluation of the impact of PACS in particular clinical contexts like a pediatric department at UCLA (Kangarloo et al., 1988), or on teleradiology applications (Seshadri and Arenson, 1988). Other studies deal with more technical aspects, from a technical or ergonomics viewpoint (Cox et al., 1988; Horii et al., 1988), for instance, communication issues (Blaine et al., 1988; Reijns et al., 1988), workstation, and the organization of archiving (Martinez and Archwamety, 1988).

2.2.2.2. First industrial PACS. The first industrial PACS have also been put on the market (by Philips/AT&T and Siemens) during this period; the CommView system (Philips/AT&T) turned out to have a very positive influence on the general development of PACS although its functions were relatively limited as a result of the mode of acquisition of image data based on frame-grabbing. The implementation approach (Stockbridge and Ravin, 1986) and the very pragmatic architectural choices (Hedge et al., 1986) as well as the concern for ergonomics (Kasday, 1986) actually did promote a number of key concepts. This system was installed at the Duke University Hospital in Durham (North Carolina) and at the Georgetown University Hospital in Washington where a wide range of aspects of the medical impact of PACS have been studied (Mun et al., 1988; Braudes et al., 1989; Levine et al., 1990). More recently, a few systems have been purchased in Europe, especially in Italy (mainly at Trieste, Ferrera, and Bologna).

The Siemens approach is quite different. The major concern is to provide a very user-friendly environment on a high performance console (diagnostic reporting console or DRC); the PACS itself mainly consists of retrieval facilities based on a hierarchical folder concept and the capability of interfacing the Siemens imaging modalities. This system is operational in several sites in Canada (Nosil et al., 1988), Japan, Europe and the U.S.A.

2.2.2.3. ACR/NEMA standard. Last, but not least, the ACR/NEMA standard was issued in 1985. Although some imperfections remain, this standard had a great influence on PACS developments around the world (Creasy et al., 1986; Hemminger et al., 1986; Good et al., 1988). Significant efforts were devoted to adapt the organization of the archives to the schema proposed in the standard (Budler and Lee Hamilton, 1988). The SPI specification, defined by Philips and Siemens, is basically an extension of the ACR/NEMA standard, which tries to find a remedy for some of the shortcomings of the standard (Herforth et al., 1989). It is a good illustration of the half-success of the standard since the nomenclature and data formats were well accepted by the PACS community, whereas the lower levels part, based on the 50 pin connector, were accepted neither by users, nor by manufacturers. The best evidence for this is the extremely small amount of equipment which actually offers this kind of interface, today.

2.3. The Sirene project in Rennes

2.3.1. Motivation and genesis of the project

The first impetus to initiate a PACS project in Rennes was given by a group of researchers and physicians working in the field of signal and image processing in medicine (GBM-SIM group), at Rennes University. The major part of this research group was already involved in *medical signals and images understanding*, especially applied to neurosurgery, which is a domain where the utilization of multi-modal images and the reference to anatomical models play a major role. In this context, PACS seemed to us able to provide the communication and data management infrastructure which is necessary to assess computer assisted procedures for diagnosis and therapy planning (fig. 1). Beyond this interest which was directly related to our research activities, the perspectives offered by PACS at the medical, economic and industrial levels seemed very exciting to us. The proceedings of the PACS I and PACS II meetings reinforced this feeling and the idea to participate in this great venture rapidly gained ground.

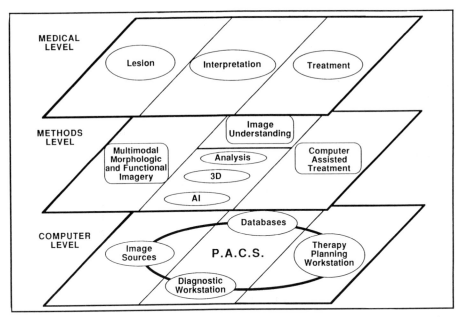

Fig. 1. A three-level schema showing the role of PACS for computer-assisted therapy planning.

The existence in Rennes of research centers like the CCETT* and the CELAR** and engineering schools like the ESE*** enabled the creation of a project definition document in June 1983 (Scarabin et al., 1983). The project was supported by the French Ministry of Research and Technology and the Regional Council of Brittany. It has been managed by the University Hospital of Rennes and the CCETT has been in charge of its technical direction.

2.3.2. Objectives

At the beginning, the approach was very ambitious since the objective was to connect all digital imaging modalities to a local area network in order to achieve the archiving of images in a central high-capacity database and to provide a range of terminals distributed throughout the hospital with access facilities to images. The project also aimed at evaluating the medical and economic impact of the system. It was supposed to be conducted in close collaboration with manufacturers in order to allow a partial or total transfer to industry of the

---

* CCETT: Centre Commun d'Etudes de Télédiffusion et Télécommunications.
** CELAR: Centre d'électronique de l'armement.
*** ESE: Ecole Supérieure d'Electricité.

developments at the end of the project. Our approach was definitively a *technology driven* one. The idea was to rely on high technology because it seemed to us to be the only way to provide durable technical solutions and to deal with the big volumes of data encountered in radiology.

(1) The *Carthage Network* was industrialized by the LCT* from research carried out at the CCETT. It was a first generation of multi-service networks (voice/data), it consisted of a digital token ring using fiber optics and, as it had been developed in the environment of telecommunications, it could offer standard interfaces and was open to public networks.

(2) The *Multimedia Copernique Server* integrated the management of images in a database management system (DBMS) offering both navigational and relational models. The multi-processor architecture provided a very high input/output throughput. This feature seemed to us very critical to make possible *real-time* image transfers and to allow future extensions of the PACS system without significant decrease of performance. The Copernique company had already had a good experience of high-capacity servers since it had been selected by the telecommunications administration to design and equip the servers of the national telephone electronic directory.

(3) Our approach to PACS terminals distinguished three kinds of systems:
   - high performance workstations with image processing capabilities, dedicated to radiologists;
   - middle range workstations allowing the integration of images with other medical records, the basic idea was that the same screen could be used to display the various features composing medical files (texts, either coded in ASCII or in facsimile, graphics, images, etc.); the objective was to manage all these data in a single structured document;
   - consultation terminals, which were supposed to be widely distributed throughout the hospital, at the beginning they were considered as simple display screens with no image manipulation and processing features.

2.3.3. Project history

The project has had three major phases: a specification phase (from January to July 1985), a realization phase (from September 1985 to April 1988) and an integration phase (from May 1988 to November 1989).

2.3.3.1. Specifications. At the beginning of this period, physicians were asked to define the capabilities they wished as far as image display and processing were concerned. The objective to allow some interworking with the HIS was

---

* LCT: Laboratoire Central des Télécommunications.

stressed at the very beginning. This led to an attempt to harmonize the PACS design with HIS projects like the development of a central patient file application, or the extension of the HIS to the management of clinics. These efforts did not succeed due to several factors:

(1) the complexity and multiple interrelationships of these problems;
(2) the very slow and tedious progress of this reflection; and
(3) the impatience of some of us to start actual development.

The major technical options of the system were chosen in a second stage. The interfaces available on the Carthage network offered a maximum data rate of 64 Kbits/s which was not suitable for image transmission in PACS. So, it was decided to 'graft' into the network a rapid interface with additional hardware and software. The SCSI interface was chosen, on the one hand because of its intrinsic performance, and on the other hand because it was increasingly available on mini-computers, workstations and medical image sources. Two communication channels would be considered on the same physical network: low-rate 64 Kbits/s channels (based on the CCITT X25 recommendation), mostly dedicated to the management of protocols, and high-speed channels (based on SCSI interface), dedicated to image transfers.

Concerning software, a *retrieval application* was designed on the central server, based on tree-menus and offering navigation tools to select and retrieve data from the database (patient data, study descriptions and image characteristics). This application was supposed to communicate with terminals by means of menus (with a VT100 or videotex presentation), managed by an access method called SATURNE, initially developed by the CCETT for videography applications. An *archiving application* was also defined. It was based on an archiving protocol allowing the creation or updating of patient, study, acquisition and image data within the central database. A file transfer protocol (based of the FTAM standard) was also designed to control the image transfer procedures.

The final choices of terminals were made later and for the high-performance workstation, we finally selected an image processor manufactured by CGR. At that time CGR wanted to develop a common hardware platform to equip all its future imaging equipments. This RGN processor (with a 512 × 512 display resolution, upgradeable to 1 K × 1 K) was supposed to be integrated in the next generation of CGR medical image sources and PACS multi-modality consoles. Regarding Faxicolor, the middle range workstation, a specification document was composed in 1986 and a contract was signed between the CCETT and the ESE to carry out the developments. Lastly, after an initial choice of the Graph16 (a videotex alpha-photographic terminal), a new orientation was taken in 1987 aiming at building a low-cost consultation terminal on a simple PC. This approach consisted of extending a medical office management software in order to provide it with facilities to display, manipulate and retrieve images from the central database.

2.3.3.2. Realization and integration phases (Gibaud et al., 1989). The PACS prototype was implemented at the CCETT between 1985 and 1988. The integration of the main components was achieved in the hospital environment and it turned out to be much longer and more difficult than expected. The most difficult aspect of the integration was the high-speed SCSI communication link as a result of the specificities induced by the interface itself and by management of the two communication channels associated with individual sessions. Moreover, only the CT scanner could actually be connected to the network, by means of a capture computer emulating the CT magnetic tape unit; the archiving application was also implemented on the image processing system host computer (VAX 11-750) in order to archive magnetic resonance and angiographic images.

This integration phase actually came to an end in November 1989, with the official reception of the prototype by the hospital administration.

Additional software development was carried out in 1989. Given the low flexibility and developmental possibilities of the current image retrieval facilities, we decided to seek a way to develop autonomous distributed applications with the ability to retrieve data from the central server. The solution we proposed implies three elements:

(1) the implementation of the retrieval application on the workstation;
(2) the utilization of software offering a remote access to the central database (provided by Copernique); and
(3) the utilization of a local commercial DBMS package in order to make the management of local data easier and to facilitate the development of applications.

This solution was implementented to provide a workstation used in neurosurgery for stereotactic procedures with image retrieval facilities (Gibaud et al., 1990).

2.3.4. Conclusion of the first phase of the Sirene project (1983 – 1989)

2.3.4.1. Negative aspects. When we look back in detail to the Sirene experience, we must realize that all the initial objectives could not be met: little implantation in the radiology department, little diffusion in the clinics, no link with the HIS. But the most critical point is that some of the major components, like the network or the terminals, turned out to be obsolete before the system was ready for use. The Carthage network configuration was purchased in 1986 and we realized in 1989 that it could no longer be extended because the manufacturer considered the technology outdated. There was very hard because the specificity of the network had required tremendous effort to be dealt with, within the network (specific hardware and software), but also on the workstations (specific device drivers, management of dual communication channels) and on the Copernique server (direct interfacing with the SCSI internal bus linking the various processors, specific access to applications). Most of this effort had been useless, at least in the long term. The Faxicolor workstation also turned out to be a dead-end, although it was based on a still up-to-date idea of integration between images and medical records; namely, the assessment of this workstation could not be achieved as the functional and operational contexts were not properly addressed (which documents? to communicate with whom? additional means to scan and hardcopy documents, etc.). There was a similar destiny for the RGN image processor based workstation but for other reasons. First, the VAX 11-750 host computer proved to be insufficient to run the enhanced man – machine interface provided by the touch screen display console and secondly, CGR was purchased by General Electric (GE) in 1987, which put an end to the industrial development of the RGN image processor and also resulted in a years uncertainty about further collaboration with this partner.

From a methodological viewpoint, we certainly committed a number of mistakes at several levels:

(1) the medical needs were not properly perceived and could only be dealt with later on, after the introduction of the system in the medical environment;
(2) the technological choices led to a complex system, with little modularity; this (often useless) complexity was not properly calculated at the beginning, which explains the two year delay with all the resulting consequences on the system hardware obsolescence; and, lastly,
(3) we certainly failed to evaluate the real motivation of our partner in the area of networks (LCT, then Matra, Communications division).

2.3.4.2. Positive aspects. Despite the significant delay we mentioned, the project did result in an operational PACS, actually used, for instance, in the preparation of therapeutic procedures in neurosurgery and radiotherapy. Besides, the system provides a communication infrastructure which is daily used for the study and assessment of three-dimensional algorithms and multi-modal registration techniques.

In a general manner, the PACS activity carried out in Rennes since 1983 has stimulated further thought in our environment, not only among doctors but also among researchers, hospital administrators and the manufacturers we work with. We certainly gained experience and this experience enables us to consider the future with confidence and lucidity.

3. The 1990 – 2000 period

3.1. General conditions at the beginning of the decade

A new tendency can be observed at the beginning of this decade, characterized by a number of new hospital-wide PACS projects, aiming at installing filmless systems in two or three years; it seems to us that such initiatives (which mark a break with the former period) reveal the beginning of a certain developmental maturity.

Four such projects can be listed. The first one results from an acquisition document (MDIS, 1990) prepared by the MDIS technical development team of the U.S. Army and aims at installing PACS in three military hospitals and to equip a teleradiology hub, in the first stage. In a second stage, the acquisition of PACS for nine other hospitals and the purchase of 12 additional teleradiology centers (accessible from 96 nodes) are anticipated. A second project concerns Hammersmith hospital in London which has the same objective of a filmless operating system in 1993 (Glass and Slark, 1991). A third similar project deals with equipping a new hospital in Vienna in Austria (Mosser et al., 1991). The PACS developed in UCLA also belongs to this category. It has been constantly developed since 1983 and its scale and integration level means that it can be considered as a hospital-wide system.

The appearance of such projects contrasts with the general tendency of the previous period. Does this new ambition reveal a new maturity or a return to unconsciousness? That is the question we will try to answer. Therefore, we are going to draw on a number of issues that people generally agree about, then examine the remaining uncertainties and lastly, we will present various possible scenarios of evolution towards a generalized PACS.

3.1.1. Maturity of technology

In his opening talk at the NATO ASI 'PACS in medicine', in October 1990, H.K. Huang declared that, 'the technology for building PACS was available'. Although we agree that a significant evolution has taken place since 1980, we believe it is necessary to further discuss what we actually mean by *maturity of PACS technology*. Let us take an example in a completely different domain of industry. Everyone would certainly agree that the Cugnot machine (1770) was only a very early prototype of what we call a car today, but when would we consider that car technology became mature? The De Dion Bouton (1905)? The Citroën Traction (1939)? Or the series 5 BMW (1990)? The concept of maturity has a completely different meaning whether technology is considered in itself (does it still evolve?) or is considered in relation with the way it is used (only affordable by a small number of people, or able to even modify the structure which makes use of it). If maturity is associated with the *steadiness of perfor-mance*, then PACS technology obviously will not be mature for many years; on the other hand, if it is judged as the *general feasibility of a functional set* using this technology (including of course the economic aspect), then a certain maturity can be considered as available. The criteria to evaluate this feasibility are that the technology involved in PACS must

(1) offer a minimum level of performance;
(2) be reliable;
(3) be able to be used together (which necessitates standards to interface them);
(4) offer enough modularity to allow a smooth evolution without modification of the overall system architecture (which is related with the steadiness of standards); and finally
(5) be available at a reasonable cost (namely consistent with the added value brought by the system).

If one assumes this latter definition, we can consider that the available hardware and software to communicate, archive and process information have real maturity.

Regarding communications, Ethernet has a very wide diffusion, on both very low cost media (like twisted pair and thin coaxial cable) or fiber optics. In the latter case, the cabling can be chosen to manage change towards higher rate networks. The relative low performance of Ethernet can be remedied by clustering the network into small functionally related sub-networks (clinics, technical units). More powerful technology like FDDI (fibre distributed data interconnect) or DQDB (distributed queuing dual buses) is becoming available and it is clear that this evolution of the performance of networks will continue in the future. As far as higher levels of protocols are concerned (3 – 4 layers of the ISO-OSI model), TCP/IP provides a general solution until ISO protocols become widespread.

A very wide range of software tools are available today to develop and integrate distributed applications. In the Unix/X-Window area, the localization of information processing becomes increasingly transparent to end-users. Besides, the great diffusion of relational DBMS makes information management much easier. Such software tools facilitate the development of distributed applications because, on the one hand, they allow the retrieval of data from local or remote databases through standard query languages (like SQL) and, on the other hand, they offer an increasing number of fourth generation languages which help designing and maintaining these applications (forms and reports generators, etc.).

The current technology of storage media, based on high-speed magnetic disks and optical disks enables short-term archives of several Gigabytes and long-term archives of several hundred Gigabytes to be built up at affordable costs.

Without entering into details, the workstations technology (like SUN Sparc-stations or DEC stations based on RISC technology) has enjoyed considerable evolution; products with a very high performance/cost ratio can now be purchased. These advances also concern the man – machine interface issues: Graphical interfaces like MOTIF (OSF) or OPEN-LOOK (SUN) and the associated toolboxes really offer very high performance tools to users and programmers.

3.1.2. Architectural issues (Meyer-Ebrecht, 1986)

The analysis of PACS problems did converge towards solutions or elements of solution. Difficult problems like the necessary integration with other information systems (HIS, RIS) have been addressed to in a comprehensive and consistent way by the whole PACS community, even if the proposed solutions are still limited to concepts. It is clear today that distributed systems offer more flexibility and developmental possibilities than monolithic centralized systems, which are also very hard to build up. The key issue is to be able to divide the system into modular sub-systems, communicating across steady and well-established interfaces. The reflection is very active in this area in the U.S.A., Europe and in Japan. Let us review some on the works currently in progress in this area.

The IEEE P1157 Medical Data Interchange Committee (MEDIX) was created in 1986 to 'specify and establish a robust and flexible communications standard for the interchange of data between heterogeneous healthcare information systems'. Similarly, the HL7 group is a consortium of users and vendors aiming at specifying and promoting a standard for the exchange of data in the area of healthcare, and especially in HIS. A joint technical working group was created to manage convergence to MEDIX. The ACR/NEMA standard (ACR/NEMA Publication, 1985, 1988) has already been mentioned in the previous paragraphs. A number of working groups are still involved in various aspects of the definition and validation of the standard; in particular, an important release (V3.0) is in discussion. The European standardization body (CEN) is also involved in standardization in the area of healthcare by means of actions carried out by the European workshop for open systems (EWOS) and the technical committee TC 251 (medical informatics). All these efforts should lead to standards in the very near future.

Given the very high investments required by such systems, obsolescence is a critical issue which needs to be tackled. Functional obsolescence can be fought against by offering flexible and rapid solutions with minimum specific developments. Software obsolescence can also be avoided by means of constant evolution of the system, module by module. In order to remedy hardware obsolescence, investments have to be decided with a short-term perspective and upgrade contracts have to be purchased, when this is possible.

The utilization of standards is another issue gathering consensus. It is generally agreed that a standard element has to be preferred to a specific one, even if it is more efficient. A good approach is to compensate inefficient features by enhanced organization. A typical example is 'pre-fetching': in order to make information immediately available for the physician, all the possibly useful data are transferred in advance; such a procedure is certainly necessary when the communication throughput offered by the network is low but it remains attractive even when a more powerful network becomes available because it allows a better distribution of the traffic and consequently a better management of the resource.

From the economic viewpoint, it is clear that integrated information systems will bring savings (decreased use of films, improved organization as a result of the immediate availability of information, medical added value, etc.) and most people no longer try to prove *a priori* the cost effectiveness of PACS. Namely, profound changes in organization, with heavy sociological consequences, are necessary to actually provide these savings. Consequently, the assessment of PACS cost effectiveness is almost impossible *in practice* since, on the one hand, PACS investments will bring significant additional costs during a probably long transition period, and on the other hand, the actual savings that can be expected are very difficult to assess.

3.2. Remaining uncertainties

Does this general agreement mean that the wide spread of PACS is near at hand? May be not, because of a number of remaining uncertainties.

3.2.1. Technology
The evolution of PACS technologies is still very strong and it is feared that jumps of generation will drastically change current expectations. In practice, the rapid evolution of the capacity of storage media will likely continue during the next decade. Will the optical disks we write today be still readable in five years? How can continuity over longer periods be ensured (as required by the regulations in some countries) without copying data on the new media as they become available? And what about the resulting costs?

The utilization of high-resolution screens (2 K × 2 K) is still subject to discussion between those who consider that a 1 K × 1 K resolution, associated with the capability to display the original pixels of a 2 K × 2 K image, is suitable for the whole primary diagnosis, and those who argue that 2 K × 2 K is actually needed, otherwise a console-based diagnosis will not be as accurate

as a film-based one. The economic consequences of this debate are very important, namely, the price of this technology (still very expensive in 1991) is not
supposed to decrease in the short term whereas the price of $1 K \times 1 K$ monitor
is now quite low as a result of the wide diffusion of workstations; besides, images requiring high resolution are numerous in hospitals (for instance, chest,
mammography, etc.).

3.2.2. Human factor

Another, much more critical uncertainty, deals with the human factor. How
will the medical staff behave facing the development of PACS? Big changes
have to be expected since almost the whole process of image utilization is currently based on films, from diagnosis to therapy planning and follow-up,
education and archiving. Will the medical community uniformly accept or re-
ject this evolution or will behavior depend upon medical specialties? The
answer is very difficult. How will the administrative authority manage this
evolution, by directing it or just leaving doctors to manage the process?

3.3. Possible evolution schemes towards a generalized PACS

Three scenarios seem possible, according to local conditions, maturity of the
medical staff, position of the administrative authority and investment
possibilities.

3.3.1. Scenario 1: imposed generalized PACS

Following the example of big projects we already discussed (MDIS, Hammersmith, SMZO, UCLA), it is likely that an increasingly large number of wide
scale projects will be issued in the future, aiming at a gradual elimination of
films. The launch of such projects may also remain limited to isolated cases or
particular circumstances (for instance, building of a new facility). The case of
the U.S. Army is a particular case, namely, the administrative authority is
strong and the investment possibilities exceed what is usually available in civil
facilities and lastly, the medical staff working in the army is generally younger
than elsewhere, which may also facilitate the changes in organization resulting
from the introduction of PACS.

Definitively, we believe that this first scenario can only be applied in particular contexts where the administration is well-established and can invest
sizable amounts of money.

3.3.2. Scenario 2: integrated digital radiology department

This second scenario consists of introducing PACS gradually, by means of integrated filmless radiology departments. The spread of computed radiology,

especially in the U.S.A. and Japan will probably catalyse the mutation towards console-based procedures, mostly for diagnosis and the management of archiving. According to this evolution, films would only remain as a communication medium between radiologists and clinicians located throughout the hospital. With this scenario, generalized PACS would result from step by step extensions of the network outside the radiology department.

3.3.3. Scenario 3: departmental PACS

According to this third scenario, the evolution towards generalized PACS would be a very gradual one. A first stage would consist of connecting together the main digital modalities (mostly CT scanners and MRI (magnetic resonance imaging) systems) in order to organize a digital archiving of these images and to establish digital links with a reduced number of clinics like in the surgery or radiotherapy departments. Regarding this scenario, any evolution would have to be justified by an expected added value, either related to diagnosis (resulting, for example, from improved communication between the radiology department and an intensive care unit) or related to therapy (previous examples). The introduction of computed radiology would also take place very gradually and would not eliminate films as a medium used for archiving and communication with clinicians, at least in the first stages. Generalized PACS would only arise in the long term, well after the year 2000, when communication technology, archiving media and high resolution monitors will be widespread.

This kind of evolution would certainly be more *undergone* rather than *conducted*; it would lead to a very smooth transition between film-based procedures and computer-based ones.

Under such assumptions, the HIS is likely to manage images as well as other medical records before the PACS itself reach real maturity.

3.3.4. Discussion

The question is what are the factors determining the kind of evolution applicable to a particular situation? Economic factors will certainly play a major role, since the transition to filmless systems will require enormous financial investments. Regarding, for instance, the second scenario, we may wonder whether the hospital administration would accept building up those integrated radiology departments which would constitute the system core from which the PACS would start to diffuse throughout the hospital. This is uncertain because the high investment costs will cumulate with operating costs related to the consumption of films for the distribution of the images outside the radiology department. In addition, little saving can be expected from this scenario since savings resulting from better organization will only concern radiology. All these factors make this solution very expensive; an alternative would perhaps arise if a consensus could be found between radiologists and clinicians in order to limit the quantities of data sent to the clinics (reduced number of images, smaller film sheets, lower quality medium like paper, etc.). This solution may be a reasonable tradeoff, however, its major drawback is that clinics could not enjoy the benefits brought by digital management of images. In conclusion, we think that this scenario is not likely to happen, especially in Europe, except in particular cases like the building of a new facility.

The human role will also be a primary factor. The PACS concept is being gradually accepted by radiologists, nevertheless, facing competing priorities like a choice between a new imaging modality and a PACS, a number of them would still make the choice of a new modality. This fact simply proves that the concern for optimizing radiology departments in not a primary one yet, or that radiologists do not really believe that PACS is able to provide this kind of optimization. Similarly, the demand for PACS among non-radiology physicians is still moderate. A study carried out at Seattle (Saarinen et al., 1990) has highlighted what clinicians actually expected from PACS. They are supportive of this technology as far as it can remedy the current system inadequacies (reduction of lost examinations, reduction of the number of trips to the radiology department). Some specialties like radiotherapy or neurosurgery are more supportive of acquiring PACS; the added value in these cases clearly justifies the installation of PACS equipments in these clinics, however, it is not sufficient to justify hospital-wide systems.

In conclusion, the medical demand remains moderate and it is highly probable that hospital administrations will adopt this argument to be *careful* towards PACS investments.

4. Perspectives of evolution of the Sirene experience

4.1. Context and assumptions

4.1.1. Departmental or generalized PACS: a dilemma to be resolved

Departmental PACS certainly offers a number of advantages, namely, a department is a functional unit and consequently most information flows remain within this entity. Besides, the setting up of a such system is easy because needs are generally well-known as a result of the proximity of the communicating parties. Finally, this approach is consistent with a gradual introduction of PACS, department by department, allowing a distribution of acquisition costs over several years.

Nevertheless, we believe that such developments have to be integrated in a comprehensive hospital-wide reflection. The reason for this is that PACS will finally be a component, actually a sub-system of the HIS, so it seems reasonable to plan the installation of the network for instance (especially the cabling), in order to harmonize it with the HIS developments. Software interworking is a desirable but not so critical issue. However, a choice for consistent solutions will facilitate the developments (specific abilities, partly integrated solutions), and the future integration process.

4.1.2. Conditions for a successful introduction of PACS

Good acceptance of PACS needs the contributions of many partners within the hospital institution. This aspect is very crucial since PACS represent different stakes for each of them, as previously mentioned:

(1) The medical community must be involved from the design, up to the evaluation of the system because PACS remain a tool to improve the quality and effectiveness of patient care which is the doctors primary concern.

(2) The administrative authority is also obviously concerned because it supports (either partly or entirely) the hospital investments. Besides, it manages the information system that PACS belongs to. This management role implies a number of tasks that cannot be dealt with by the rather small teams involved in system design and integration: daily operation of the system, reliability and security issues, maintenance, medium and long term planning.

(3) Researchers and physicists have often been involved in PACS developments and assessment. As long as no suitable industrial PACS are available, these scientists will have a major part to play, since they facilitate exchanges between industrialists and doctors and help to find solutions. They have been able to convince their own administrations and regional communities of the interest of PACS-related research and they succeeded in getting some support from them to carry on experiments.

(4) The collaboration with manufacturers is also a necessity; in spite of real advances, the interfacing of imaging modalities remains very difficult, or even impossible without the agreement of the manufacturers. Besides, they have not always a precise perception of PACS requirements and may hesitate between completely integrated solutions and simple PACS components, interfacable by means of existing standards. Lastly, PACS acceptance requires user-friendliness which cannot be reached without a deep understanding of the medical procedures the PACS is supposed to assist. Consequently, the development and assessment of PACS equipments needs close collaboration between end-users and manufacturers.

The creation of CERIUM* is the solution we have found in Rennes to create

---

* CERIUM: Centre Européen de Recherche en Imagerie à Usage Médical.

194   *B. Gibaud et al.*

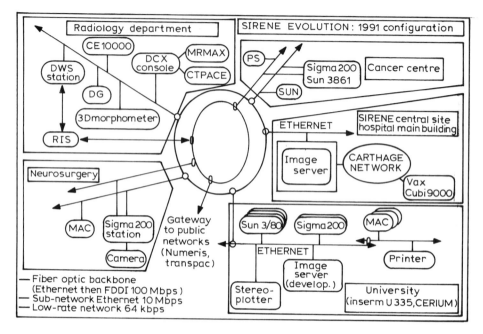

Fig. 2. Sirene configuration expected at the end of 1991.

this collaboration. This entity groups together several institutions (university, hospital administration, manufacturers) to carry out common interest projects. Six such projects are defined for the 1989–1993 period. CERIUM is supported by the French Ministry of Research and Technology, the Regional Council of Brittany and contributions of each partner. It is composed of engineers either coming from the partners or directly employed by CERIUM. Its role consists of participating in the projects at different levels (discussion on specifications with doctors, researchers and manufacturers, specific developments especially related to user interface, technical and medical assessment), with the objective of an optimal transfer to industry of the technology developed or integrated during the projects.

4.2. Short- and medium-term plans

The kind of PACS evolution we expect in Rennes is likely to be in accordance with what we called the third scenario, for both financial reasons and reasons related to the general level of maturity of the medical staff.

The extension of the system should be based on departmental sub-systems, federated by a global network (fig. 2). The development we want to carry out aims at making the communication and management of images easier within the sub-networks and to provide access facilities with the central archives. The application field has been intentionally limited to medical domains where the PACS is supposed to bring a concrete added value. Three medical specialties are concerned at the first stage:

(1) the radiology department;
(2) the neurosurgery department; and
(3) the Cancer Centre (radiotherapy and nuclear medicine departments).

The evaluation will also be limited to a specific population of patients, suffering from disorders of the central nervous system (tumors, epilepsy, etc.). Namely, such cases require an intensive use of images for diagnosis, therapy planning and follow-up. All the specialties we mentioned are interested in this pathology at various levels of patient care and also need to communicate with each other.

A significant configuration will be installed in the radiology department, in partnership with GE. All GE modalities will be connected to the network: two CTs (CT-PACE and CE10000), a digital angiography system (DG200) and a MRI system (MR-MAX). The CT-PACE and MR-MAX are products of the Japanese subsidiary of GE (YMS) and will be interfaced by means of a bi-modality console called DCX, provided by the same manufacturer. The other modalities will be directly interfaced to the network. A second GE multi-modality console (diagnostic workstation, DWS) will also be installed and evaluated; it will be used for the selection of the images to be archived or retrieved from the Sirene central archive. We also expect to develop an interface with the future RIS, with a primary aim to allow the pre-fetching of data related to returning patients. Appointments will be available from the RIS so that the image data and related reports can be retrieved. This feature seems to us especially relevant in our particular applicative context.

Extensions to the neurosurgery and radiotherapy departments will be conducted step by step: a PACS workstation is already in use in neurosurgery and applications should rapidly start in radiotherapy and in nuclear medicine.

The connection with the 'research' sub-network has also to be highlighted since it seems necessary, to us, to ensure good cooperation between clinicians, researchers and computer scientists from the CERIUM and the INSERM unit.

Regarding technology, the departmental networks should be based on Ethernet, at least at the beginning; the backbone network will also be Ethernet but should rapidly be upgraded to FDDI, when the medical needs make it necessary.

4.3. Long-term perspectives

Our current perspectives regarding PACS research mostly deal with medical image databases; this reflection is carried out in collaboration with our partners of the NRV* group. We believe that the current implementations are too strictly limited to administrative descriptions of studies and image acquisition parameters and consequently are not sufficient to properly represent the whole study data set (medical meaning of the successive series, role and representation of processed images, diagnosis related features, etc.). Our objective is to try to integrate such features in a comprehensive, generic and evolutive object-oriented model (Bizais et al., 1991); this reflection disregards the current frontiers between the different information system components (PACS, RIS, HIS). Consequently, the actual implementation of this scheme is not realistic in the short term. Nevertheless, the solutions we propose open interesting prospects for a more explicit presentation of examination data, including the medical context, and may bring significant help for the design of computer-aided image interpretation systems.

5. Conclusion

Integrated medical information systems will certainly emerge in the long term and the big new PACS projects created in 1990 confirm this. Nevertheless, the question of *when* such systems will really be available has not been given a sound answer yet. In 1983, PACS was supposed to appear in the near future. One can measure the long distance covered since that time: technology has enjoyed a considerable evolution and PACS issues are much more deeply understood. However, PACS costs remain very high and are not relevant with the immediate added value which can be expected. Consequently, investments are not likely to occur, at least in Europe in the present economic climate. Another critical issue is the human factor, given the profound changes in organization which would undoubtedly result from the introduction of PACS.

In conclusion, we believe that, in the same way that wide diffusion of workstations in industrial enterprises has not eliminated paper and has also failed to provide the productivity increases which were anticipated, it is highly probable that the integration of images in medical information systems will be very gradual and closely conditioned by the changes in organization it will induce.

---

* Collaboration between the PACS teams of Nantes, Rennes et Villejuif (DIMI project: Y. Bizais, Inserm U335: J.M. Scarabin, Inserm U66: R. Di Paola, respectively).

Acknowledgements

The authors gratefully acknowledge the CCETT and R. Renoulin, who played a major role in the initiation and development of the Sirene project, as well as all partners who have contributed to this project. We also would like to thank the Regional Council of Brittany for its constant support.

References

ACR-NEMA Publication 300-1985 (1985) Digital Imaging and Communication (NEMA, Washington D.C.).

ACR-NEMA Publication 300-1988 (1988) Digital Imaging and Communication (NEMA, Washington D.C.).

Arenson, R.L., D.E. Morton and J.W. London (1982) Fiber optic communication system for medical images. In: Duerinckx, A.J. (Ed.), Picture Archiving and Communication Systems (PACS) for Medical Applications, First International Conference and Workshop, *Proc. SPIE* 318, 74–79.

Arenson, R.L., D.E. Morton and J.W. London (1983) Early experience with fiber optic PACS for medical images, In: Dwyer III, S.J. (Ed.), Picture Archiving and Communication Systems (PACS) for Medical Applications, Second International Conference and Workshop, *Proc. SPIE* 418, 116–121.

Bakker, A.R. (1991) HIS and RIS and PACS. In: Huang, H.K., (Eds.), Picture Archiving and Communication Systems (PACS) in Medicine, *NATO ASI Series F* 74, 157–162 (Springer, Berlin).

Barneveld Binkhuysen, F.H., F.P. Ottes, B.M. ter Haar Romeny, P.L.M. Klessens, C.G. Vos, L.H.L. Winter, P.J. Calkoen and J.H.T.H. Andriessen (1989) First results of the diagnostic evaluation studies and the clinical efficacy evaluation in the Dutch PACS project. In: Schneider, R.H., S.J. Dwyer III and R.G. Jost (Eds.), Medical Imaging III: PACS System Design and Evaluation, *Proc. SPIE* 1093, 13–19.

Bizais, Y., F. Aubry, B. Gibaud, J.M. Scarabin and R. Di Paola (1991) A comprehensive model for medical image data bases. In: Demongeot, J., and A. Sousa Pereira (Eds.), Proc. Meeting COMAC-BME ISCAMI 1, Aveiro (P), 73–81 (Springer, Berlin).

Blaine, G.J., R.L. Hill, J.R. Cox and R.G. Jost (1983) PACS workbench at Mallinckrodt Institute of Radiology (MIR). In: Dwyer III, S.J. (Ed.), Picture Archiving and Communication Systems (PACS) for Medical Applications, Second International Conference and Workshop, *Proc. SPIE* 418, 80–86.

Blaine, G.J., R.L. Hill, A.P. Rueter, E. Senol and J.W. Studt (1988) Image transmission studies. In: Schneider, R.H., and S.J. Dwyer III (Eds.), Medical Imaging II, *Proc. SPIE* 914, 953–960.

Braudes, R.E., S.K. Mun, J. Sibert, J. Schnizlein and S.C. Horii (1989) Workstation modelling and development: clinical definition of a picture archiving and communication system (PACS) user interface. In: Schneider, R.H., S.J. Dwyer III and R.G. Jost (Eds.), Medical Imaging III: PACS System Design and Evaluation, *Proc. SPIE* 1093, 376–386.

Budler, D.M., and C. Lee Hamilton (1988) A prototype relational implementation of the NEMA schema. In: Schneider, R.H., and S.J. Dwyer III (Eds.), Medical Imaging II, *Proc. SPIE* 914, 1066–1068.

Bulatek, D.E., and S.B. O'Connell (1983) Working PACS prototype. In: Dwyer III, S.J. (Ed.),

Picture Archiving and Communication Systems (PACS) for Medical Applications, Second International Conference and Workshop, *Proc. SPIE* 418, 144–111.

Cox, J.R., G.J. Blaine, R.L. Hill and R.G. Jost (1982) Study of a distributed PACS for radiology. In: Duerinckx, A.J. (Ed.), Picture Archiving and Communication Systems (PACS) for Medical Applications, First International Conference and Workshop, *Proc. SPIE* 318, 133–142.

Cox, J.R., R.G. Jost, T. Monsees, S. Ramamurthy and M. Karlsson (1988) An inexpensive electronic viewbox. In: Schneider, R.H., and S.J. Dwyer III (Eds.), Medical Imaging II, *Proc. SPIE* 914, 1218–1224.

Creasy, J.L., D.D. Loendorf and Hemminger B.M. (1986) Initial experience with a prototype storage system at the University of North Carolina. In: Schneider, R.H., and S.J. Dwyer III (Eds.), Medicine XIV/PACS IV, *Proc. SPIE* 626, 631–636.

Cywinski, J.K., L.M. Cywinski and L. Lee (1983) Medical image distribution, storage and retrieval network: the M/NET. In: Dwyer III, S.J. (Ed.), Picture Archiving and Communication Systems (PACS) for Medical Applications, Second International Conference and Workshop, *Proc. SPIE* 418, 74–79.

Dwyer III, S.J., A.W. Templeton, W.H. Anderson, M.A. Tarlton, K.S. Hensley, K.R. Lee, D.F. Preston, S. Batnitzky, E. Levine, S.J. Rosenthal, N.L. Martin and L.T. Cook (1982) Salient characteristics of a distributed diagnostic imaging management system for a radiology department. In: Duerinckx, A.J. (Ed.), Picture Archiving and Communication Systems (PACS) for Medical Applications, First International Conference and Workshop, *Proc. SPIE* 318, 194–204.

Gibaud, B., F. Picand, A. Benslimane, P. Grassin, L. Urbano, C. Toumoulin, F. Fresne, M. Rouvière and J.M. Scarabin (1989) Sirene: desin and evaluation of a PACS prototype, Proc. CAR 89 (Springer, Berlin), pp. 484–488.

Gibaud, B., S. Rodriguez-Pereira, A. Benslimane and J.M. Scarabin (1990) A distributed approach for the development of distributed applications in PACS. In: Dwyer III, S.J., and R.G. Jost (Eds.), Medical Imaging IV: PACS System Design and Evaluation, *Proc. SPIE* 1234, 568–577.

Glass, H.I., and N.A. Slark (1991) PACS and related research in the U.K. In: Huang, H.K., O. Ratib, A.R. Bakker and G. Witte (Eds.), Picture Archiving and Communication Systems (PACS) in Medicine, *NATO ASI Series F* 74, 319–324 (Springer, Berlin).

Good, W.F., J.M. Herron, G.S. Maitz and D. Gur (1988) ACR-NEMA standard: the reality vs the ideal. In: Schneider, R.H., and S.J. Dwyer III (Eds.), Medical Imaging II, *Proc. SPIE* 914, 1081–1086.

Hegde, S.S., A.O. Gale and J.A. Giunta (1986) AT&T PACS architecture. In: Schneider, R.H., and S.J. Dwyer III (Eds.), Medicine XIV/PACS IV, *Proc. SPIE* 626, 618–625.

Hemminger, B.M., B.G. Thompson, S.M. Pizer and P. Stancil (1986) The ongoing implementation of a prototype medical communications system at the University of North Carolina. In: Schneider, R.H., and S.J. Dwyer III (Eds.), Medicine XIV/PACS IV, *Proc. SPIE* 626, 574–580.

Herforth, M., K. Müller and C.F.C. Greinacher (1989) What are the ACR/NEMA standard and the SPI specification, Proc. CAR 89 (Springer, Berlin), pp. 548–552.

Horii, S.C., J.H. Schimpf, G.Q. Maguire, M.P. Zeleznik and M.E. Noz (1983) Broadband coaxial cable image viewing and processing for radiology, In: Dwyer III, S.J. (Ed.), Picture Archiving and Communication Systems (PACS) for Medical Applications, Second International Conference and Workshop, *Proc. SPIE* 418, 247–257.

Horii, S.C., H.N. Horii and P. Kowalski (1988) An eclectic look at viewing station design. In: Schneider, R.H., and S.J. Dwyer III (Eds.), Medical Imaging II, *Proc. SPIE* 914, 920–928.

Huang, H.K., Z. Barbaric, N.J. Mankovich and C. Moler (1983a) Digital radiology at the University of California, Los Angeles: a feasibility study. In: Dwyer III, S.J. (Ed.), Picture Archiving and Communication Systems (PACS) for Medical Applications, Second Internatinal Conference and Workshop, *Proc. SPIE* 418, 259 – 265.

Huang, H.K., N.J. Mankovich, Z. Barbaric, H. Kangarloo and C. Moler (1983b) Design and implementation of multiple digital viewing stations. In: Dwyer III, S.J. (Ed.), Picture Achiving and Communication Systems (PACS) for Medical Applications, Second International Conference and Workshop, *Proc. SPIE* 418, 189 – 198.

Kangarloo, H., M.I. Boechat, R.B. Dietrich, T. Hall, R.K. Taïra, N.J. Mankovich and H.K. Huang (1988) Clinical experience with a PACS module in pediatric radiology: clinical viewpoint. In: Schneider, R.H., and S.J. Dwyer III (Eds.), Medical Imaging II, *Proc. SPIE* 914, 1036 – 1045.

Kasday, L.R. (1986) Human factors considerations in PACS design. In: Schneider, R.H., and S.J. Dwyer III (Eds.), Medicine XIV/PACS IV, *Proc. SPIE* 626, 581 – 592.

Levine, B.A., S.K. Mun, H.R. Benson and S.C. Horii (1990) Assessment of the integration of a HIS/RIS with a PACS. In: Dwyer III, S.J., and R.G. Jost (Eds.), Medical Imaging IV: PACS System Design and Evaluation, *Proc. SPIE* 1234, 391 – 397.

Lodder, H., B.M. van Poppel, H. Wilmink, B. Scharnberg, J.P.J. de Valk and A.R. Bakker (1988) HIS/PACS coupling, BAZIS/ZIS and Philips/Marcom speaking terms, *Med. Inform.* 13, 361 – 367.

Maguire, G.Q. (1986) Looking back at PACS attempts – What has happened since PACS I. In: Höhne, K.H. (Ed.), Pictorial Information Systems in Medicine, *NATO ASI Series F* 19, 391 – 399 (Springer, Berlin).

Maguire, G.Q., M.P. Zeleznik, S.C. Horii, J.H. Schimpf and M.E. Noz (1982) Image processing requirements in hospitals and an integrated systems approach. In: Duerinckx, A.J. (Ed.), Picture Archiving and Communication Systems (PACS) for Medical Applications, First International Conference and Workshop, *Proc. SPIE* 318, 206 – 213.

Martinez, R., and C. Archwamety (1988) Image migration in a three level data base archive system. In: Schneider, R.H., and S.J. Dwyer III (Eds.), Medical Imaging II, *Proc. SPIE* 914, 1122 – 1127.

Medical Diagnostic Imaging Support System (MDIS) (1990) US Army Engineer Division, Acquisition document.

Melrose, J.P., and R.P. Ericson (1981) Integrated medical information services: a resource management view of automated hospital information system. *Proc. IEEE EMBS*, 824 – 829.

Meyer-Ebrecht, D. (1986) On the architecture of pictorial information systems. In: Höhne, K.H. (Ed.), Pictorial Information Systems in Medicine, *NATO ASI Series F* 19, 151 – 179 (Springer, Berlin).

Mosser, H., A. Mandl, M. Urban, H. Hradil and W. Hruby (1991) The Vienna SMZO project. In: Huang, H.K., O. Ratib, A.R. Bakker and G. Witte (Eds.), Picture Archiving and Communication Systems (PACS) in Medicine, *NATO ASI Series F* 74, 247 – 250 (Springer, Berlin).

Mun, S.K., H.R. Benson, C. Welsh, L.P. Elliott and W.J. Davros (1988) Baseline study of radiology services for the purpose of PACS evaluation. In: Schneider, R.H., and S.J. Dwyer III (Eds.), Medical Imaging II, *Proc. SPIE* 914, 978 – 987.

Nosil, J., G. Justice, P. Fisher, G. Ritchie, W.J. Weigl and H. Gnoyke (1988) A prototype multimodality PACS at Victoria General Hospital. In: Schneider, R.H., and S.J. Dwyer III (Eds.), Medical Imaging II, *Proc. SPIE* 914, 1362 – 1378.

Ottes, F.P., J.P.J. de Valk, H.M. Kroon, F.H. Barneveld Binkhuysen, G.W. Seeley, L.H.L. Winter and L.J. Schultze Kool (1989) Diagnostic image quality evaluation chain applications of FEASIBLE package in practice. In: Schneider, R.H., S.J. Dwyer III and R.G. Jost (Eds.), Medical Imaging III: PACS System Design and Evaluation, *Proc. SPIE* 1093, 2 – 9.

Parrish, D.M., J.L. Creasy, B.G. Thompson, D.C. Rogers, E.R. Johnston, J.R. Perry and E.V. Staab (1986) Functional requirements for interfacing PACS to RIS. In: Schneider, R.H., and

S.J. Dwyer III (Eds.), Medicine XIV/PACS IV, *Proc. SPIE* 626, 597 – 602.

Reijns, G.L., A.R. Bakker and J.P.J. de Valk (1988) Simulation and communication aspects of PACS. In: Schneider, R.H., and S.J. Dwyer III (Eds.), Medical Imaging II, *Proc. SPIE* 914, 1153 – 1158.

Rienhoff, O. (1989) PACS – RIS – HIS, the demand for communication management. Proc CAR 89 (Springer, Berlin), pp. 597 – 601.

Rogers, D.C., R. Wallace, B.G. Thompson and D.M. Parrish (1986) Information flow analysis as a tool for PACS development. In: Schneider, R.H., and S.J. Dwyer III (Eds.), Medicine XIV/PACS IV: PACS System Design and Evaluation, *Proc. SPIE* 626, 690 – 697.

Saarinen, A.O., G. Youngs, D.R. Haynor and J.W. Loop (1990) Clinical determinants of PACS acceptance. In: Dwyer III, S.J., and R.G. Jost (Eds.), Medical Imaging IV: PACS System Design and Evaluation, *Proc. SPIE* 1234, 817 – 822.

Scarabin, J.M., B. Gibaud, J. de Certaines and J.L. Coatrieux (1983) Projet Sirene, Serveur d'Imagerie médicale accessible via un Réseau Numérique Expérimental. Université de Rennes I.

Seshadri, S.B., and R.L. Arenson (1988) Satellite transmission of medical images. In: Schneider, R.H. and S.J. Dwyer III (Eds.), Medical Imaging II, *Proc. SPIE* 914, 1416 – 1423.

Stockbridge, C., and C.E. Ravin (1986) Phased implementation of AT&T PACS at Duke University Medical Center. In: Schneider, R.H., and S.J. Dwyer III (Eds.), Medicine XIV/PACS IV, *Proc. SPIE* 626, 570 – 573.

ter Haar Romeny, B.M., J. Raymakers, P.F.G.M. van Waes, J.C. Helder, C.N. de Graaf, P.P. van Rijk, H. Schuttenbeld, K.J. Zuiderveld, J. Tiemann and B. Scharnberg (1987) The Dutch PACS project: philosophy, design of a digital reading room and first observations in the Utrecht University Hospital in the Netherlands. In: Schneider, R.H., and S.J. Dwyer III (Eds.), Medical Imaging, *Proc. SPIE* 767, 787 – 792.

ter Haar Romeny, B.M., J.M.M. van der Wielen, A.J. Acherberg, F.H. Barneveld Binkhuysen, K.J. Zuiderveld, J.H.T.H. Andriessen and A.R. Bakker (1989) PACS efficiency: a detailed quantitative study of the distribution process of films in a clinical environment in the Utrecht University Hospital. In: Schneider, R.H., S.J. Dwyer III and R.G. Jost (Eds.), Medical Imaging III: PACS System Design and Evaluation, *Proc. SPIE* 1093, 259 – 271.

Integrated Diagnostic Imaging
Editor: J.P.J. De Valk
© *Elsevier Science Publishers B.V., 1992*

Chapter 10

PACS – demands on spatial and contrast resolution for digital workstations

W. Wiesmann, P. Vassallo and P.E. Peters

1. Introduction

Digital radiography enables the replacement of conventional radiographs with digital data which are computed and projected as an image on a cathode ray tube (CRT).

The development of digital image processing such as computerized tomography, digital subtraction angiography and magnetic resonance tomography has led to a parting of ways between recording and reproduction media. Film has been replaced as receptor by detectors which produce electrical signals in response to incident quanta of ionizing radiation or coils which receive tissue-specific signals in response to radiofrequency impulses. The CRT has to some extent replaced film as an interface between the user and these new investigative techniques for presentation of results. The images are saved as raw binary data on diskettes, magnetic tapes, optical disks or other forms of digital storage.

Through the development of fast, high-performance computers and novel optoelectronic storage and networking techniques, the problems of transfer and storage of these large volumes of digital visual data may eventually be overcome. Such systems were initially described in the late 1970s. In 1981, Duerinckx coined the acronym PACS for 'picture archiving and communications system' to describe an essentially all-electronic imaging system (Duerinckx and Pisa, 1982).

2. The workstation

The term 'workstation' essentially implies an all digital image display terminal at which the radiologist may process images accessed from an electronic archive on a CRT. One general consensus among experts is that the workstation represents a very critical component of a PACS. According to Meyer-Ebrecht, the display of high-resolution, high-contrast gray-scale images and their digital processing in 'real time' places high technological demands (Meyer-Ebrecht, 1988).

The advantages of a PACS described in the literature (Mun et al., 1989b,c) should not overshadow the numerous problems still left unsolved. The construction of a workstation requires a profound understanding of ergonomic and functional design with an insight into the daily requirements of a radiological department. The studies presented below analyze several of the various components of the workstation. Numerous studies were performed to assess the diagnostic value of digital images of the chest and hand displayed on workstations. The diagnostic accuracy of reports obtained from CRT images was evaluated by comparison with the film-based diagnosis. The diagnostic value of the various procedures was then assessed using the ROC-method (receiver operation characteristic), a measurement procedure originating from the field of cognitive theory. ROC investigations were performed at a workstation with a matrix of 1024×1024 pixels. Additional investigations were conducted on a prototype unit with a image matrix of 2048×2048 pixels. Both units transferred and stored the optical density data on an 8-bit gray scale.

3. Diagnostic efficiency of low-contrast images

3.1. Material and methods

120 p.a. (posterior/anterior) chest radiographs of healthy individuals with no history of disease undergoing routine examination for employment purposes were selected for the investigation. Only radiographs from patients with normal initial and follow-up examination a year later were chosen. All films included were correctly exposed and focused and were taken at 125 kVp with a film – focus distance of 1.8 m on a chest radiographic unit (Thoramat, Siemens). A film – screen combination [T-Mat-L/Lanex medium (Kodak)] optimized for chest radiography was employed. Optimal exposure with adequate penetration of the mediastinum was achieved using a mediastinal filter and automatic exposure (Stender, 1989). All 120 radiographs were reviewed by two radiologists who agreed with the initial reports. The images were randomly divided into two groups of 60 films each. The *first* group of images was left unprocessed and represented the negative group (controls). Single lung nodules were produced in the second group of radiographs (positive films).

A new technique for lesion simulation was developed for this investigation. The pulmonary nodules were generated using a subtractive photographic agent (potassium-hexacyanoferrateIII), also known as Farmer's solution. The ferric ions contained in this reagent oxidize elemental silver to silver ions and are themselves reduced to the ferrous state. The silver ferrocyanide, formed in the film emulsion, reacts with the sodium thiosulphate forming a water soluble silver – thiosulphate complex, which can be washed away (Mutter, 1955). When applied to the emulsion, Farmer's solution thus removes silver and can be used to create shadows of any size and shape. If left sufficiently long, the entire silver content can be removed from the film in the area of application. Subtractive agents affect all grey tones to the same degree, so that image gradation remains unaltered. The density of the lesion can be controlled by rapidly washing away or reapplying the agent. A thorough washing of the film arrests the process at any given time. A number of techniques, such as dispersion with a cotton swab and varying application time or concentration can be used to create lesions of differing density, size, shape and definition. The nodules were produced on the reverse side of the original film, as shown in fig. 1. This prevented the observer from detecting the change in luster of the emulsion in the zone of application.

The protocol for generating an ROC-analysis emphasizes the requirement for two approximately equal numbers of negative and positive cases with all

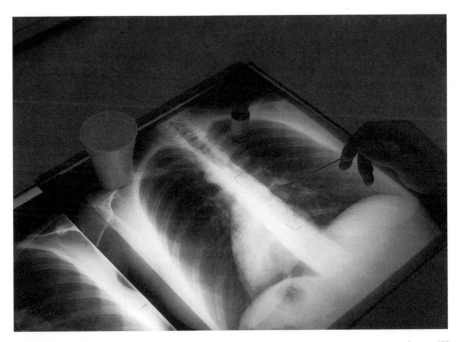

Fig. 1. Creating pulmonary lesions on the reverse side of the film with potassium-hexacyanoferrate III.

degrees of diagnostic difficulty in order to cover the whole spectrum of diagnostic thresholds with an adequate number of false positive and false negative results. The distribution of the lesions included central and peripheral lung fields, as well as hilar, mediastinal and diaphragmatic regions. Figure 2 illustrates the distribution of the artificial pulmonary nodules. The nodules measured 0.5 – 2.3 cm in diameter, were round to oval and showed sharp to gradual transitions to normal surrounding structures. The optical density of the lesions ranged between 0.3 and 2.5.

Only one nodule was produced on each film since the multiple lesions in the same radiograph would have lead to problems of signal localization during evaluation of the results (Chakraborty et al., 1986; Chan et al., 1987; Oestmann and Galanski, 1989). In a preliminary investigation with artificial and true pulmonary nodules, two experienced radiologists, who were not participants in the ROC-study, were unable to differentiate the two, confirming the credibility of the artificial lesions.

All 120 films were then digitized with a matrix of 1024 × 1024 pixels and an 8-bit gray scale (256 gray-steps) using a film digitizer. The digitized images were stored without data compression or loss.

Distribution of nodules

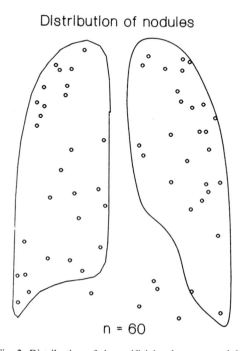

n = 60

Fig. 2. Distribution of the artificial pulmonary nodules.

3.2. Reporting sessions

The images were evaluated by five observers: three staff radiologists (4 – 15 yr experience) and two senior residents. All images were presented to the observer in five separate sessions; in the first session, the conventional films were assessed at the viewing box under optimal conditions, i.e., with adequate illumination and shuttering and dim ambient lighting. After an intervening period of at least two weeks, the conventional radiographs were reviewed in a second session in order to assess the intra-individual variation. In the third session, the images digitized with a 1024 × 1024 matrix were reported at the CRT workstation. No image processing was allowed at this stage. In the fourth sitting, the digitized (1024 × 1024) radiographs were reviewed on the workstation with the possibility of image processing, which included gray-scale windowing, magnification (factor 2 and 4) with capability to scroll across the image and electronic gray-scale inversion between a positive and negative image.

Prior to the digital image reading sessions the observers were allowed to familiarize themselves with the controls on each workstation. The settings for monitor contrast and brightness were standardized for all sessions at the workstation.

All reporting sessions on the workstations were conducted with dim ambient lighting arranged so as to avoid reflection on the CRT.

In cooperation with the research laboratories Philips Medical Systems (PMS) Hamburg, we were also able to evaluate another interactive workstation (PMS prototype unit). This viewing station was designed by the group of Meyer-Ebrecht and Wendler. Their views regarding the design and requirements of a workstation have been presented at many meetings and appeared in the medical literature (Meyer-Ebrecht and Wendler, 1983; Wendler et al., 1986). However, no studies assessing CRT quality and the diagnostic value of digitized images had been conducted on this system.

This interactive workstation was furnished with a video board handling 1024 × 1024 pixels, an 8-bit gray scale (256 gray-tones) and a display refresher-rate of 50 Hz. The same set of 120 chest radiographs were scanned by a drum laser scanner (Optronix) with a pixel size of 50 μm, digitized and stored with a 2048 × 2048 pixel matrix on hard disk.

During each session the observer's diagnostic confidence level, the localization of the nodule and viewing time were recorded. Confidence levels were rated by the observer on a 5 point scoring scale (table 1).

In order to utilize the full resolution of images (2048 × 2048 pixels) at the CRT (display matrix 1024 × 1024 pixels) zoom and scroll functions were employed. Additional image processing options included grey-scale windowing. No histogram equalization or other image processing algorithms were used. The reading session at the PMS prototype workstation was designated as session 5.

An intervening period of at least 14 days was allowed between each of the five reporting sessions in order to limit image recognition and learn effects.

The localization of a lesion was recorded according to quadrant, the four quadrants were separated by vertical median line and a horizontal line at the level of the dorsal portion of the seventh rib bilaterally. The localization data were not utilized for a localization-ROC-analysis (LROC), since no validated statistical methods exists to determine the significance of these ROC-curves and their differences (Oestmann and Galanski, 1989). The localization data however, served to verify whether the correct signal (lesion) had been detected and to estimate the true degree of accuracy.

ROC-curves were fitted from the true and false positive results obtained for each observer and session using a non-linear regression procedure and the area under the curve was determined with a least square fit available on standard software (Mun et al., 1989b).

3.3. Results

3.3.1. Viewing time
A total of 3000 chest images were reviewed by the five observers. The average reading time required for all participants was 33 s per image with a standard deviation of 23.

The average viewing times for all five participants are listed in table 3.

The average viewing time in session 5 was clearly longer than for sessions 3

Table 1

Confidence levels used for evaluation of chest radiographs.

Confidence thresholds for assessing pulmonary nodules
(1) = definite lesion
(2) = probable lesion
(3) = equivocal
(4) = probably *no* lesion
(5) = definitely *no* lesion

Table 2

Overview of the 5 reporting sessions.

Session 1	Reading of conventional chest radiographs at the light-box
Session 2	Reviewing of conventional chest radiographs at the light-box for assessment of intraobserver variation
Session 3	Reading of CRT images with a 1024 × 1024 pixel matrix without image processing
Session 4	Reading of CRT images with a 1024 × 1024 pixel matrix and image processing
Session 5	Reading at the CRT with an image matrix of 2048 × 2048 pixels and image processing

Table 3
Average viewing times (in seconds) for sessions 1 – 5.

Viewing time (sec)	Session 1 (Conv. film I)	Session 2 (Conv. film II)	Session 3 (Dig. 1024)	Session 4 (Dig. 1024)	Session 5 (Lab.-model PMS)
Observer A	45	33	20	39	55
Observer B	40	34	38	42	55
Observer C	25	27	19	39.5	42
Observer D	40	39	39	43	58
Observer E	36	25	22	43	53

and 4. The differences in viewing time between session 5 and sessions 3 and 4 are statistically significant (Student's T-test) ($p < 0.01$).

Figure 3 shows the box-and-whisker plot of viewing times of conventional film reading sessions and the sessions on the CRT with a matrix of 1024×1024 and 2048×2048 pixels.

3.3.2. ROC analysis

The ROC-curves for sessions 1 and 2 showed only minor interobserver variance which was not statistically significant. Intraobserver variation was also not statistically significant, so that both image recognition and learn effect could be discounted.

There were obvious differences in diagnostic accuracy obtained between reading sessions at the viewing box and those at the workstation. The decrease in area under the curve (AUC) in the third viewing session reflected a reduction in diagnostic accuracy with digitized chest radiographs on the CRT. This reduction was evident with all observers and was statistically significant ($p < 0.01$). The comparison of ROC-curves for sessions 3 and 4 yielded no significant differences in AUC and thus no change in diagnostic value. Hence, the poorer

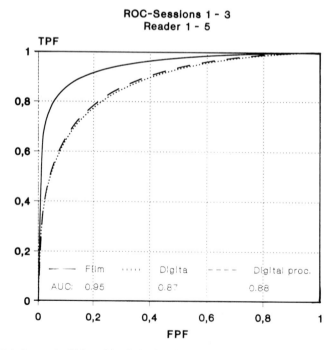

Fig. 3. Multiple box-and-whisker plot of viewing time for the conventional film reading sessions (1 + 2) and the CRT reading sessions (3 + 4, 5).

diagnostic value of images read at the workstation compared with those viewed at the lightbox was not influenced by image processing.

The ROC curves for session 5 yielded an averaged AUC value of 0.75. In comparison with sessions 1 and 2, session 5 showed clearly inferior diagnostic performance. When compared with sessions 3 and 4, session 5 showed a similar AUC value. Thus digitization with a matrix size of 2048 × 2048 pixels provides no diagnostic advantage over a 1024 × 1024 matrix. Table 4 summarizes the AUC values for the five reading sessions.

The significances of the differences in AUC between the reading sessions are summarized in table 5. Student's T-test with a probability level of 1% was used for assessing significance.

4. Diagnostic value of digitized CRT images in high-contrast radiographs

The diagnostic value of the digitized thoracic image has already been the subject of several trials. The major discussions currently involve matrix size and grey-

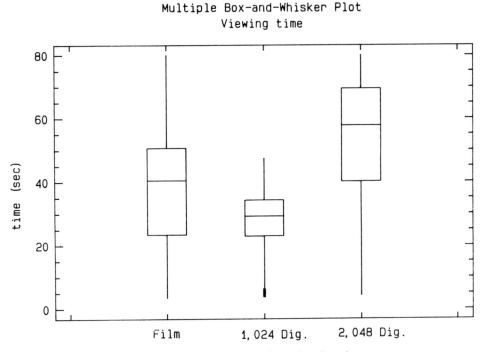

Fig. 4. ROC-curves for session 1 – 5 and for all readers.

scale depth required, and image processing algorithms. The internal annual analysis conducted at our institute shows that between 1986 and 1990, chest radiography accounted for 30% of all radiological investigation performed. Plain skeletal radiographs also comprised 30% of the total number of investigations.

In comparison with digital chest imaging, however, little is said regarding digital skeletal radiography (Sartorius and Sommer, 1984; Braunstein et al., 1988; Galanski et al., 1990; Wiesmann et al., 1990a,b). No data is available regarding the necessary matrix size and gray-scale depth, both of which are crucial factors for the integration of skeletal radiography into PACS. Certain requirements described for chest radiography may also hold true for skeletal radiography when considering its integration into PACS (Marceau, 1982; Crowe and Perrignon, 1991).

4.1. Technical requirements

Comparing chest and skeletal radiographs shows fundamental differences in their spectral composition. Chest radiographs contain the full spectrum of spatial frequencies and require high contrast resolution (Johnson and Ravin,

Table 4

Average areas under the ROC curves and their standard deviations for the viewing sessions 1 – 5

Session	Average value AUC	Stnd.dev.
1	0.91	0.04
2	0.92	0.05
3	0.76	0.07
4	0.76	0.02
5	0.76	0.03

Table 5

Statistical significance of the differences in the AUC for sessions 1 – 5 averaged for all observers (s = significant; n = not significant) (significance level: $p < 0.01$).

	Session 1	Session 2	Session 3	Session 4	Session 5
Session 1	–	n	s	s	s
Session 2	n	–	s	s	s
Session 3	s	s	–	n	n
Session 4	s	s	n	–	n
Session 5	s	s	n	n	–

1983). Skeletal images contain mainly high-frequency structures (bone contours) and a relatively small proportion of low frequency (soft tissue structures) and require high spatial resolution.

The design of the study presented below was based on theoretical and clinical considerations and several preliminary trials. The hand radiograph is a suitable object for testing the quality of image display and the diagnostic value of such an imaging system. The spatial resolution required for hand radiography should also be sufficient for other skeletal regions. The radiographic changes occurring in the bones of the hand can be occasionally very discrete and are certainly well suited for exploring the limits of spatial resolution of an imaging system. There is also little doubt about the clinical relevance of these subtle osseous lesions of the hand.

4.2. Material and methods

A total of 80 conventional film-screen radiographs (film format 18 × 24 cm) were digitized with a matrix size of 1024 × 1024 pixels and 8-bit gray scale (256 gray tones). Patient data and examination date were removed from the original films which then received a randomized identification number. Half of the films showed abnormal findings including discrete fractures or minimal inflammatory or degenerative joint disease. The films were chosen and the 'truth' data (gold standard) established by an expert panel of three skeletal radiologists, who were not involved in subsequent ROC analyses. Each radiologist on the panel reviewed the films independently and only those cases in which all three experts were in unanimous agreement about the findings were included in the study. In order to assist in establishing the 'gold standard', old or subsequent films were provided when required for all of the fractures and fissures and for most of the inflammatory and degenerative changes. For the ROC analysis, all 80 images were read by five radiologists (three board certified radiologists and two senior residents) in three sessions, which were separated by an intervening period of at least three weeks. All five readers were aware of the fact that equal numbers of pathological findings and normal films were presented. In session 1, the original films were read at the lightbox. In session 2, the unprocessed digitized images were reported at the CRT. Interactive post-processing including grey-scale windowing, zooming, grey-scale inversion and various lookup tables (LUT) was only provided on the workstation in session 3. High- or low-pass filtering or histogram transformation was not provided.

Reading sessions at the viewbox were conducted under the same conditions as in the chest study.

Prior to the image reading session at the CRT, the aim of the study was explained and each observer allowed to familiarize himself with the operation of the workstation. Skeletal test films with and without abnormal findings were provided for this purpose. In the course of viewing sessions, 80 images (40 films and 40 digitized images) were presented in random order.

Viewing time for all reading sessions was not limited, but was recorded for each image and observer. Confidence levels of the radiographic findings were scored on a 5 point scale (table 1).

The location of each finding was documented using area codes in a hand diagram. Both this diagram and the list of confidence levels were provided for reference during all reading sessions. The location data was only used to ensure correct lesion detection. A conventional ROC analysis was performed using software designed by Metz (1986) for curve fitting and estimation of AUC. The significance of the differences between results obtained for the different sessions was assessed using Student's T-test.

4.3. Results

4.3.1. Viewing time
The average viewing time was 27 s for the film-screen radiographs and 22 s for digitized images on the CRT without postprocessing (table 6). The difference in viewing times between sessions 1 and 2 was statistically significant ($p < 0.01$).

Image processing (session 3) further prolonged viewing time to 38 s. The differences between session 3 and sessions 1 and 2 were also statistically significant ($p < 0.01$)

4.3.2. ROC analysis
A total of 1200 hand images were read and the results evaluated in a ROC study. Reading the conventional films at the lightbox yielded an average AUC

Table 6

High-contrast skeletal radiographs − average viewing times and standard deviation for sessions 1−3.

For all observers	Session 1	Session 2	Session 3
Average viewing time	27	22	38
Standard deviations	19	15	30

of 0.95. The interobserver variation in diagnostic accuracy in session 1 was not statistically significant.

An obvious deterioration in diagnostic accuracy was noted with the digitized images; average AUC for session 2 dropped to 0.87 with large interobserver variation. The differences in average AUC between session 1 and 2 were statistically significant ($p < 0.01$). The average AUC value obtained for session 3 was 0.88, which was not significantly different from that of session 2 (fig. 5).

As indicated earlier, skeletal radiographs are essentially high-contrast images. The abnormal findings which were analyzed in our study (hairline fractures and inflammatory and early degenerative joint disease) were often very discrete and therefore required high spatial resolution for adequate demonstration. The use of such clinical material appears justified for evaluating spatial resolution of an imaging system. Trials with artificial cortical lesions in isolated

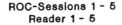

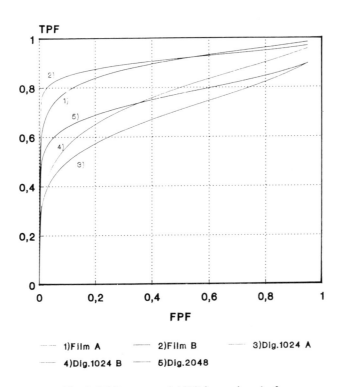

Fig. 5. ROC-curves and AUC for sessions 1–3.

bones, such as those by Galanski et al. (1990), were more suited for investigating contrast resolution than spatial resolution with different imaging parameters.

One crucial factor for the success and validity of a ROC analysis is the strength of its truth data (gold standard). For this reason, all films repeatedly read false positive were reevaluated with knowledge of the observers localization data. No lesions were found which had not been recorded in the truth data.

In a ROC study, values over 0.95 mean that the findings were too obvious and thus identified correctly by the observers in nearly all cases. However, the significant reduction in the diagnostic validity of the digitized films in the present study indicates that the lesions were not too obvious using that mode of presentation. The high specificity and sensitivity in evaluating the conventional films may also be attributed to the expertise of the reader.

5. Summary of the results

The reading sessions with digitized images were conducted using different monitors on two workstations designed for a PACS.

ROC methodology was used to assess the diagnostic value of the systems employed. The area under the ROC curve quantified the degree of the diagnostic accuracy of the display modality. The significance of the differences in AUC were calculated using Student's T-test and the method described by Hanley and McNeil (1983).

For assessment of the conventional radiographs, AUC values of 0.92 to 0.91 were obtained for the 'low-contrast' (chest) images and 0.95 for the 'high-contrast' (skeletal) images. The AUC values obtained for the sessions at the workstation (digitized images) were significantly lower with 0.76 for the 'low-contrast' images and 0.87 for the 'high-contrast' images. The differences in the AUC between the film reading sessions and the reading sessions at the workstation were statistically significant ($p < 0.01$). Image processing at the workstation provided no statistically significant improvement in the diagnostic accuracy (AUC = 0.76 and 0.88, respectively).

The viewing sessions conducted on the prototype unit in Hamburg resulted in an average AUC of 0.75. The AUC values for the individual observers ranged from 0.66 to 0.83. No statistically significant improvement in diagnostic accuracy was observed with images digitized with a 2048 × 2048 matrix compared with those with a 1024 × 1024 pixel matrix.

For the *chest images*, the average viewing times for the film sessions were 34 s (session 1) and 32 s (session 2), whereas those on the 'standard' workstation without image processing averaged 28 s. The viewing times at the CRT were thus significantly shorter than those of the lightbox ($p < 0.01$).

For the *hand images*, viewing times averaged 27 s for film reading session and 22 s for reading sessions at the CRT with no image processing; a difference which was also statistically significant ($p < 0.01$).

For both *chest* and *hand* images, image processing prolonged viewing times to 41 and 38 s, respectively, with both values being significantly different from their counterparts without processing ($p < 0.01$).

Viewing times on the workstation in Hamburg proved to be the longest; with this unit on which image processing was also allowed, the average viewing time (52 s) required was significantly longer than that at the 'standard' workstation with image processing ($p < 0.01$).

6. Discussion

6.1. PACS − technical aspects

To date, no exclusively digital radiologic imaging department with digital archiving and image transmission exists. PACS installations described in the literature are few and essentially closed circuit constructions (Taira et al., 1988; Mun et al., 1989b). The concept of a 'filmless' imaging department, or still better, a 'filmless' hospital remains hypothetical.

Mun et al. postulate that one can only start to seriously consider the introduction of a totally digital imaging department in about 2−3 years (Mun et al., 1989b). Bauman showed greater insight into the problems involved when stating that it will take at least five, but probably nine or more years for the concept of a completely 'digital department' to become reality (Bauman, 1986). The author sees more problems in design and construction of workstations than in the availability of basic hardware.

6.1.1. The resolution
Adequate resolution is one of the basic requirements of a PACS, however, the definition of standard minimum requirements to ensure inclusion of all image information is a complex task. Three different aspects of this issue shall be discussed: the definition of resolution requirements, technological solutions available, and financial consequences.

Resolution requirements of a system depend on the imaging technique and the size and contrast of the structure to be documented.

Regarding spatial resolution, several authors are of the opinion that a matrix of 1024 × 1024 pixels is perfectly adequate to reproduce diagnostically relevant spatial definition. Due to the perception threshold of the human eye, the full resolution of a conventional radiograph can only be appreciated if the viewing distance is greatly shortened. This phenomenon was demonstrated by Brogdon et al., who showed that the detection of pulmonary lesions on chest radiographs at the viewing box can be improved by shortening viewing distance ('Every abnormality has its own specific viewing distance'; Brogdon et al., 1983).

The minimum angle subtended by an object on the retina required for its detection may be determined by $\check{S} = 2 \arctan(h/2d)$, where d is the viewing distance and h is the size of the object in question. This minimal angle required for object discrimination at the retina is 1', so that an optimal viewing distance of approximately 70–90 cm is required to appreciate pulmonary structure (Grewer et al., 1985; Widoff et al., 1989). Closer viewing with digital images may lead to discrimination of the individual pixels, a phenomenon called 'pixel artifact' or 'pixel clutter', which is probably based on a particular sensitivity of human visual perception to structured patterns and may affect contrast resolution and global image perception (Kundel, 1986; Pizer, 1986).

One possible method for improving resolution involves image sampling* with a large matrix (e.g., 2048 × 2048 pixels) and displaying it on CRT with a smaller size (e.g., 1024 × 1024); when required, the full resolution can be employed by zooming in parts of the image. Our ROC study evaluating this capability, however, yielded no statistically significant improvement in diagnostic accuracy. The extensive use of zooming by all observers was reflected by the marked increase in viewing time.

Similar reports evaluating the effects of pixel size on lesion detection rate appeared in the literature (Kelsey et al., 1981). Lams and Cocklin observed no change in the detection rate of pulmonary nodules with pixel sizes less than 0.8 mm (Lams and Cocklin, 1986). Foley et al. report an improvement in detection rate of pulmonary nodules, despite large interobserver variation, with increasing resolution till 0.5 lp/mm, but no significant advantage beyond this limit (Foley et al., 1981). Our results also showed large degrees of interobserver variation at the workstation. The detection of disseminated lesions seems to be generally easier than solitary lesions, which are frequently difficult to delineate from overlying ribs and pulmonary vessels. This factor was also confirmed by Kundel et al. for the assessment of conventional chest radiographs (Kundel et al., 1969).

Most pulmonary lesions are readily detectable with a matrix size of 1024 × 1024 pixels, but this resolution is insufficient for subtle changes. Our experience showed that displaying higher resolution images (2048 × 2048) at a workstation with a 1024 × 1024 matrix and scrolling through portions of the magnified image is both complicated and very time consuming. Other authors

---

* For example, Imlogix.

evaluating the perception of pulmonary lesions also critized the piecewise viewing of chest radiographs. Through their analysis of eye tracking movements, Kundel et al. demonstrated that 15% of all undiagnosed pulmonary nodules were missed due to incomplete visual sampling of the image. In a supplementary study by the same group, parts of the chest radiographs containing the missed nodules were presented to the observers; the number of lesions detected under these conditions remained unchanged and an increase in false-positive fraction was noted (Carmody et al., 1980). Our experience with digitized chest radiographs reviewed on a prototype workstation has produced similar results with an increase in the false-positive fraction occurring through the use of zooming; the ROC curves for these sessions exhibited a lower plateau segment.

Other authors suggested that a global impression of the whole image and comparison with the contralateral region by rapid jumps of the eyes assist in the detection and interpretation of radiographic findings (Kundel et al., 1969; Kundel, 1986). One reasonable solution to this problem would be a monitor which displays the whole image in full resolution (2048 × 2048 pixels). Recently, a CRT (Megascan*) with the necessary resolution performance has become available. This monitor can display images with a matrix size of 2560 × 2048 pixels in a 12 bit gray scale and should be virtually flicker-free with a refresher-rate of 72 Hz. Preliminary investigations conducted on this new CRT show a diagnostic quality comparable with that of conventional film for the detection of septal lines and nodules (Frank et al., 1989; Hayrapetian et al., 1989; Widoff et al., 1989).

In a large study by Cox et al., ROC studies were used to investigate the diagnostic validity of digitized images (containing nine different pulmonary lesions) on a workstation. The CRT images were compared with original films and with digitized hard copies (image matrix 2048 × 2048). The three methods yielded similar results for pulmonary atelectases, shadows in the lung fields and diaphragmatic recesses, hilar and mediastinal masses and apical pleural thickening. The changes of obstructive lung diseases were clearer on the hard copy than on the CRT. For detecting interstitial pulmonary disease and pneumothorax, original films were superior to CRT images. In contrast, both on the CRT and as hard copy, digitized images were superior for the detection of pulmonary nodules.

The authors attributed the decrease in detection rate of obstructive lung disease at the workstation compared to hard copy to lack of observer experience with this new display medium. They also suspect that inadequate edge definition and insufficient display luminance may play a role in limiting diagnostic

---

* Megascan Technology Inc., Boston, MA.

performance. They consider a resolution of 2048 × 2048 pixels to be adequate for chest imaging, since the diagnostic value of such images as hard copy was comparable to that of conventional films in their study. For most radiographic findings, the digitized hard copy was in fact superior to the conventional radiograph possibly due to improved contrast (Cox et al., 1990).

The manufacturers of the Megascan workstation announced new developments in the fluorescent layer of the monitor, which may possibly improve image quality.

Another factor affecting lesion detection on the CRT besides matrix size is image size. Radiologists improve their detection of smaller lesions by changing the eye-to-image distance, thus magnifying certain details (Brogdon et al., 1983). Since conventional radiographs display details more or less in its original size, it is conceivable that smaller lesion may be detected by this maneuver. Digital images presented on a CRT are usually smaller than conventional radiographs. Fisher and Brauer as well as other authors have shown a positive correlation between total image size and the perception of signals of diagnostically relevant size (Kundel, 1986; Fisher et al., 1989). For this reason, CRTs should be large enough to guarantee adequate object perception. For a given resolution, however, the necessary viewing distance can conflict with the magnification of the CRT. As discussed above, a minimum viewing distance is required to avoid the pixel detection and eliminate pixel artifacts. Increasing monitor size without increasing matrix size would result in poorer perception of details. By enlarging the CRT while simultaneously improving its resolution, the viewing distance can be maintained or even reduced, thus improving in spatial resolution.

Mammography places the greatest demands on spatial resolution. The digitization of mammograms without loss of image information has not been successful. Mammogram digitization with a pixel size of 0.1 μm is accompanied by a lower detection rate of microcalcifications. Image processing using filtering techniques such as unsharp masking may increase sensitivity at a given matrix size, but is paralleled by an increase in false-positive rate (Chan et al., 1986, 1987; Behrman et al., 1989). Systems with resolutions of 5 lp/mm were recommended for digitizing such images; this would essentially mean a matrix size of at least 4096 × 4096 pixels.

6.1.2. The grey scale

The grey-scale gradation required for displaying an image essentially depends on its grey tone content and consequently on its contrast. Images which primarily contain a greater dynamic range of optical densities than can be perceived by the human eye are optimally displayed on CRT. The possibility to 'window' on structures with widely differing intensities allows the observer to evaluated all parts of an image to advantage: this capability is not possible with film-based images. The trained human eye can differentiate approximately 100 grey tones (Pizer et al., 1984). Through adaption to various levels of brightness, 485 different grey tones can be distinguished (Krestel, 1988). High-quality CRTs specially manufactured for diagnostic image viewing can display 256 gray levels (8 bit). Kasday considers an 8-bit gray scale to be sufficient for diagnostic purposes whereas Kundel feels that 10-bit gray scale is necessary (Kasday, 1986). The basic limiting factor is essentially not grey-scale size, but the limited linearity of the CRT, which makes it difficult to transform different signal strengths into discrete densities. In our own investigations, we were able to confirm similar nonlinear dynamic ranges in both of the systems tested. In the higher and lower optical densities, the markedly lower gradient of the dynamic curve corresponded with a decrease in contrast resolution.

This limitation in dynamic range may influence diagnostic values of images displayed on CRT. In our study with radiographs, the majority of pulmonary lesions missed had optical densities located within the lower and upper portion of the dynamic range. Consequently, it may be favorable to alter the form of an optical density curve using appropriate image processing algorithms such as known as LUT (look-up tables). The design and application of LUT are still the subject of discussion (Pizer et al., 1984, 1986; Mitchell and Sorensen, 1986).

One LUT suggested by Kundel involves contrast enhancement. The effect of contrast enhancement is to improve the discrimination of smaller differences in gray tone, which would otherwise not be perceived on the CRT due to low luminance levels. Psychophysical analyses showed that discrete contrast is better discriminated at higher luminance levels such as those provided by a lightbox (ten-fold luminance of most CRTs).

The use of simple manipulation methods such as windowing are employed routinely in CT and MRI and such image processing possibilities should also be provided for projection radiography.

Depending to the requirements, narrowing and shifting of the dynamic curve should be achieved using nonlinear transformation tables. Several other helpful image processing algorithms have been described, such as histogram equalization* and its variants as well as gray-scale rating techniques such as JND (just noticeable difference) scaling, power law scaling and de-facto power law** (Pizer et al., 1984; Lehr and Capek, 1985; Wolschendorf et al., 1985;

---

* Histogram equalization essentially involves the spreading of pixel intensities within a region of interest over the whole gray-scale spectrum to enhance contrast (Pizer et al., 1984).

** JND scaling = just noticeable difference scaling — the intensities are distributed over the gray scale, so that all intensity differences reach the barely visible limit required for the human eye; power law scaling and de-facto power law are modified methods of gray-scale processing.

Kasday, 1986; Barnes and Lauro, 1989; Plessis et al., 1989; Zimmermann et al., 1989).

6.2. Other factors

In addition to spatial and contrast resolution, there are yet other factors which affect the image quality of a CRT. The perception of image flicker caused by low refresher rates varies from individual to individual and depends on total image brightness and viewing angle. Both factors must be considered in the design of a CRT workstation. The endeavor to increase display luminance results in an increased awareness of the human eye to image flicker, and may therefore prove detrimental. Consequently, an increase in luminance must be accompanied by higher CRT refresher rates.

A further factor preventing the replacement of the lightbox by the CRT is the increased sensitivity of the eye to image flicker towards the periphery of the visual field, which induces a subconscious suppression of image information reaching these portions of the retina. Thus the ideal CRT refresher rate can only be determined by also considering luminance, brightness and viewing angle.

In a series of trials evaluating image quality on different monochrome CRTs with differing fluorescent layers of short persistence, Bauer recommended a refresher rate of 91 Hz for word and data processing purposes. At this frequency, 95% of the observers reported no perceivable flicker (Bauer, 1984). In our series of investigations, the prototype model used for viewing chest images had the lowest frame frequency (50 Hz) of all the workstations tested. With this monitor none of the readers were conscious of any image flicker, which may have been due to low luminance levels and a limited viewing angle (only one monitor was used on this workstation).

A number of factors, which cannot be quantified, also determine the perceptive capabilities of the observer and his acceptance of a digital workstation. Kundel has named these factors 'attractivity' and 'esthetics' of an image (Kundel, 1986). Radiologists have shown the tendency to over-emphasize the requirement for high spatial resolution above all other parameters, however, signal – noise ratio is probably a more important factor in diagnostic imaging.

In our studies, the average viewing times at the workstation without post-processing were shorter than those for conventional films. This could be due to the lack of 'attractivity' and 'esthetics' of the workstation image, which was confirmed by most observers during the reading sessions. Another possible cause for shorter viewing times on the CRT could be the image size. One trial by Brogdon et al. on the detection of pulmonary lesions showed the zone of foveal vision to be only 2°; (Brogdon et al., 1983) and that approximately 300 fixations are necessary to scan a whole chest film*. The small size of the CRT image may result in a reduction in the number of fixation points required and a shortening of the viewing time.

The analysis of eye tracking movements could provide valuable data in this respect. A further point made by Brogdon et al. (1983) in the same study was that true-positive findings were detected within the first seconds of image viewing, whereas false-positive lesions were reported towards the end of a longer viewing period.

Our studies have shown similar results for both film and CRT image reading sessions with viewing times being twice as long with those images in which false-positive lesions were reported.

7. A synopsis

At present, the integration of *digital* imaging procedures and *digital* subtraction angiography into a PACS is both possible and recommendable. The workstation is superior to film as a medium for displaying these images. The integration of *projection* radiography into a PACS is currently hindered by the limited diagnostic value of the systems developed so far. Most authors consider a matrix size of 2048 × 2048 pixels to be sufficient, however, this may only a compromise between the matrix of 4096 × 4096 pixels with its staggering data content and the inadequate resolution of 1024 × 1024 pixels.

The production of hard copies from digitized projection radiographs for reviewing and communication purposes is only a transitional solution and does not fulfill the aims of a PACS. High-quality workstations for diagnostic image viewing are still very expensive and require further evaluation.

8. Summary

The studies presented concentrate on the evaluation of an important component of an electronic PACS − the CRT − on which investigations assessing diagnostic values of digitized radiographs were conducted. These results were analyzed using ROC methodology.

The ROC investigations were conducted on two units with different spatial resolutions. On the standard unit, the films were reviewed on a workstation with a resolution of 1024 × 1024 pixels; on the protype unit, the films were

---

* In practice, however, only 80 − 120 fixations are employed.

digitized with a matrix of 2048 × 2048 pixels and reviewed with a matrix of 1024 × 1024. Both workstations provided grey scales of 256 gray tones. 120 thoracic radiographs prepared with artificial lesions were presented to five observers both as original films and as digitized images on the CRT in separate reading sessions. The results showed that an image matrix of 1024 × 1024 pixels was insufficient to display pulmonary nodules. The loss of diagnostic accuracy is not only due to the spatial resolution of the system, but also to lesion contrast with surrounding structures. The analysis of lesion detection with regards to its location showed that the lesions overlooked were mostly localized in the zones of high or low optical density where lesion contrast was low.

The evaluation of the chest images with an image matrix of 2048 × 2048 pixels on a display matrix of 1024 × 1024 pixels with zooming to allow full use of their resolution showed poorer diagnostic accuracy than that obtained with the original films. These results were similar to those obtained using an image matrix of 1024 × 1024 pixels. This differences in diagnostic accuracy between the reading sessions with film and digitized images on CRT were all statistically significant. Zooming markedly prolonged viewing times through an attempt by all observers to utilize the full resolution in all portions of the image.

In another study, hand radiographs were digitized and both original film and digitized CRT images were read by five radiologists. In contrast with chest radiographs, the image information of hand films lies predominantly in the upper and lower portions of the optical density curve resulting in high image contrast. A loss in diagnostic value was also observed with digitized CRT images of the hand compared to the original films. Allowing processing of the CRT images achieved no improvement in diagnostic accuracy and markedly prolonged viewing times.

In summary, the following conclusions can be made from our results:

(1) A matrix of 1024 × 1024 pixels or smaller is inadequate for storage and display of image information contained in conventional chest and skeletal radiographs.

(2) On our prototype system a digitized image with an image matrix of 2048 × 2048 pixels displayed with a matrix of 1024 × 1024 pixels is of no advantage over an image matrix of 1024 × 1024 pixels even with a zooming facility.

(3) The image digitization techniques available are unable to transform grey-scale information without loss of contrast, which is diagnostically essential.

Thus, we infer that:

(1) A minimum matrix size of 2048 × 2048 pixels is necessary for storing and displaying projection radiographic images.

(2) Entire images should be displayed in full resolution at the workstation.

Such systems are already available but still require testing.

(3) More accurate grey-scale transformation techniques are required for image digitization. Change gray-scale gradation of a digital display may improve perception of diagnostically valuable image information at the CRT.

9. Conclusion

At present, it may be not financially feasible nor medically useful to replace the radiographic film with electronic image storage, display and transmission for *all* imaging techniques.

The development of larger CRTs with improved luminance and contrast levels should, however, provide the necessary hardware required to display digital projection radiographs in the future.

References

Barnes, G.T., and K. Lauro (1989) Image processing in digital radiography: basic concepts and applications, *J. Digital Imaging* 2, 132–146.

Bauer, D. (1984) Causes of flicker at VDUs with bright background and ways of eleminating interference. In: Grandjean, E. (Ed.), Ergonomics and Health in Modern Offices (Taylor and Francis, London), pp. 364–370.

Bauman, R.A. (1986) The future of digital computers in medical imaging. In: Höhne, K.H. (Ed.), Pictorial Information Systems in Medicine, *NATO ASI Series F* 19, 381–389 (Springer, Berlin).

Behrman, R.H., R.G. Zamenhof and K.M. Blazo (1989) Evaluation of a commercial mammography image-enhancement system, *J. Digital Imaging* 2, 163–169.

Braunstein, E.M., P.Capek, K. Buckwalter, P. Bland and C.R. Meyer (1988) Adaptive histogramm equalization in digital radiography of destructive skeletal lesions, *Radiology* 166, 883–885.

Brogdon, B.G., C.A. Kelsey and R.D. Mosely (1983) Factors affecting perception of pulmonary lesions, *Radiol. Clin. North Am.* 21, 633–654.

Carmody, D.P., C.F. Nodine and H.L. Kundel (1980) Global and segmental search for lung nodules of different edge gradient, *Invest. Radiol.* 15, 233–244.

Chakraborty, D.P., E.S. Breatnach, M.V. Yester, B. Soto, G.T. Barnes and R.G. Fraser (1986) Digital and conventionale chest imaging: a modified ROC study of observer, performance using simulated nodules, *Radiology* 158, 35–39.

Chan, H.P., C.I. Vyborny, H. MacMahon, C.E. Metz, K. Doi and E.A. Sickles (1986) Evaluation of digital unsharp-mask filtering for the detection of subtle mammographic microcalcifications. In: Schneider, R.H., and S.J. Dwyer III (Eds.), Medicine XIV/PACS IV, *Proc. SPIE* 626, 347–348.

Chan, H.P., C.J. Vyborny, H. MacMahon, C.E. Metz, K. Doi and E.A. Sickles (1987) Digital mammography ROC studies of the effects of pixel size and unsharp-mask filtering on the detection of subtle microcalcifications, *Invest. Radiol.* 22, 581–589.

Cox, G.G., L.T. Cook, J.H. McMillan, S.J. Rosenthal and S.J. Dwyer III (1990) Chest radiography: comparison of high resolution digital displays with conventional and digital film,

Radiology 176, 771 – 776.

Crowe, B.L. and A. Perrignon (1991) Introduction of digital imaging archiving system at John Hunter Hospital, Newcastle, Australia. In: Lemke, H.U., M.L. Rhodes, C.C. Jaffe and R. Felix (Eds.), Proc. Computer Assisted Radiology CAR'91 (Springer, Berlin), pp. 407 – 413.

Duerinckx, A.J., and E.J. Pisa (1982) Filmless picture archiving and communication in diagnostic radiology. In: Duerinckx, A.J. (Ed.), Picture Archiving and Communication Systems (PACS) for Medical Applications, First International Conference and Workshop, *Proc. SPIE* 318, 9 – 18.

Fisher, P., B. Grover, G. Brauer and G. Ritchie (1989) Digital image display station performance requirements based on physician experience with a prototype system, *J. Digital Imaging* 2, 150 – 155.

Foley, W.D., C.R. Wilson, G.S. Keyes, F.A. DiBianca, G.T. Scanion, D. Schleuter and T.L. Lawson (1981) The effect of varying spatial resolution on the detectability of diffuse pulmonary nodules, *Radiology* 141, 25 – 31.

Frank, M.S., R.G. Jost, G.J. Blaine, S.M. Moore, R.A. Whitmann and R. Hagge (1989) Interpretation of mobile chest radiographs from a high-resolution CRT display, RSNA '89 Chicago (Abstract), 401, Supplement to *Radiology* 173(P), November 1989.

Galanski, M., M. Prokop, J.W. Oestmann, S. Reichelt and U. von Falkenhausen (1990) Anwendung der digitalen Lumineszenzradiographie (DLR) in der Skelettdiagnostik: ROC-Studie zur Erkennbarkeit kortikaler Läsionen. In: Schneider, G.H., E. Vogler and K. Kocever (Eds.), Digitale Bildgebung – Interventionelle Radiologie – Integrierte digitale Radiologie (Blackwell & Ueberreuther Wissenschaft, Berlin), pp. 234 – 241.

Grewer, R., K.J. Mönnich, J. Schmidt, H. Svensson and Th. Wendler (1985) Design of interaktive workstations for the interactive interpretation of medical images in pictorial information systems. In: Lemke, H.U., M.L. Rhodes, C.C. Jaffe and R. Felix (Eds.), Proc. Computer Assisted Radiology CAR'85, (Springer, Berlin).

Hanley, J.A., and B.J. McNeil (1983) A method of comparing the areas under receiver operating characteristic curves derived from the same cases, *Radiology* 148, 839 – 843.

Hayrapetian, A., D.R. Aberle, H.K. Huang, R. Fiske, C. Morioka, D. Valentino and M.I. Boechat (1989) Comparison of 2048-line digital display formats in conventional radiographs: an ROC study, *Am. J. Roentgenol.* 152, 1113 – 1118.

Johnson, G.A., and C.E. Ravin (1983) A survey of digital chest radiography, *Radiol. Clin. North Am.* 21, 655 – 665.

Kasday, L.R. (1986) Human factors considerations in PACS design. In: Schneider, R.H., and S.J. Dwyer III (Eds.), Medicine XIV/PACS IV, *Proc. SPIE* 626, 581 – 592.

Kelsey, C.A., R.D. Moseley, F.A. Mettler and D.E. Briscoe (1981) Observer performance as a function of viewing distance, *Invest. Radiol.* 16, 435 – 437.

Krestel, E. (1988) Bildgebende Systeme für die medizinische Diagnostik (Siemens-Aktienges., Berlin).

Kundel, H.L. (1986) Visual perception and image display, *Radiol. Clin. North Am.* 24, 69 – 78.

Kundel, H.L., G. Revesz and H.M. Stauffer (1969) The electro-optical processing of radiographic images, *Radiol. Clin. North Am.* 7, 447 – 459.

Lams, P.M., and M.L. Cocklin (1986) Spatial resolution requirements for digital chest radiographs: an ROC study of observer performance in selected cases, *Radiology* 158, 11 – 19.

Lehr, J.L., and P. Capek (1985) Histogramm equalization of CT images, *Radiology* 154, 163 – 169.

Marceau, C. (1982) What is a picture archiving and communication system (PACS)? In: Duerinckx, A.J. (Ed.), Picture Archiving and Communication Systems (PACS) for Medical Applications, First International Conference and Workshop, *Proc. SPIE* 318, 24 – 29.

Meyer-Ebrecht, D. (1988) PACS oder der zukünftige Arbeitsplatz des Radiologen, *Radiologe* 28,

195 – 199.

Meyer-Ebrecht, D. and Th. Wendler (1983) Concept of the diagnostic image workstation. In: Dwyer III, S.J. (Ed.), Picture Archiving and Communication Systems (PACS) for Medical Applications, Second International Conference and Workshop, *Proc. SPIE* 418, 180 – 188.

Metz, C.E. (1986) ROC methodology in radiologic imaging, *Invest. Radiol.* 21, 720 – 733.

Mitchell, C.R., and J.A. Sorensen (1986) Digital image processing in chest radiography. In: Schneider, R.H., and S.J. Dwyer III (Eds.), Medicine XIV/PACS IV, *Proc. SPIE* 626, 259 – 267.

Mun, S.K., H. Benson, C. Welsh, L.P. Elliott and W. Davros, (1989a) Baseline study of radiology services for the purpose of PACS evaluation. In: Mun, S.K., and S. Horii (Eds.), Digital Imaging Network Systems, Projekt Papers, Department of Radiology, Georgetown University Hospital, Washington, Chapter 4.

Mun, S.K., H. Benson, S. Horii et al. (1989b) Completion of a hospital-wide comprehensive image management and communication system. In: Mun, S.K., and S. Horii (Eds.), Digital Imaging Network Systems, Projekt Papers, Department of Radiology, Georgetown University Hospital, Washington, Chapter 1.

Mun, S.K., H. Benson, L.P. Elliott, F. Goeringer, A. Saarinen and D. Haynor (1989c) Total digital department: implementation strategy. In: Mun, S.K., and S. Horii (Eds.), Digital Imaging Network Systems, Projekt Papers, Department of Radiology, Georgetown University Hospital, Washington, Chapter 21.

Mutter, E. (1955) Die Technik der Negativ- und Positivverfahren. In: Michel, K. (Ed.), Die wissenschaftliche und angewandte Photographie (Springer, Berlin).

Oestmann, J.W., and M. Galanski (1989) ROC: Methodik zum Vergleich der diagnostischen Leistung bildgebender Verfahren, *RöFo* 151, 89 – 92.

Pizer, S.M. (1986) Psychovisual issues in the display of medical images. In: Höhne, K.H. (Ed.), Pictorial Information Systems in Medicine, *NATO ASI Series F* 19, 211 – 248 (Springer, Berlin).

Pizer, S.M., J.B. Zimmermann and E. Staab (1984) Adaptive grey level assignment in CT scan display, *J. Comput. Assist. Tomogr.* 8, 300 – 305.

Pizer, S.M., J.D. Austin, J.R. Perry, H.D. Safrit and J.B. Zimmermann (1986) Adaptive histogram equalization automated contrast enhencement of medical images. In: Schneider, R.H., and S.J. Dwyer III (Eds.), Medicine XIV/PACS IV, *Proc. SPIE* 626, 242 – 250.

Plessis, B., M. Goldberg, R. Dillon, J. Tombaugh, J. Robertson, G. Bélanger and N. Hickey (1989) Context-dependent enhancements for radiological images, *J. Digital Imaging* 2, 114 – 122.

Sartorius, D.J., and F.G. Sommer (1984) Digital film processing: applications to the musculoskeletal system, *Skeletal Radiol.* 11, 274 – 281.

Stender, H.-St. (1989) Qualitätssicherung bei Röntgenuntersuchungen – Leitlinien der Bundesärztekammer zur Qualitässicherung in der Röntgendiagnostik, *Dt. Ärztebl.* 86, 1437 – 1444.

Taira, R.K., N.J. Mankovich, M.I. Boechat, H. Kangarloo and H.K. Huang (1988) Design and implementation of a picture archiving and communication system for pediatric radiology, *Am. J. Roentgenol.* 150, 1117 – 1121.

Wendler, Th., R. Grewer, K.J. Mönnich and H. Svensson (1986) Design considerations for multi modality image workstations. In: Höhne, K.H. (Ed.), Pictorial Information Systems in Medicine, *NATO ASI Series F* 19, 401 – 420 (Springer, Berlin).

Widoff, B., D.R. Aberle, K. Brown, D. Hansell, P. Batra, A. Hayrapetian and H.K. Huang (1989) Hard copy versus soft copy display of 2 000 digital chest images: ROC study with simulated lung nodules., RSNA '89, Chicago (Abstract), 401.

Wiesmann, W., M. Reiser, Th. Pauly, M. Fiebich, U. Bick and P.E. Peters (1990a) Darstellung von Metallimplantaten mit der digitalen Lumineszenzradiographie, *Fortschr. Geb. Röntgenstr.* 152, 687 – 692.

Wiesmann, W., M. Reiser, Th. Pauly, N. Roos and P.E. Peters (1990b) Untersuchung von Hüftgelenksendoprothesen mit einem digitalen Radiographiesystem — Vergleich mit der konventionellen Film Folien-Radiographie. In: Schneider, G.H., and E. Vogler (Eds.), Digitale Bildgebung (Blackwell, Berlin), pp. 241–248.

Wolschendorf, K., K. Vanselow and J. Lindner (1985) Hybride Histogrammequalisation bei der Digitalisierung von Röntgenbildern mit einem Halbleiter-Zeilensensor. In: Lemke, H.U., M.L. Rhodes, C.C. Jaffee and R. Felix (Eds.), Proc. CAR '85 (Springer, Berlin), pp. 232–236.

Zimmermann, J.B., S.B. Cousins, K.M. Hartzell, M.E. Frisse and M.G. Kahn (1989) A psychophysical comparison of two methods for adaptive histogram equalization, *J. Digital Imaging* 2, 82–91.

Integrated Diagnostic Imaging
Editor: J.P.J. De Valk
© *Elsevier Science Publishers B.V., 1992*

Chapter 11

The Trieste PACS project: now and the future

L. Dalla Palma, P. Giribona, F. Stacul and W. Ukovich

1. Introduction

In order to assess the impact of PACS technology on health structures, a project of experimentation of a PAC system has been planned in 1987 at the Local Health Unit of Trieste which administers the four public hospitals of Trieste (2500 beds, 4 Radiology Departments, about 250 000 imaging examinations/year) delivering health care services to a population of about 260 000 inhabitants.

The PACS facility is presently installed in the Radiology Department of the University Hospital of Cattinara with a remote connection to the Maggiore General Hospital (the second largest hospital of the city).

The University Hospital of Cattinara has been operational since May, 1984. It has 840 beds for eight surgical and seven medical departments. The Radiology Department provides the diagnostic imaging facilities for the inpatients as well as for the outpatients. About 100 000 examinations are performed yearly in the 21 examination rooms (14 conventional and 7 new modality ones: 4 ultrasonographies (US), 1 computed tomography (CT), 1 magnetic resonance (MR) and 1 angiography).

The present ensemble of workers consists of 19 radiologists, 31 technicians, 17 trained nurses and 13 administrative clerks.

Most activities operate on a single eight-hour shift for five days a week. Two partially overlapping shifts, with a cumulative coverage of about twelve hours, are normally applied to some critical activities. An emergency X-ray room connected to the first-aid department operates twentyfour hours a day, seven days a week.

As far as the operation management is concerned, the main functions of the department are examination processing and diagnostic reporting. Besides them, a number of secondary level functions are required (scheduling, reception, radiological data retrieval, statistical reporting, archive management).

2. The Trieste PACS project

The 'Trieste project' of the Trieste Local Health Unit (U.S.L. n.1 Triestina), had four main objectives in the assessment of PACS technology on health structures:
(1) to install and operate a commercial PACS in the Radiology Department;
(2) to evaluate technical and clinical key aspects of the system in routine operation;
(3) to experiment a connection between two major hospitals and a research institution in the neighboring (Area di Ricerca), by a digital link (T2-2.048 Mbps (Mbit/s) and V35-48/64 kbps);
(4) to issue general guidelines and specifications for an operational PAC system, suitable for national deployment in the health care system.

Steps (1) to (3) are quite advanced, and some results from these researches will be described in the following. Some experimental investigations are in progress, comparing the usual operations carried out for some diagnostic modalities with the corresponding ones performed using the PACS.

The present geographical topology of the Trieste PACS installation is shown in fig. 1.

The system configuration presently installed in the hospitals of Trieste is shown in fig. 2.

A data management system (DMS) is devoted to system communication and arbitration, archive management and long-term information storage on a juke box of optical disks.

An acquisition module (AM) collects all images produced from five different radiological modalities (CT, MRI, DSA, US1 and US2), converts them into a digital format, and sends them to the DMS.

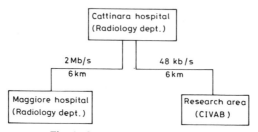

Fig. 1. Current network topology.

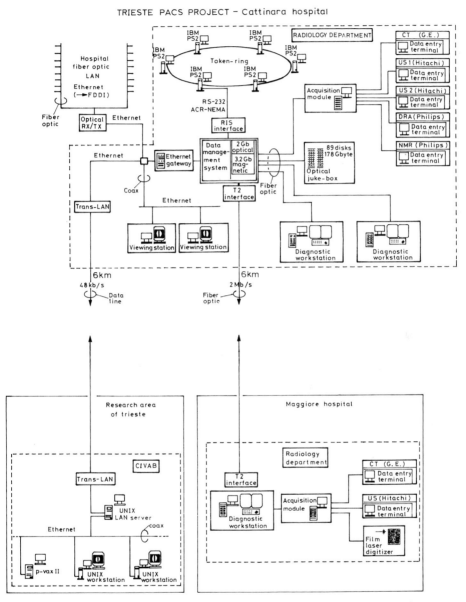

Fig. 2. Gateway under development to connect radiology network to clinical and research areas.

Two display workstations (DW) are connected in order to represent images and demographic data acquired from the AM and coming from the RIS interface.

Two results viewing stations (RVS) are connected via an Ethernet gateway to the DMS. In particular, the Ethernet gateway potentially allows a distribution of images in the whole hospital by means of a fiber-optic Ethernet LAN which connects all the hospital departments.

A consulting workstation (CW) is installed in the Radiology Department of the Maggiore Hospital (connection via optical fiber link), enabling the access to the DMS archive and the acquisition of images from three modalities (CT, ultrasound, laser film digitizer).

3. Research activities

Several research activities have been carried out and some other ones are under development in order to assess the PACS technology. The Trieste project involves people belonging to different institutions:
- Administration of Public Hospitals of Trieste;
- University of Trieste;
- Research Area of Trieste;
- Economy University 'Bocconi', Milan.

Research activities are related both to the evaluation of PACS technology and to the development of the PACS already installed.

The main topics covered by these research activities are the following:
- analysis of the organization of the radiology departments;
- analysis of the work volumes;
- clinical evaluations;
- technical evaluations;
- economic evaluations;
- development of a RIS/PACS interface;
- integration of PACS in the Hospital LAN;
- connection to Trieste Metropolitan Area Network (MAN).

Some of these research activities are developed in the framework of national and European projects:
- advanced informatics in medicine (A.I.M.): Research Project A 1030;
- concerted action on bio-medical equipment (COMAC-BME): integrated systems for computer assisted management and manipulations of medical images (ISCAMI);
- Italian Ministry of Health, Department for Health Planning: PACS technology assessment project.

The main results of the research activity have been presented in the scientific literature (Bravar et al., 1987; Giribona et al., 1989; Ukovich et al., 1989; Bouillier et al., 1990; Dalla Palma et al., 1990a; Ukovich et al., 1990) and can be summarized as follows.

3.1. Analysis of the organization of radiology departments

In order to evaluate the impact of PACS in a radiology department, a general model of the radiology system has been developed using the IDEF0 technique (Bravoco and Yadav, 1985a,b). Functions, actions and flows affected by PACS have been identified. Quantitative evaluations have been carried out in order to compare PACS and non-PACS situations.

In particular times for consecutive activities of the image flow (from image acquisition to archiving) were collected: the results show that for this class of operations the most relevant improvements in productivity and use of resources could be rather achieved from an adequate management of the operations than from simply transferring them to a new technology. Nevertheless, the mere availability of such technologies may trigger a rationalization of the existing procedures.

3.2. Analysis of work volumes

Static and dynamic work volumes have been analyzed in order to quantify the amount of data generated by the diagnostic imaging activity. Global data (on yearly basis) have been collected over a period of five years (1985 – 1989) in order to estimate the first-order approximation of the archival system requirement.

Furthermore, data have been collected during a period of some weeks and a dynamic description of the image generation process during an average weekday has been obtained. Preliminary results show that in a medium-sized radiology department (100 000 procedures/year) uncompressed data peak rates rise up to 1.27 Mbps.

3.3. Clinical evaluations

Some experiments of comparison of diagnostic efficacy on CRT screen versus conventional film have been carried out by a group of four radiologists on CT cases (100 brain CTs, 100 spine CTs, 2 observations of the same case with a time interval of 1 month).

The results of tests pointed out the relevance of reporting experience of the radiologist on CRT-based systems (and, as a consequence, the need of an adequate training). A substantial equivalence of film and PACS as far as diagnostic efficacy is concerned has been demonstrated by the tests carried out. However, reporting times were longer because of the low system speed.

3.4. Technical evaluations

Technical evaluations are mainly addressed to the analysis of workstation performances.

Some computer-generated images and test patterns have been developed in order to evaluate the contrast – detail perception curve of diagnostic workstations and of remote low-cost viewing stations.

A protocol for a complete performance evaluation (image quality, image management capability, response times, etc.) is under development and experiences and results will be shared in the framework of the ISCAMI concerted action.

3.5. Economic evaluation

An economic evaluation of PACS technology has been carried out in cooperation with the Bocconi Economic University of Milan in the framework of A.I.M. Research Project A1030.

Cost items connected to the introduction of PACS in a health care institution have been determined and quantified. About 25 cost items have been analyzed covering six cost areas:
– costs of the technology;
– costs of acquisition;
– related costs;
– operational costs;
– personnel costs;
– savings.

Furthermore, a new approach in the economic evaluation of PACS has been proposed trying to assess the feasibility of the 'PACS choice' for an health institution not only on the basis of monetary evaluations but also analyzing non-monetary issues that can justify the very large investment related to PACS acquisition (i.e., strategic relevance, improvement of management, improvement of operational activities, improvement of institution's prestige, etc.).

3.6. Integration of PACS in hospital environment

In order to proceed torwards the direction of a full integration of PACS within the existing hospital information system facilities, a RIS/PACS interface has been developed. The interface allows a one-way data communication (RIS to PACS) through an asynchronous line with ACR-NEMA protocol (ACR-NEMA, 1989).

By means of an Ethernet gateway, the PACS has been connected to the fiber-optic Ethernet LAN which connects all the hospital departments, potentially allowing the distribution of images in the whole hospital.

Furthermore, LAN translators have been installed connecting the Ethernet hospital LAN to the geographic data network. Dedicated and switched 64 kbps lines, provided by the national telephone company (SIP), have been experimented in order to evaluate their applicability to diagnostic image distribution in the Trieste metropolitan area.

4. Impact of PACS in the clinical practice

Different groups of people are involved in handling medical images using modern technology (radiologists, physicians, engineers, administrators, legislators and even politicians). However, each group has established different perceptions and patterns of thinking when comparing issues relating to computer and communication technology in medicine (Lemke, 1989). Interrelating and collating these perceptions is a difficult task.

From the radiological point of view, it is possible to assess the impact of PAC systems on the clinical practice on the basis of the four years experience with PACS of the Trieste site.

There are four broad areas to be considered relating to the implementation of PACS throughout a hospital: technology, diagnostic accuracy, organization of a radiology department (RD), impact on hospital design and practices (Glass, 1989).

We have focused on the impact of PACS on the organization of RDs, with minor attention to technical problems. The following steps have been approached:

– analysis of the 'manual' (pre-PACS) organisation structure of the RD;
– analysis of the actual impact of PACS.

4.1. Analysis of the 'manual' (pre-PACS) organization structure of the RD

This analysis has involved:
(a) the identification of the significant activities and of their functional relations;
(b) a quantitative analysis of each activity, with special emphasis on resources and time sequences and/or durations.

These features were already analyzed in details in previous papers (Ukovich et al., 1989; Dalla Palma et al., 1990b; Ukovich et al., 1990). The interested reader is referred to them. However, the relevance of this analysis must be stressed, for two reasons.

First, it allowed to identify the bottlenecks among the radiological activities, and then possibly to improve the organization, without PACS.

For example, Mun et al. (1988a) reported a mean time between typing and report signing of 3.2 days. We experienced long delays as well. Therefore in our department the radiologist who is on duty during the night presently signs his colleagues' reports. This implies that images and reports are now available for delivering in the early morning of the day following the procedure. This is a result of an organizational change following a baseline study in the department, before PACS.

Secondly, it allows to forecast the actual impact of PACS in different RDs.

For example, the number of times the retrieval of old radiological examinations was successful changes remarkably in different RDs. Retrieval was not successful in 243/417 (59%) requests according to Hedgcock Jr. and Kehr (1989), in 84/826 (10%) according to Mun et al. (1988a), and in 11/280 (4%) according to ter Haar Romeny et al. (1989). In our experience previous exams were required in 81/434 (19%) patients referred for US, CT or MR and retrieval was unsuccessful in 10 of them (10/81 = 12%; 10/434 = 2%). These percentages can be expected to be reduced with PACS and of course the impact of the system will be much greater where retrieval is a major problem.

4.2. Analysis of the actual impact of PACS

A simplified model of the radiological process consists of five stages:
– preparation (patient identification, scheduling, radiological chart and previous images retrieval);
– image acquisition;
– reporting;
– communication of diagnosis;
– archiving.

PACS was expected to influence three of these stages above all (preparation, communication of diagnosis, archiving). Some data available from other sites and from our actual experience in this regard will be discussed.

4.2.1. Preparation

PACS is involved in the final part of the preparation only, i.e., previous images retrieval. PACS allowed to reduce the percentage of unsuccessful old examinations retrieval up to 1% (Choyke et al., 1985). Human errors (i.e., typing of data) account for the remaining number of cases that cannot be found.

In our experience, radiologists looked for previous digital exams at the display workstation 60 times during a period of 6 months (i.e., about once every 2 days). However, we estimated that such search is required about 9 times a day: the present lack of a long-term archive on the juke box and the effectiveness of the manual ongoing procedure explain this difference. Retrieval times with PACS are very short. In our experience the retrieval of one case from the temporary or from the permanent archive (juke box) takes 1'45'' and 3'30'', respectively.

The integration with the radiological information system (RIS) is very useful, because it allows a common management of the archives.

4.2.2. Image acquisition
This is not affected by PACS.

4.2.3. Reporting
We monitored a set of brain and spine CT cases in order to reveal different performances in the diagnostic process and conclusions using the PACS viewing console versus conventional CRT film images on alternators. We concluded (Dalla Palma et al., 1990a,c) that the image quality provided by the PACS was adequate for routine CT reporting. The opportunity of an adequate training period on the PACS monitor was stressed. Moreover the effectiveness of the image processing facilities of PACS was appreciated.

However, reporting times turned out to be significantly increased (20 – 30%), mainly due to the low speed of the system in retrieving the requested images. This feature prevented routing reporting on the PACS monitor.

4.2.4. Communication of diagnosis
Three methods are commonly used for communication of the procedure diagnosis to the referring physician: written reports, unscheduled consulting (phone or in person), and scheduled clinical radiological meetings (Taira et al., 1989). PACS is expected to influence the first two methods above all.

As to the distribution of images and written reports to the departments within the hospital, PACS can provide appealing solutions with the location of workstations in the departments, thus allowing an almost instantaneous availability of images and of the reports as well, when approved. However, extensive studies were not carried out (De Simone et al., 1988; Horii and Mun, 1989; ter Haar Romeny et al., 1989): workstations were located in a few departments (intensive care units above all) and could alter patterns of communication between the radiologist and the referring physicians: in fact, according to De Simone et al. (1988), images were viewed without a radiologist's interpretation only 5% of the time before PACS installation but this percentage raised to 40% when the workstation became available.

We feel that the possibility of loosing the relationship with the clinicians is an actual danger and therefore images should be available when the report is approved only. Again the effectiveness of the system is limited by reporting and typing times. Moreover we feel that selected cases should become available only following a consultation to perform a clinically oriented diagnosis.

As to unscheduled consulting, in our experience the immediate availability of images was perceived as a distinct advantage of the system, when referring clinicians reached the RD for informations on previous digital examinations.

The impact of PACS on the distribution process should allow a reduction of films consumption. Definite savings are expected because a limited number of images can be reproduced and because extra copies are not needed (Chiesa et al., 1990).

However, in our experience the film consumption was not reduced for some reasons. First, a video output for hard copies was not available in our system until September, 1991, and then it was not possible to photograph selected images. Moreover a wide distribution of workstations in the departments should be carried out. Finally, film will continue to be an optimal tool for diagnosis communications of outpatients.

4.2.5. Archiving

A definite reduction of the archive size can be achieved with PACS. The size of our juke box, comprising 89 optical disks, 2 Gbytes each, and the management system, is $1.90 \times 0.83 \times 2.05$ m. About 700 000 digital images can be stored in it. The size of the corresponding traditional archive is about 53 linear meters. However, it should be stressed that presently the two archives coexist, because the distribution of images to hospital wards is still film-based. This is the key factor that presently prevents the shifting to the digital archive alone. As a consequence costs do not decrease but are even higher. A reduction of personnel devoted to archiving can be achieved too, but considerations about the present coexistence of the two archives apply to this issue as well.

In the Trieste PACS project we faced several limits of the system, such as: operational overhead, slow image presentation, operational complexity of some functions, no video output from the workstation, a closed commercial system to work with.

Moreover an economic justification of PACS was hard to achieve until now: costs for a global PACS seem to be ten times higher then savings and only a shorter length of the hospitalization stay could overcome this problem (Andriessen et al., 1989).

Presently, we face large investment costs, personnel costs (one full-time unit) and material costs (one optical disk every 15 days). No savings were registered.

However, a PACS offers definite advantages such as a quicker and more efficient retrieval of old examinations, the reduction of archive size and of devoted personnel, a more efficient communication within the RD.

5. Future

None of the PAC systems to date has claimed to be fully usable on the department level (Baumann, 1989). It means that there are only 'partial' PACS available on the market. However, it must be pointed out that now those partial systems may be more attractive from a financial point of view (Mun et al., 1987; Chiesa et al., 1990).

Therefore, even if PACS are said to offer several advantages over the traditional organization of RDs (Cannavo, 1988a,b), many of these advantages should be considered as potential at the moment, such as the reduction of hospital costs, the reduction of films consumption, and a more efficient communication within the hospital.

As PAC systems mature technologically, benefits will become clearer and it will be possible to do careful assessments. However, it seems clear that PACS represent the future of radiology and medical imaging, and their introduction in the hospital environment in the next few years will be unavoidable (Mun and Benson, 1987; Van Beekum and Banta, 1987; Mun et al., 1988b).

However, some fundamental requirements for the development of PACS have been identified:
− systems must be 'open';
− systems must suit needs of different users;
− systems must be integrated with the radiological information system (RIS) and the hospital information system (HIS).

As to the PACS project in Trieste, we are forecasting the following developments.
− Reporting: faster DWs have already been achieved and therefore the main drawback of this function could be overcome, thus allowing routine reporting of digital modalities at the DW.
− Archiving: since 1991 a video output from the DW for hard copies is available, progressively allowing the archiving of images from digital modalities on optical disks only, thus avoiding the coexistence of two archives, at least for digital modalities.
− Communication within the hospital: the PACS has already been connected to the fiber optic Ethernet LAN that connects all the hospital departments. We plan a gradual connection, beginning with two departments with a low rate of requests for digital modalities, then moving to the connection of other departments with higher rates, such as neurosurgery and abdominal surgery. The relationship with physicians is a key factor for us: therefore we plan to deliver images and reports of cases which don't require consultation. The latter ones (about 10% of the cases) should be available for transmission only following a clinical radiological meeting. Moreover we planned connections between Radiology and Pathology and between Radiology and one operating theatre. The availability of radiological images will provide a guide to pathologists performing necroscopies. On the other hand the availability of specimen images will improve the understanding of radiological images. Clinical and teaching advantages are obvious. Same concepts apply to the connection between Radiology and one operating

theatre. Moreover in such cases the availability of three-dimensional images will allow tailored surgical approaches.

– Communication with other hospitals: LAN translators have been installed connecting the Ethernet hospital LAN to the geographic data network, with the aim of connecting all the hospitals of the Trieste area on the same network and of implementing a common archive for digital modalities.

In conclusion the PACS experimentation in the Hospital of Trieste through the collection of data concerning clinical technical, organizational and economic aspects represents the first step for the definition of a reasonable strategy at a national level for the introduction of PACS in Italy.

References

ACR-NEMA Publication 300-1988 (1989) Digital Imaging and Communication (NEMA, Washington D.C.).

Andriessen, J.H.T.H., B.M. Ter Haar Romeny, F.H. Barneveld Binkhuysen and I.E. Van Der Horst-Bruinsma (1989) Savings and costs of a picture archiving and communication system in the University Hospital Utrecht. In: Schneider, R.H., S.J. Dwyer III and R.G. Jost (Eds.), Medical Imaging III: PACS System Design and Evaluation, *Proc. SPIE* 1093, 578–584.

Baumann, R.A. (1989) Possible social implication of PACS on radiology in the United States. In: Lemke, H.U., M.L. Rhodes, C.C. Jaffe and Felix R. (Eds.), Computer Assisted Radiology (Springer, Berlin), pp. 833–839.

Boullier, D., J. de Certaines, M. del Vecchio and P. Giribona (1990) PACS technology assessment on pilot sites, Commission of the European Communities, A.I.M. Project A-1030, W.P. 1040 Final Report.

Bravar, D., et al. (1987) Costi ed attivita' di alcuni servizi di radiodiagnostica, Rapporti Finali AC-MAGEST, Consiglio Nazionale delle Ricerche, Roma.

Bravoco, R.R., and S.B. Yadav (1985a) Requirement definition architecture – an overview, *Computers in Industry* 6, 237.

Bravoco, R.R., and S.B. Yadav (1985b) A methodology to model the functional structure of an organization, *Computers in Industry* 6, 345.

Cannavo, M.J. (1988a) Low-risk strategy for PACS calls for modular phase-in, *Diagn. Imaging* 7, 135–140.

Cannavo, M.J. (1988b) Fitting the PACS technology into the hospital of tomorrow, *Diagn. Imaging* 10, 188–190.

Chiesa, A., G. Battaglia, G. Moscatelli and R. Maroldi (1990) Economic justification of a 'partial PACS', Abstracts 8th EuroPACS Meeting, Trieste, May 3–4.

Choyke, P.L., S.K. Mun, H. Benson, P. Wang and F. Fahey (1985) Reliability issues in digital image archiving. In: *Proc. SPIE* 536, 21–25.

Dalla Palma, L., W. Ukovich, R. Cuttin-Zernich, P. Giribona and F. Stacul (1990a) The Trieste PACS project: one year experience. In: Schneider, G.H., E. Vogler and K. Kocever (Eds.), Digitale Bildgebung, Interventionelle Radiologie, Integrierte Digitale Radiologie (Blackwell, Berlin), pp. 541–546.

Dalla Palma, L., W. Ukovich, F. Stacul, R. Cuttin-Zernich, N. Carbi and P. Giribona (1990b) Sistema PACS a progetto modulare. Esperienza operativa preliminare, *Radiol. Med.* 80, 9–17.

Dalla Palma, L., W. Ukovich, F. Stacul, R. Cuttin-Zernich, R.S. Pozzi Mucelli, S. Magnaldi, P. Cassetti, N. Carbi and P. Giribona (1990c) Sistema PACS a progetto modulare. Esperienza clinica preliminare, *Radiol. Med.* 80, 18 – 23.

De Simone, D., H.L. Kundel, R.L. Arenson and S.B. Seshadri (1988) The effect of a digital imaging network on physician consultations. In: Chiesa, A., R. Gasparotti and R. Maroldi (Eds.), Planning Considerations in Diagnostic Imaging and Radiation Therapy (Clas International, Brescia), pp. 231 – 234.

Giribona, P., D. Bravar, C. Giuricin, N. Carbi, R. Cuttin, L. Dalla Palma, F. Stacul and W. Ukovich (1989) A global project for the assessment of a PACS system, Proc. of the Annual International Conference of the IEEE Engin. in Med. and Biol. Society, Seattle WA, 789 – 790.

Glass, H. (1989) The impact of PACS on hospital information and practice. In: Schneider, R.H., S.J. Dwyer III and R.G. Jost (Eds.), Medical Imaging III: PACS System Design and Evaluation, *Proc. SPIE* 1093, 354 – 361.

Greinacher, C.F.C. (1988) System architecture and functionality of the structured Siemens PACS. In: Chiesa, A., R. Gasparotti and R. Maroldi (Eds.), Planning Considerations in Diagnostic Imaging and Radiation Therapy (Clas International, Brescia), pp. 212 – 224.

Hedgcock Jr., M.W., and K. Kehr (1989) Assessing the impact of computed radiography and PACS. In: Schneider, R.H., S.J. Dwyer III and R.G. Jost (Eds.), Medical Imaging III: PACS System Design and Evaluation, *Proc. SPIE* 1093, 558 – 562.

Horii, S., and S.K. Mun (1989) Radiology operations with a large scale diagnostic network, Abstracts 7th EuroPACS Conference, Brussels, March 6 – 7.

Lemke, H.U. (1989) Imaging, communication and perceptions. In: Lemke, H.U., M.L. Rhodes, C.C. Jaffe and R. Felix (Eds.), Computer Assisted Radiology (Springer, Berlin), pp. 793 – 798.

Mun, S.K., and H.R. Benson (1987) Fast-paced progress in computers ensures feasibility of PACS, *Diagn. Imaging* 4, 106 – 116.

Mun, S.K., D. Stauffer, P. Choyke, H. Benson and R. Zeman (1987) PACS workstation, Invited manuscript to AAPM Summer School, Digital image processing and PACS, Ann Arbor, Michigan.

Mun, S.K., H. Benson, C. Welsh, L.P. Elliot and W. Davros (1988a) Baseline study of radiology services for the purpose of PACS evaluation. In: Elliot, L.P., and S.K. Mun (Eds.), Progress Report, Digital Imaging Network Project, Selected paper, March.

Mun, S.K., L.P. Elliot and H.R. Benson (1988b) Development and operational evaluation of PACS network at Georgetown University, Progress report, Georgetown University, Washington D.C.

Taira, R.K., P.S. Cho, H.K. Huang, N.J. Mankovich and M.I. Boechat (1989) Performance evaluation of a clinical PACS module. In: Schneider, R.H., S.J. Dwyer III and R.G. Jost (Eds.), Medical Imaging III: PACS System Design and Evaluation, *Proc. SPIE* 1093, 406 – 415.

ter Haar Romeny, B.M., J.M.M. Van Der Wielen, A.J. Achterberg, F.H. Barneveld Binkhuysen, K.J. Zuiderveld, J.H.T.H. Andriessen and A.R. Bakker (1989) PACS efficiency: a detailed quantitative study of the distribution process of films in a clinical environment in the Utrecht University Hospital. In: Schneider, R.H., S.J. Dwyer III and R.G. Jost (Eds.), Medical Imaging III: PACS System Design and Evaluation, *Proc. SPIE* 1093, 259 – 271.

Ukovich, W., D. Bravar, R. Cuttin-Zernich, P. Giribona, M. Maffessanti, F. Stacul and L. Dalla Palma (1989) An experimental evaluation of the impact of a PAC System on the operations of radiology department. In: Lemke, H.U., M.L. Rhodes, C.C. Jaffe and R. Felix (Eds.), Computer Assisted Radiology (Springer, Berlin), pp. 537 – 540.

Ukovich, W., D. Bravar, N. Carbi, R. Cuttin-Zernich, P. Giribona, F. Stacul and L. Dalla Palma (1990) Trieste PACS project: a functional assessment, *Med. Inform.* 15, 31 – 37.

van Beekum, W.T., and H.D. Banta (1987) Policy implications of picture archiving and communication systems, *Proc. Documed Europe 87, Amsterdam*, 827 – 835.

Integrated Diagnostic Imaging
Editor: J.P.J. De Valk
© *Elsevier Science Publishers B.V., 1992*

Chapter 12

Integrated diagnostic imaging: digital PACS in medicine 1980 – 2000

R. Maroldi, G. Battaglia, G.L. Moscatelli and A. Chiesa

1. Introduction and definitions

To look at the state of art of picture archiving and communication systems (PACS) in 1991 is like being in the middle of a river ford; the starting edge is far away, the crossing has been long, nevertheless the target looks quite easy to reach.

Why this metaphor? The edges represent two different ways of conceiving the diagnostic imaging department: one relying on conventional radiological techniques (and therefore on films as display and storage media), the other based on digital imaging, where information and images are shown on video displays and where data are stored on electronic media.

Up to now the path between the two edges was difficult and complex, therefore some people were skeptical on judging PACSs feasibility. On the other hand, all indications coming from informatics and medical industry show PACS as an evolution in the management of radiological activities. These indications are quite important, since PACS' concept begins as a direct consequence of present development of informatics and digital imaging. In fact, the need of dealing with an increasing volume of digital images produced by new diagnostic procedures has led to the idea of PACS (table 1). During the 1980s, these procedures acquired a more and more significant clinical role, and gradually became a substantial share of radiological activity.

Up to date, PACS are still in an evolutionary stage; proof of this evolution are several complex problems, which have not yet been solved in both technological and economical aspects. Some problems which arose at the beginning of the 1980s, are solved today through the changes of informatics (such as reproduction of digital images by laser camera and storage on optical discs); moreover, some PACS aspects, thought to be relevant at the beginning, have

Table 1
Definitions.

PACS (picture archiving and communication system) is an interconnected computer network that
   interfaces with existing diagnostic imaging units to acquire, process, display and store digital images as an alternative to film.
Partial PACS encompasses only the digital imaging modalities − computed tomography, magnetic
   resonance, digital subtraction angiography, computed radiography, ultrasound and nuclear
   medicine.
Total PACS encompasses not only the digital units but also the analog imaging modalities −
   radiography and fluoroscopy.
IMACS (image management and communication system) encompasses local and long-distance
   teleradiology, digital image archives, computer-based radiology education, consolidation of image display capabilities for digital imaging devices, radiology information systems, and filmless
   image management networks.

been gradually postponed to the future (e.g., digital image processing). On the
other hand, even today not anybody justifies an introduction of PACS based
only on diagnostic or managerial advantages which these systems could produce.

During the 1980s, the research concerning PACS was focused on complex
technical problems and one was worried for the impact of these systems on activity and people involved with radiology. On the other hand, very little attention was given to the real need for the attending physicians to access the
radiological information. For this reason, today, the integration between PACS
and hospital information systems (HIS) is a must for the clinical acceptance of
any system. Therefore, the PACS concept actually covers a wide area which
deals with the management of images and of clinical data (IMACS) (table 1).

In the effort to foresee the near future of image storage and management
systems, there is a need − in our opinion − for a very careful analysis of papers
on PACS written during the last decade.

By means of such an analysis it is possible to identify some 'frontier centres'
where pilot projects are tested and implemented.

Since the analysis of PACS literature in the 1980s shows that there are well
defined and continuous trends (fig. 1), it is possible to foresee the next PACS
developments through the extrapolation of present figures and the evolution of
digital technologies.

2. PACS 1980 – 1990

PACS was born in the beginning of the 1980s. During this decade, radiologists,

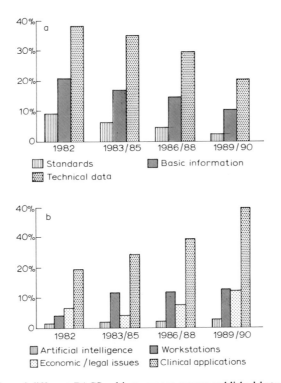

Fig. 1. Distribution of different PACS subjects among papers published between 1980 – 1990.

Table 2
Surveyed papers on PACS.

Period	Surveyed papers
1980 – 1982	82
1983 – 1985	76
1986 – 1988	77
1989 – 1990	183
Total 1980 – 1990	418

medical/clinical physicists, manufacturers and informaticians were showing great interest in PACS.

In order to analyze the state of the art and the trends of PACS, a revision was carried out on more than 400 articles published between 1980 and 1990. The information was obtained from some specialized reference sources (SPIE,

CAR, SCAR, ISPRAD) and from articles published in radiological journals
(Radiology, Am. J. Roentgen., J. Digital Imaging, etc.).

The analysis of the chronological distribution of these references reveals that
the number of papers was quite constant during the periods 1980 – 1982,
1983 – 1985 and 1986 – 1988 (table 2).

In accordance with this analysis, it is possible to identify some centres which
are more active in studying and testing PACS systems; these centres are belonging to universities, to equipment manufacturers, or to informatics companies;
some of them derive from a direct co-operation between university and industry
(tables 3, 4, 5).

Only three out of 14 of these centres have their main activity in Europe
(Bazis, Philips and Siemens); the major projects in the universities are still
North American.

2.1. PACS issues

In order to evaluate the development of PACS during the 1980s, the papers
were grouped in seven categories (table 6) each of them considered as an 'in-

Table 3

Most active research groups on PACS

Research groups	Number of papers
Univ. of Washington and Georgetown Univ.	22
Univ. of California/Los Angeles	12
Univ. of Ottawa	9
Univ. of Pennsylvania, Philadelphia	8
Mallinckrodt Inst. of Radiology, St.Louis	8
Univ. of Utah, Salt Lake City	8
Univ. of North Carolina, Chapel Hill	6
Univ. of California/S.Francisco	6
Univ. of Pittsburgh	5

Table 4

Manufacturers involved with PACS clinical research.

Companies	Number of papers
AT&T	19
Siemens	16
Philips	11
IBM	5

Table 5
Main cooperations manufacturer/university.

Research groups	Number of papers
AT&T and Georgetown Univ.	29
Philips and Bazis/Utrecht Univ. Hospital	19

dicator' suitable to prove the interest of different 'pilot centres' towards specific aspects and problems of PACS. These 'indicators', on the other hand, point out significant steps of PACS evolution, from the theoretical starting phase to the clinical application phase.

2.1.1. The starting phase
The leading papers at the initial phase of PACS are based mainly on technical and preliminary aspects; particular emphasis is given to standardization and communication problems. In the early 1980s, since these subjects represent 60% of all studies, it is clear that they are characterizing an approaching phase (table 6). At the end of the 1980s, on the other hand, there exists a phase of increased clinical applications, and the above percentage is reduced to 30%.

2.1.1.1. PACS solutions. At the beginning of the 1980s, several centres foresee a PACS which could share some common features: the system is presented as a global solution to the radiological imaging management and is economically justified mainly by reducing film-production and film-archiving costs.

Later in the decade, because of the complex economic, technological and organization problems of PACS, a new proposal becomes popular; this proposal is based on a modular approach, which gradually overtakes the conven-

Table 6
Distribution of different papers according to the subject and to the time of publication.

Subject	1980 – 1982	1983 – 1985	1986 – 1988	1989 – 1990
Basic information	20.9%	17.1%	14.6%	10.3%
Technical data	38.3%	35.1%	29.9%	20.2%
Standards	9.0%	5.9%	4.3%	2.3%
Workstations	4.2%	11.7%	12.0%	13.1%
Clinical application	19.4%	24.3%	29.6%	39.8%
Economic/legal issues	6.7%	4.1%	7.4%	11.6%
Artificial intelligence	1.5%	1.8%	2.2%	2.7%

tional (analog) imaging modalities. The present trend of PACS tries to develop a system which could integrate radiological activities in a wider context, through a PACS/RIS/HIS interface. This solution has the advantage of improving radiological activity's efficiency (waiting-time reduction and improvements of communication speed).

2.1.1.2. Technological aspects. In the early 1980s, the main emphasis was on technological aspects (storage devices, communication media, image reproduction and processing systems, etc.). Later in the 1980s, these aspects are slowly and continuously disregarded or modified. The criticisms and the discussion limited, at first, to the devices to be utilized (optical discs, optical fibres, displays), move later on how these devices could be integrated (databases architecture, networking).

In PACS technology, many problems modify their consistence and some others are completely solved, e.g., the digital images reproduction by means of laser cameras.

2.1.1.3. Standards. The debate on standards (message formats and protocols for transmission of data and images among compatible equipment) was fo-

Table 7
Characterization and change of sessions content at 'SPIE-PACS' meetings.

1982	1990
1. Introduction to PACS	1. PACS issues
2. Picture archiving devices	2. Systems and components
3. Picture communication	3. High-resolution displays
4. Architectures for PACS	4. Network issues
5. Teleradiology	5. Image filling and retrieval schemes
6. Hard and soft pictures	6. Hardware and software issues
7. Digital images acquisition	7. PACS workstations
8. Standardisation of PACS	8. Interfaces: man and machine
9. Prototype PACS	9. Clinical evaluation of PACS
10. Picture archiving systems	10. PACS experience I
11. The need for PACS in medical imaging	11. PACS experience II
12. Legal, human and marketing aspects of PACS	12. PACS experience at the University of Pittsburgh
	13. Planning, expectation and image evaluation for PACS at the University of Iowa
	14. Siemens experience with PACS
	15. Implementation experiences of the CommView System PACS applications

cused, at first, on the need of defining these standards; later on, a standard was chosen (the ACR-NEMA and SPIE standard), and it was more or less accepted by many manufacturers. The general interest on the standards was rapidly reducing, during the decade, with a prevalent contribution of the manufacturers.

2.1.2. Present phase

The present status of PACS (1989 – 1991) is characterized by a growing interest for implementing prototype systems and their clinical application (nearly 40% of papers surveyed) (tables 6, 7).

More than 30 centres are involved in the clinical application of different PACS, most of them in the U.S.A., only part of them in Europe and Japan. These clinical trials mostly arise from cooperation between universities and medical manufacturers.

Most of the studies are still involved with the technical engineering of the different prototypes and their activation modalities. At the present stage, PACS can be considered in the initial clinical phase, an important issue, in this step, is the integration of the different components of PACS, i.e., databases, local area networks, workstations, interfaces with RIS and HIS.

Many of the preliminary experiences come from projects of 'partial PACS'. This solution is generally considered as the most convenient in order to develop and test the most suitable solutions towards a total digital department. A partial PACS is certainly a compromise which does not allow to obtain all the advantages of 'total PACS'. However, it is the only option economically feasible today.

2.1.2.1. PACS/RIS/HIS integration.

The present research on databases is focused on obtaining differentiated storage devices (with major or minor capacity and access rate) and on the possibility to integrate PACS in intelligent networks. An intelligent network should be able to automatically perform some operations (such as the retrieval of clinical data and images of a patient) under the supervision of expert systems. This solution improves the efficiency of PACS and therefore increases their clinical acceptance because intelligent networks can be used not only within the diagnostic imaging department but also with and within other hospital departments.

The integration factor – an 'intelligent link' between PACS, RIS and HIS – appears to be one of the key points for developing IMACS, where the network of the diagnostic imaging department is a part of the global communication system within the hospital. In this view all the advantages of PACS will be available to every user of the information network. The improvements obtained can be so relevant that the high costs inherent to PACS could be justified.

For this reason it is quite important – especially in the phase of PACS projects implementation – that the specific needs of radiological information (images and data) of the different referring physicians could be evaluated. Data obtained from our survey show that the need of diagnostic images can be divided into two subsets: highly specialized departments (neurosurgery, heart surgery, etc.) mostly demand the visualization of digital images (with low-resolution matrix); not specialized departments, on the other hand, still require a great number of conventional analog images (high-resolution digitized images). For this reason, it is possible to foresee a system where departmental displays have different resolution power (and different cost) according to the real need of the department.

2.1.2.2. Workstations. The increasing clinical use of PACS has developed a large interest for all technological and design characteristics of the workstations. Workstations are, in fact, the real interface – the physician's window to PACS – between the system and the radiologist. It has been stated that the only way for PACS to be successful is that the primary interpretation performed by the radiologist should be done at the workstation, if resolution is sufficient ($\geq 2 \text{ K} \times 2 \text{ K}$). At present, this activity is very time consuming. The reasons are essentially two: it takes too much time to retrieve images from the database and to complete the radiological report.

The first problem could be solved with the introduction of larger memories and communications systems based on optic fibres. The second problem will be probably solved by means of voice recognition devices.

Highly sophisticated programs for image processing and three-dimensional reconstruction should be limited to dedicated workstations for orthopedic or facial surgery.

2.1.2.3. The economic justification. During the last decade one of the main problems was the high cost of PACS. This aspect is still particularly important. During the survey of the reference papers, a similarity was observed between papers dealing with the technological problems of the early 1980s and papers dealing with the present economic issues. All of them emphasize some particular and restricted aspects of problems, probably because we are still in the phase where there are no global solutions to meet the economic implications of PACS.

However, this specific issue of PACS gained an increasing interest in the last years from several researchers.

3. PACS 1990 – 2000

During the 1980s the most important question on PACS was about its technology: 'Will all technical instruments and systems be able to control and work out digital images (LANs, databases, workstations, etc.)?'

At the beginning of the next decade, the most important question is different: 'Is it worthwhile to realize PACS?' This question can be answered in different ways.

3.1. The answer of people who already have PACS

All people who are using PACS are somehow convinced of its usefulness. The same people, nevertheless, are not convinced that these systems will diffuse in the near future. This consideration is particularly important because these people are directly involved in clinical research and are using PACS of different manufacturers.

3.2. The answer of people who have not yet PACS

The answer of radiologists who do not have PACS is quite different. In fact, these people do not conceive these systems as an expensive proprietary solution settled in the department from outside, but as a system that has to be integrated into the department from a free market where the best solution can be chosen.

This hypothesis is based on the previous experience of many office automation implementations, where only compatible hardware and software products succeeded.

Such a scenario may be considered possible because of the explosion of production, acquisition and management of medical data. This trend will force administrators to create high-speed communication networks that could allow fast retrieval of archived data and images. In this view PACS becomes only a part of the HIS. In this perspective the basic elements of PACS consists of networks, workstations and storage devices, while equipments that produce digital images have to be considered only peripheral devices. Many predictions about the future development of computers strengthens this hypothesis. Personal computers and workstations are becoming parts of one single entity. Both systems are becoming able to process different kinds of information (data, images, sound). Moreover, the computing power of these microprocessor based machines is constantly increasing, from 0.1 MIPS in the 1980s to 5 – 10 MIPS today. In the next decade, most probably, systems with 100 – 300 MIPS with RAMs upgraded to 8 – 16 Mbytes will be available (this feature will certainly improve graphic interfaces); this goal will be achieved by new multiprocessing technologies. The resolution capacity of the displays will also be improved. Particularly important will be the expansion of storage memories based on technological innovation of magnetic and optical hardware. This technology will allow reduced access times and larger memory capacities that will meet almost all the requirements of a total PACS at acceptable costs.

3.3. Future perspectives

From the comparison between the growth of PACS and that of office automation it is possible to extrapolate some considerations. The first consideration foresees that tomorrow computers in an imaging department should be able to exchange any type of information in standard code and to transmit it through the local hospital network.

Data and images obtained can consequently be processed by means of different softwares, according to the specific requirements of each diagnostic problem.

PACS are going to change dramatically their configuration from the experimental phase of the 1980s to the present clinical phase; in the meantime the unitary and proprietary concept evolves in the portable concept. At the present phase, therefore, it is desirable that the different groups working on the clinical validation of PACS could focus their interest on the extra-radiological application of systems rather than on an 'inward-directed' attraction to imaging technologies.

4. PACS here and now

The Department of Diagnostic Imaging at the University of Brescia was opened in 1984, therefore it is younger than PACS.

In these first years of operation, great interest had been in, and considerable efforts had been made for, the automation of procedures management. This effort had led to the realization of a RIS, evolving over the years into the present configuration.

The introduction and realization of a RIS allowed some well-known advantages, such as a better organization of the patient management and a reduction of the total time required for performing the whole radiological cycle.

A useful extension of the capabilities of a RIS is the possibility to access not only to the personal data of each patient or to the reports of his previous exams, but also to some of his archived images. Starting from this assumption, the first approach to the development of PACS at our institution has been the interfacing of a source of digital images (two ultrasound units) with the RIS.

In this solution, images are being considered similarly to a report, and are filed on optic discs together with the report.

The transition from RIS to PACS, according to our opinion, should be limited to the department of diagnostic imaging at this preliminary phase; only in a second phase it can be an extensive project of computerization within the hospital. This initial phase concerns predominantly technical characteristics (e.g., how to integrate data and images), while its broader extension is mostly concerned with clinical application.

At this moment we have not realized PACS, nor do we intend to develop one in the near future. Essentially this is due to economic and strategic reasons.

4.1. The economic reason

The total PACS and the partial PACS are not economically justified at this moment, nor regarding the reduction of costs of the radiologic films, nor regarding the shortening of the patient stay at the hospital. The main reasons of this negative cost/benefit evaluation can be attributed to the high costs of the 'proprietary systems' and to the prevalent utilization of PACS in a restricted hospital area, within the radiology departments.

4.2. The strategic reason

Currently, no system is available which could present all the requirements that we consider essential for the implementation of PACS at acceptable costs; e.g., PACS with elevated performances and with the possibility of upgrading it at low cost. These specifications identify, according to our opinion, PACS based on personal computers/workstations, capable of multiprocessing; these units will probably be available at acceptable costs by the end of the 1990s. It is our opinion, moreover, that the benefit of a system of acquisition, transmission, storage, and communication of radiological images and reports can not leave apart the distribution and the utilization of intelligent terminals at the different wards of the hospital.

Only in this second configuration, sufficient advantages can be obtained to justify the economic and organizing efforts which are needed for the realization of PACS.

Integrated Diagnostic Imaging
Editor: J.P.J. De Valk

Chapter 13

PACS as an infrastructural essential element in an advanced digital imaging department

Bart M. ter Haar Romeny and Frits H. Barneveld Binkhuysen

1. Introduction

Picture archiving and communication system (PACS) experiments were started enthusiastically on many sites over the world, but now we see as a general picture a more pragmatic stepwise approach towards a full-scale introduction. Lessons from the first experimental sites have learned that the requirements regarding image quality, speed and user-interface are not yet met for primary reading and daily clinical routine, that the capacity of storage and transmission lines is on the edge of what is available today, and that the complexity of the local logistic and procedural organization makes that a substantial investment in manpower and money is required for introduction of PACS. Sofar the money for the larger projects was in general supplied by governmental programs with substantial industrial on-site testing and developing. The number of full-scale installations is still small, however. Japan, taking the lead in their government-supported pilot-site in Sapporo, for example, has the advantage of having a different role of radiology, and a greater need for distribution of the images throughout the hospital without radiological review, and a less critical (in juridical sense) attitude towards image quality (and compression). This book gives many substantial accounts of the many important PACS studies all over the world. In the Netherlands, we learned much from the 'Dutch PACS project' (1986 – 1989), a collaboration of a large university hospital, a major electronics company, and a hospital information systems (HIS) developer/supplier, funded by the Dutch government.

Despite the initial complexity and high cost, the overall outcome from these projects regarding the usefulness of PACS, either towards the radiology department or towards the referring clinical wards, was throughout positive. A parallel trend of increasing quality and capacity with decreasing overall costs gave food to a deep trust that PACS is on its way and finally will be a similar infrastructural element in the distribution of (pictorial) information as is the HIS for the complementary data.

In the long run we will see that next to the basic storage and distributive *logistic* function of PACS, PACS will become *intelligent*. There is an enormous potential in the images being *digital* and the progress we see in the capacity of modern hardware and software. The advent of computer vision techniques, recognition based on neural networks, interactive three-dimensional display, etc. will result in highly sophisticated viewing stations. The clinical acceptance of these advanced techniques, and to focus these developments to real practical problems, is greatly stimulated and facilitated through the use of gateways between PACS and the research groups working in these areas.

This chapter focuses on two fields: the experience with the logistic aspects of PACS, as acquired in the Dutch PACS project (1986–1989); and the integrative aspects of PACS, related to the facilitation of advanced processing and visualization techniques, and the way we are working on this particular future. We will give many examples to illustrate this additional potential of PACS.

2. Experiences in the Dutch PACS project

During the period 1986–1989, the Dutch PACS project had been carried out (ter Haar Romeny et al., 1987; de Valk et al., 1988a,b; Ottes et al., 1990). This project had been financially supported by the Dutch Ministry of Health Care (WVC). The project was jointly performed by three partners:
- The Utrecht University Hospital (UUH).
- BAZIS, central development and support group HIS, Leiden.
- Philips Netherlands/Philips International B.V., product division medical systems.

The project had the objective to achieve a presentation of *integrated* information, i.e., *all* available images, new and old, coupled with other patient-data from the HIS/RIS (radiology information system).

Philips provided and maintained the prototype PACS equipment used in the clinical evaluation in the UUH. The clinical evaluation was rather unique because in daily clinical routine *all* images of *all* modalities (digital and conventional) were handled in a PACS for a 15-bed ward of internal medicine and intensive care units of cardiology (ten beds) and cardiosurgery (ten beds). This small number of patients was chosen to keep the storage capacity manageable, and to be able to focus on *completeness*. A coupling from this PACS to a HIS/RIS has been established, based on the ACR/NEMA standard and extensive research has been carried out on diagnostic image quality, user interface, modeling/simulation and technology assessment (de Valk et al., 1988a,b).

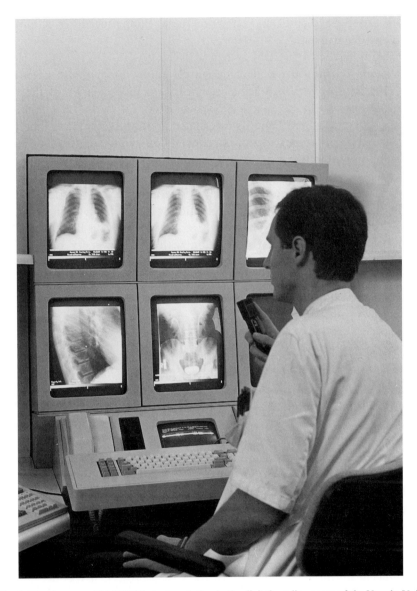

Fig. 1. The six-screen MARCOM viewing station in the digital reading room of the Utrecht University Hospital, as used in the Dutch PACS project.

2.1. Project design

Within the project a number of subprojects were accomplished:
- The clinical evaluation of the prototype Philips-PACS (called MARCOM, see fig. 1) in the UUH environment, in terms of user satisfaction, speed,

logistic benefits and costs, and effects on the working procedures within the radiology department.

– The linking of the MARCOM system with the BAZIS-HIS in the UUH by BAZIS and drafting the general design for future linking with a generic RIS/HIS. This project included a study of the standardization of file formats and interfaces.

– The modeling of a PACS and its use, aimed to allow performance analysis beforehand on different scales of implementation and to support the PACS design and construction process by computer modeling and simulation.

– Image quality studies: the analysis of the differences in diagnostic quality of identical series of images by 'receiver operating characteristic' (ROC) studies, presented under different conditions (1 K × 1 K viewing station, images scanned by video or laser-digitizer, versus film on lightbox). This problem was addressed in co-operation with the University of Arizona (Tucson). This study also included analysis of the user-interface of all workstations used.

– Technology assessment with respect to PACS in Dutch hospitals: cost – benefit analysis.

2.2. Findings and results

With the premature stage of PACS development at the beginning of the project in mind, it is no surprise that the project did not always develop as was expected. In December 1986, a digital viewing room was realized in the UUH (ter Haar Romeny et al., 1987). Soon after the installation of the Philips prototype equipment in this room, the first problems came up. The PACS technology appeared indeed still in its infancy. Not only did problems arise concerning reliability, it also appeared that the design of the PACS prototype had serious limitations. These limitations concerned the resolution and the accuracy of the images. Studies were carried out using the evaluation method and software developed for this purpose by BAZIS. The results showed that the diagnostic image accuracy of the prototype equipment was insufficient for primary diagnosis. Due to these findings and the fact that it was impossible to improve the equipment during the first phase of the PACS project, it was decided to shift the focus from the radiology department towards the referring departments.

During the period that PACS was used in clinical routine in the referring department of internal medicine (where a four-screen viewing station was placed), the initial skepticism of the physicians turned into a growing enthusiasm about the possibilities of PACS. Especially the fact that the results of new examinations are readily available and the presence of the patient's radiological history, including the radiological reports, was much appreciated. The permanent availability (24 hours/day, 7 days/week) of the images on the department itself, close to the patient, was especially appreciated because it facilitated discussion and consultancies about the patient, it was fast, no images were lost or had to be retrieved with much delay. The lower image resolution of 1 K × 1 K was sufficient for reference purposes, because the report from the radiologist was available with all images.

An analysis of the conventional, film-based working method within the UUH, based on accurate timing studies on 1000 patients in the PACS pilot, showed that some 25% of the old pictures that had to be viewed for reference in combination with the new images, were not easily traced for legitimate reasons, e.g., being somewhere in the reporting process, or being loaned (ter Haar Romeny et al., 1989). It could be derived that this caused a delay of, on average, 1.5 days, in the retrieval of these old images. In the case of a PACS, it might be possible to reduce this delay to several minutes, depending on the efficiency of the image management system.

All the images for the target group were digitized with a laser scanner, thus simulating computed radiography (or phosphor-stimulated luminescence radiography) which was at that time not available. Images were scanned within one hour after acquisition. The PACS pilot study was embedded within the organization of the radiological department.

The performance of the prototype equipment was, despite the efforts of Philips, insufficient. A potential possibility to use HIS data for a more efficient image management within the PACS could not be explored, because the required software was not available within the MARCOM system. At the end of the project Philips decided to discontinue the MARCOM line of PACS equipment, and to focus on the AT&T CommView family of PACS components.

The coupling between the Philips PACS and the BAZIS HIS in the UUH was realized as one of the world's first clinically fully operational systems (Lodder et al., 1989). A PC functioned as a protocol converter between PACS and HIS in order to implement the ACR/NEMA interface standard. The coupling is from HIS towards PACS. The patient identification from the HIS was used within MARCOM. The radiological reports and full radiological history were available on the MARCOM workstations. Although the appointment data of the radiology department were transferred to MARCOM, the software for management of the images in the database did not make use of this information to prefetch data, a necessary extension for proper speed requirements, as we found by manual simulation.

The working methods on a number of radiology departments were thoroughly analyzed (ter Haar Romeny et al., 1986, 1988). This analysis gave a good insight into the present handling of images, which formed a basis for

Table 1

Parties involved in the different phases of image handling in a hospital.

	Radiologists	Referring physicians	Hospital management	Patients	Health costs insurance	Technologists
Preparation	x	x		x	x	x
Acquisition	x					x
Reporting	x					
Communication	x	x				
Archiving	x	x	x	x		
Diagnostic effectiveness		x		x		
Therapeutic effectiveness		x		x		
Patient stay		x	x	x	x	

a simulation model. A special software package was developed by BAZIS to describe the entity relations and procedures by the different professionals and groups involved in the image handling (MIRACLES: medical image representation, archiving and communication learned from extensive simulation (Stut Jr et al., 1989a,b)). Several bottlenecks in the prototype PACS could be detected. This allowed for technical measures as well as measures concerning the organization, which limited the hampering effects.

For the systematical analysis of image quality software was developed that could support the set-up, realization and results of evaluation experiments. This package (FEASIBLE: feature evaluation and system inspection by logged experiments, MS-DOS compatible (Ottes et al., 1989)) is based on ROC analysis. Experiments based on CT (computed tomography), phantom thorax (Winter et al., 1989) and mammography studies showed that the accuracy of the prototype equipment with 1 K × 1 K resolution was insufficient for primary diagnosis.

Methods for compression were evaluated. This evaluation made use of CT images of the upper abdomen, provided by the Leiden University Hospital. The conclusion was that compression is possible up to a factor 20 for CT images of the upper abdomen. The interest in compression is decreasing, due to legal questions and the large computer capacity that is consumed by compression algorithms. Another drawback of datacompression is that digital manipulation of compressed images can lead to artifacts. We should wait for clarity in the legal field and special hardware and/or software that can support the algorithms. There are, however, good reversible algorithms available (i.e., the compressed data can be recovered into its original form without loss of information, e.g., Roos and Viergever, 1989).

It appeared from the image quality experiments that the convenience and 'performance' (in terms of speed) of the MARCOM system were still much less than those of the traditional lightbox. Reading the digital images on a monitor still takes far more time than evaluating films on lightboxes (Barneveld Binkhuysen et al., 1989).

Special attention was paid to the direct financial consequences (i.e., the costs and benefits) of the introduction of PACS in Dutch hospitals (Andriessen et al., 1989a,b; van Gennip et al., 1990; van Poppel et al., 1990) as part of the technology assessment (TA) study. An analysis of the available literature shows that opinions on the costs of PACS, as compared to the costs of the film-based system, differ greatly (van Gennip et al., 1990). According to Arenson (DeSimone et al., 1988; Arenson et al., 1989), a hospital-wide PACS would allow financial savings at this moment. Andriessen et al. (1989a,b), on the other hand, report that a hospital-wide PACS would now be three times as expensive as the film-based system. A cost model for PACS as compared to the traditional situation was set up (by BAZIS, available as PC software package;

CAPACITY: cost and critical analysis of picture archiving and communication indicating its true yield, Bakker et al., 1989; van Poppel et al., 1990). This model takes future price changes into account, which is of importance in cost analyses, as prices of PACS components are expected to fall. The model predicts the costs of PACS (as compared to the costs of the film-based system), depending on the moment of the introduction of PACS. The first results indicate that the break-even point, i.e., the moment the costs of PACS will equal those of the film-based system, is expected between 1995 and 2000. It is to be expected that using PACS will lead to quicker diagnoses and to an earlier start of the therapy. This will most probably lead to a shorter length of stay. This might be a substantial cost-saving factor, stimulating the discussion on what level PACS generates the most financial benefits.

2.3. Conclusions

In the referring department the use of this PACS prototype has, despite its still valid serious limitations, led to great enthusiasm. It appeared that offering *all* images through a workstation 24 hours/day, 7 days/week does indeed increase the speed and availability of images for the physicians. Also the fact that data from the HIS/RIS (report and full radiological history) were available together with the old and new images was highly appreciated.

We learned much from this project. In the sequel of this chapter, we will discuss the impact of PACS for the radiologist, *and* the impact of PACS on advanced imaging techniques, as well as the infrastructural role it has to play to enable/facilitate the many developments, which are separate today, but need integration to be fully exploited.

3. Impact of PACS from a radiologist's point of view

PACS is not restricted to radiologists or radiology departments, because PACS is part of a HIS and a management tool. Therefore, it is difficult to foresee what the impact of PACS will be in daily practice. From our own and other clinical experiences with PACS we try to oversee the impact of PACS on several phases of the radiological imaging process starting from the preparation of a radiological procedure to the effects of this procedure on average in patient stay (see table 1).

Describing these phases we assume a full-scale PACS, including a coupling between RIS, HIS and PACS.

The *preparation* phase of a radiological procedure can be divided in an initial decision phase of a referring physician and in the phase of the radiological preparation of the required procedure.

In the decision phase of requesting a radiological procedure, the referring physician has an updated radiological overview and is well informed about the radiological procedures which have already been ordered by consulting physicians. Duplication of similar radiological procedures can be prevented in this way. It is clear that the avoidance of unnecessary duplication is medically attractive for patients and financially for health cost insurers.

In the radiological preparation phase (patient identification, scheduling, etc.) PACS makes the retrieval of old images easy. There are no lost old images anymore.

The image *acquisition phase* is not effected by PACS. Concerning the impact of PACS there is no difference between getting the radiological information by digital modalities (CT, MR (magnetic resonance), computed radiography) or by digitized images from 'conventional' procedures.

In the *reporting phase* there are two important items namely:
– the accuracy of radiological diagnosis and
– the user interface.

Radiological diagnosis depends very much upon image quality. PACS in its fullest concept only makes sense when concerning the image quality, the use of films (hard copies) can be replaced by digital PACS workstations (soft copies). When the image acquisition is digital (such as CT and MR), the image quality on a workstation is no problem. Most of the monitors which are used for PACS nowadays have 1024 × 1280 lines. These monitors (if flickerfree) are perfectly adequate to display images of CT, MR, ultrasound (US) and digital subtraction angiography (DSA). A problem is still the mere number of images and how to develop 'navigational' techniques for image browsing. As we will see in the last section, one way of 'information overload compression' is the use of three-dimensional techniques.

However, for primary diagnosis a 1024 × 1280 display is insufficient in the majority of clinical settings. 2000 or more lines (dependent on the kind of examination) will be necessary to reach equal image quality compared to conventional film. A number of ROC studies proved this statement (Barneveld Binkhuysen et al., 1988, 1989). Except for digital modalities, there is no radiologist worldwide who is doing primary radiological diagnosis on a digital workstation routinely. For digital modalities there are a few places where radiologists start to use PACS workstations in daily clinical routine (e.g., Sapporo-Japan (Irie et al., 1989), Brussels (Mattheus et al., 1990), Washington (Mun et al., 1989), Los Angeles (Lou et al., 1989), Graz (Gell et al., 1988), see also a special issue on PACS of Medical Informatics, 1988). Although in these situations the image quality is no problem, working routine is heavily restricted by the still immature user interfaces. It can be concluded that the image quality of digitized films is generally not good enough for primary diagnosis, though computed radiography with 2 K × 2 K resolution, printed on film, gets widely accepted. The most important consequence of this is that at this moment PACS can only sparsely be used by a radiologist in daily clinical routine. The problem of image quality will probably be solved automatically in the future by the use of more digital modalities and higher resolution of the displays. For reference purposes by referring physicians the image quality is mostly satisfactory (Wilmink et al., 1990).

The current user interface is generally characterized by user unfriendliness. For radiologists PACS display stations have many disadvantages. The most important complaints are:
- the systems are much too slow;
- there is no good overview of an investigation;
- the comparison with previous examinations is very difficult; and
- there is often no information about the amount of work that is or has to be done.

The question arises of how users, radiologists and referring physicians can maintain control in order to be able to choose the functions which are necessary in a particular situation rapidly and straightforwardly (Schuttenbeld and ter Haar Romeny, 1987).

Communication between the radiologist and the referring physicians is getting more and more important because of the multimodality possibilities, the choice of right acquisition parameters and algorithms and the continuously increasing impact of radiology on diagnosis and therapy. After reporting the radiological procedure there are three ways of communication between radiologists and referring physicians.
(1) Written reports. PACS offers the advantage to have the reports always available together with the images.
(2) Scheduled conference. This it not really affected by PACS, although the preparation by the co-workers of the radiology department is completely different.
(3) Unscheduled consulting. Here PACS offers the biggest advantage to have images always available at many places (but this dramatically influences system performance requirements).

Clinical experiences with hospital-based PACS showed that referring physicians accept and appreciate PACS rapidly. PACS showed real advantages in daily working such as:
- fast availability of radiological information;
- more information about more procedures (overview);
- information always available; and
- more fruitful conferences with several physicians.

The question arises: 'Who is responsible for the *archive* of digital images?'

In the conventional way of working it is the radiologist who is responsible but this will not be likely in the digital future. To what extent data compression will be legally allowed? Will the radiological information be a part of the medical case history? Maybe the referring physician will be responsible or the hospital management, who now is responsible for the HIS as well.

Because PACS offers the possibility to use the radiological information as fast as possible, *diagnostic* and *therapeutic effectiveness* can be improved. Clinical experiences proved this statement already. The possibilities of fast radiological information are being used in clinical settings and this is translated in an improved diagnostic and therapeutic effectiveness. This is very important because improved patient care is one of the main goals of PACS.

It is clear that an improved effectiveness makes it possible to decline the average *in-patient stay* which involves the financial management of the hospital management and the health costs insurers.

4. Possible impact of PACS on the future of radiology

Radiologists must be able to work with PACS in daily routine as accurately and as efficiently as they do with conventional films and until now this is not possible. However, the ergonomical and technical problems will be solved. The radiological experiences with PACS generated several unsolved questions such as:

- What will be the impact of PACS upon the way radiologists are used to work?
- How will the relationship between radiologists and clinicians change?
- When should an image be accessible at every display station? After it is taken, after reporting or after an agreed period of time?
- Who controls the image?
- Who is responsible for the radiological information?

History, however, could learn that new communication systems have always a broader impact then originally considered. Going back in radiological history we can see that the origin of central radiological departments has three important reasons:

(1) the use of 'dangerous' X-rays required special skills;
(2) the efficient use of increasing costly apparatus justified centralization; and
(3) the extra-ordinary complex logistics of images (archiving, registration, availability) also required a central department.

What do we foresee in the near future? There are several trends: the use of non-X-ray modalities as US and MRI (magnetic resonance imaging) is increasing more and more. An increasing number of referring physicians likes to do the imaging itself. Imaging modalities are getting smaller and cheaper and their future development is focused at different specialisms, e.g., very small MRI's for joints. We start to see the first fully digitized nuclear medicine department (UUH, ter Haar Romeny et al., 1990), feasible and economic. The complexity of logistics will be solved when a full-scale PACS is integrated in the HIS/RIS.

The two main reasons for realizing a HIS – PACS coupling are concerned with proper image management, e.g., in order to achieve acceptable waiting times and the user need of having all patient-relevant diagnostic and therapeutic data available in the same workstation. To decrease the need for unrealistically high network capacity it is most effective to include prefetching of image data and to generate within the HIS elaborate teaching files that combine diagnostic and demographic keys.

The role of the HIS – PACS coupling cannot be underestimated. It has become clear now, that HIS and PACS must be intimately connected. Hospitals without a HIS with a sufficient RIS section should not consider PACS before installing a proper RIS. Many vendors realize this important aspect and have started either full integration of their own RIS system, or developed good interfaces to a number of important HIS/RIS systems. The HIS must be the intelligence in the system. The HIS/RIS knows about the patient, his demographics, his history, his scheduled program in the hospital, and knows about prefetching: *where* do *which* images have to be a *what* moment and for *how long*. PACS is just storage, internally intelligent and optimizing storage order and transmission speeds, etc., but a slave of the HIS, carrying out the commands from the worklists generated. The contribution from the Japan National project at Hokkaido University (Irie) clearly shows this philosophy. In the Netherlands we have a particular situation, where one vendor has many identical systems installed in 30% of the number of acute beds, the system being completely integrated and performing almost any function necessary in a hospital within a large single (mirrored) system. In the UUH (900 beds) we have now 1000 terminals connected to a single (with mirrored backup) system.

The role of computed radiography is steadily increasing, the main bottlenecks being its costs and the lack of a PACS able to handle the digital data. As is evident from the Japanese contribution to this book, and from de Valk et al. (1988a,b), Japan takes the lead in implementation of CR.

Summarizing, we see that PACS will be an essential part in the changing function of radiologists and radiology departments. Radiologists will (super)specialize more and more and maybe will be partly integrated in other clinical specialisms. Until now the main function of radiologists is processing, evaluation and representation of image data. This will change in a more general approach to medical imaging and patient care. Herefore, also more knowledge of (patho)physiology and biochemistry is required. So we see that PACS is more than only digitization of radiological information. Many parties are concerned and especially radiologists have to be aware of the possibilities and possible changes when introducing PACS (ter Haar Romeny et al., 1990).

PACS will be one of the main changes which will influence radiology in the near future. Some radiologists consider one or more of these changes as a danger, others as an opportunity. Whatever the impact will be, radiologists will have to be flexible and try to consider these changes as an opportunity to strengthen their position so the future radiological imaging department can function as a nerve center of health care.

5. *PACS and advanced computer vision techniques*

PACS takes care of the logistics of the images, with all the well-known advantages as speed, no lost films, etc. As we found in the Dutch PACS project, a major aspect was the improved communication to the referring wards. At the moment of this writing, however, the costs of PACS and the necessary hardware/software prohibit a widespread implementation, in at least the Netherlands, but it is felt as a certainty that PACS will break through. PACS introduction needs a long time, not only because it needs adaptation of a department to change existing procedures, but also it is realized now that a full-scale turn-key PACS is prohibitively expensive while rapid improvements take place in short times. Therefore, as we will elaborate on below, a step-by-step approach with feasible steps is the most commonly seen approach.

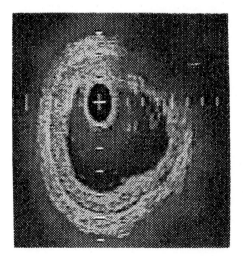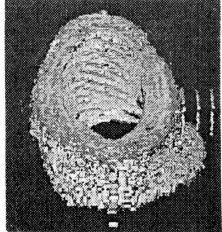

Fig. 2. Three-dimensional view of a vessel (right) from 20 consecutive images (left) from an intravascular ultrasound catheter.

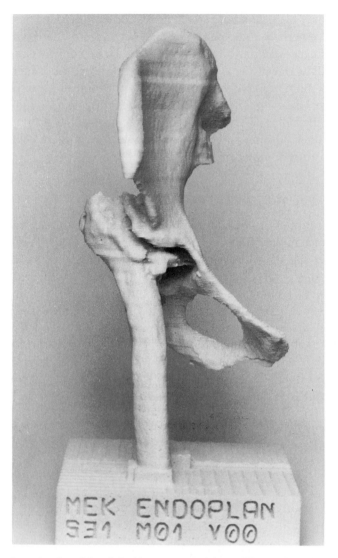

Fig. 3. Three-dimensional model tooled with a computer-driven milling machine from consecutive high resolution CT data from a patient with complicated fractures [with kind permission of prof. P.F.G.M. van Waes, UUH].

A tremendous potential is available in the fact that the images are digital. New modalities are emerging rapidly, e.g., vascular ultrasound (see fig. 2) for a three-dimensional view from 20 slices, produced with the' software package 'ANALYZE' (Robb, 1990). Not only the anatomical detail is important, but also the intrinsic quantitative information, which can be extracted now with computer assistance.

However, computer analysis has turned out to be very complicated, especially in the area of image segmentation and recognition. Techniques that has been solved to a great extent and now available are, e.g.,

- the use of three-dimensional computer graphics in surface- and volume rendering, with shading models, cut-away or transparent views, etc,
- tooling of the three-dimensional data (e.g., bone voxels from CT data) for surgery planning and even pre-operative exercises (see fig. 2),
- dynamic display, in, e.g., MR flow studies, joint movements (mandibular, knee, elbow, etc.).

We are now in a stage that the arousal about the esthetic value of the images has passed away, and much emphasis is placed on the question what is necessary: Where are these techniques successful?

In the UUH a special project was launched in 1989 to further develop these capabilities, with special emphasis on three-dimensional visualization: the 'three-dimensional computer vision' project is a collaboration of the university hospital, three universities and five industrial companies, and collaboration with a number of international groups, active in this area. Key issue is the close link between the researchers in this group and the radiologists, facilitated through the fact that the project is located within the radiology department. The project (now 22 full time equivalents per year) focuses on visualization, database management and user-interfacing, interactive manipulation, multiscale segmentation, datacompression and the use of 'front-end vision'-techniques for segmentation and feature detection.

Why are interactive techniques so promising? The answer can be given by some explanation of the notion of 'active vision'. The advent of PACS in the radiological setting brings the possibility of dynamically displaying computer-generated images, derived from the patient, on the workfloor: the radiological department. It is more and more realized that for our optimal perception of the three-dimensional structure in the patient we should make a natural use of the fact that we are observers that are able to move freely in the three-dimensional space around us. These movements induce specific changes in the images we get on our retina. Already Gibson (1952) realized the importance of this phenomenon, and coined the term 'ecological optics'. Our visual perception has evolved to optimally use this information. From this we realize the most important role for interactive display and manipulation of our data: we must move the objects we are studying *ourselves* or move *ourselves* for optimal perception of the three-dimensional structure. Passive rotation on a display is not optimal; we need to *update our internal representation* of 'what' is 'where' in space through the afferent information of our own movements. In the future we may see new user-interfaces emerge for interactive manipulation of medical volume data: head mounted display, where a stereo image is presented on a binocular LCD TV set with head translations and rotations updating the viewing angle of the displayed image so that the viewer can 'walk through' the data. He may manipulate separate parts of these virtual data with a three-dimensional mouse, or with a 'data glove', registering very finger and wrist manipulation. In this way, e.g., a radiotherapy treatment beam may be positioned manually with direct feedback of the three-dimensional isodose distribution visible in the transparent image of the relevant part of the patient. Several laboratories in the world (e.g., University of North Carolina, Chapel Hill, Department of Computer Science; MIT Media Labs) are currently working on these developments.

'Active vision' is only perceived well (smoothly) if the generation of new images is real time, i.e., within about 1/30 second per frame. This needs enormous computer power which is not yet generally available. There is an important role for the new generation of parallel computers. (Inter-)active vision techniques are used in other areas as well: architects design their new creations in the computer memory, and the customer can walk through his building, see the space from any viewpoint, and get a very realistic impression of the final product. Similarly, in flight simulators the images are updated according to the movements of the (pupil-)pilot.

The major problem is *segmentation* the definition of the contour of objects to be visualized or measured in some way. Much can be learned from the human visual system (Pizer and ter Haar Romeny, 1991). It turns out that on our retina a dynamic geometric analysis is made from the outside world, and this can be modeled in the computer and lead to modern perception theories (ter Haar Romeny and Florack, 1991).

6. Integration through PACS

PACS is seen as an essential infrastructure for an advanced medical imaging department. Apart from the obvious and proven *logistic* benefits, PACS should become *intelligent* and fully exploit the potential from digital imaging, and *make this potential available*. The number of advanced visualization techniques is rapidly increasing, but the major bottleneck in many hospitals is the problem how to get the data from A to B in a fast, automatic (background) fashion. There exist many different dataformats of the scattered optical disks, tape drives, etc. Speed is, next to effectiveness, a crucial success factor for the actual application of these techniques in a busy ongoing department. PACS should play this essential role in delivering the image-stacks to the right processors from the database it maintains.

The implementation of PACS should be done in a stepwise manner and needs a substantial commitment in terms of money and manpower (project management, ter Haar Romeny, 1989). Images are needed at many places, by many different groups/users and at different levels of resolution.

A suggested stepwise road to this goal might be (in this order), see fig. 4:
- Database for digital modalities only. Jukebox, database management system, viewing stations at radiology. Start with 256 × 256 or 512 × 512 images only. Previous and new images can be viewed at the CT/MR acquisition site directly. Laser-imagers can be shared in a mutual backup configuration. Coupling to HIS can be developed and tested. This basis system should comply with industry standards with off the shelf components.
- CR, connected to this database. Intensive care units, emergency units.
- Connection to end-users of digital images:
  - radiotherapy needs CT and MR data for three-dimensional treatment planning;
  - nuclear medicine wants anatomical references for their functional imagery;
  - three-dimensional groups/clinical platforms need stacked volumes of CT and MR data for visualization and possibly tooling;

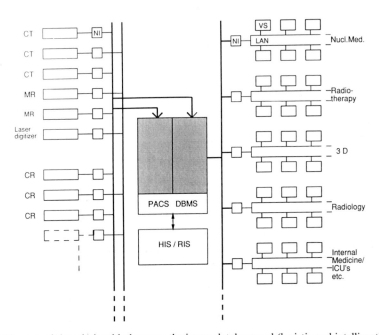

Fig. 4. Diagram of the relationship between the image database and (logistic and intelligent) users of the images. NI denotes network interface; LAN, local area network; VS, viewing station.

- teleradiology should work in an automatic fashion, both send and receive from/to the central DBMS;
- Research groups and specialized centers (universities, Dutch Eye Orbit Center, e.g., etc.).

In this phase, reporting from screen at radiology might be feasible.

- Connection to referring wards, to bring *reference* images with the report. Start of teleradiology for evening/weekend staff services, mobile systems, advices to other hospitals, etc.
- Primary diagnosis from screen. This is the most technical (and financial) demanding and not yet available option. At this stage it should be considered last.

More and more companies, traditionally large in the conventional photographic process, see this phased approach to an advanced department. A full-scale PACS will be reached in a later stage, after using PACS as a multimodality backbone for only part of the available images. We need some time to get the high-definition displays to become affordable, the introduction of faster standards, like FDDI (fiber-optic digital data interchange, a 100 Mbit/s network), and to get the problem solved of the intelligent HIS, driving a slave PACS.

An interesting possibility for a fast network through PACS might be the use of 'remote computing', allowing a number of CT/MR scanners to share over the network one (mini-super) computer for reconstruction and display only, thus enabling faster and *cheaper* front-ends. We see strong developments in the acquisition devices, many in the direction of being faster (continuous rotating CT, fast ME sequences).

7. Conclusion

We are in the very early stages of PACS. The major role for PACS is two-fold: on the short run the solving of the logistic and management problems regarding image communication; on the long run PACS will be the backbone for the availability of the possibilities due to the images being digital. Dynamic display, interactive three-dimensional display and manipulation and quantitative analysis are already introduced. When hardware makes real-time updates possible we will see a boom in interactive visualization and manipulation techniques. They all will be focused to solve the problem of the 'information overload' that may arise with the increasing resolution, speed and non-invasiveness: the data should be handled automatically, compressed in, e.g., three-dimensional presentations, one should be able to interactively manipulate the (anatomical and quantitative) information from the patient, and this should be efficiently stored and kept. For the integration and facilitation of these coherent set of functions in an imaging department, PACS is the essential carrier/medium.

It is important to be prepared for this future. In the training of residents a place must be reserved for getting acquainted with these developments, and a well-coached introduction to the techniques involved. We have only just begun with the computer-era in advanced digital imaging.

References

Andriessen, J.H.T.H., B.M. ter Haar Romeny, F.H. Barneveld Binkhuysen, and I. van der Horst-Bruinsma (1989a) Savings and costs of a picture archiving and communication system in the Utrecht University Hospital. In: Schneider, R.H., S.J. Dwyer III and R.G. Jost (Eds.), Medical Imaging III. PACS System Design and Evaluation, *Proc. SPIE* 1093, 578–584.

Andriessen, J.H.T.H., I.E. van der Horst-Bruinsma and B.M. ter Haar Romeny (1989b) Methodology of PACS effectiveness evaluation as part of a technology assessment, the Dutch PACS project extrapolated. In: Schneider, R.H., S.J. Dwyer III and R.G. Jost (Eds.), Medical Imaging III: PACS System Design and Evaluation, *Proc. SPIE* 1093, 585–588.

Arenson, R.L., S.B. Sashadri, S. Hiss and D.N. DeSimone (1989) Cost analysis of operating an all-digital radiology department, Hospital of the University of Pennsylvania, Philadelphia.

Bakker, A.R., B.M. van Poppel, I. van der Horst-Bruinsma, W.J.J. Stut Jr., J.P.J. de Valk, G.L. Reijns and B.M. ter Haar Romeny (1989) Cost modelling of PACS. In: Schneider, R.H., S.J. Dwyer III and R.G. Jost (Eds.), Medical Imaging III: PACS System Design and Evaluation, *Proc. SPIE* 1093, 545–550.

Barneveld Binkhuysen, F.H., A. Achterberg, B.M. ter Haar Romeny, J.H. Andriessen, J.A. Raymakers, K.J. Zuiderveld, P.F.G.M. van Waes and J.P.J. de Valk (1988) Setup of a clinical evaluation of a PACS system. In: Schneider, R.H., and S.J. Dwyer III (Eds.), Medical Imaging II, *Proc. SPIE* 914, 1169–1170.

Barneveld Binkhuysen, F.H., F.P. Ottes, B.M. ter Haar Romeny, P.L.M. Klessens, C.G. Vos, L.H.L. Winter, P.T. Calkoen and J.H.T.H. Andriessen (1989) First results of the diagnostic evaluation studies and the clinical efficacy evaluation in the Dutch PACS project. In: Schneider, R.H., S.J. Dwyer III and R.G. Jost (Eds.), Medical Imaging III: PACS System Design and Evaluation, *Proc. SPIE* 1093, 13–19.

DeSimone, D.N., H.L. Kundel and R.L. Arenson (1988) Effect of a digital imaging network on physician behaviour in an intensive care unit, *Radiology* 169, 41–44.

de Valk, J.P.J., A.R. Bakker, W.J.J. Stut Jr., H. Lodder and B.M. ter Haar Romeny (1988a) The Dutch PACS project: past, present and future. In: Zentralblatt Radiologie, Band 136, Heft 8–9 (Springer, Berlin), pp. 681.

de Valk, J.P.J., A.R. Bakker, K. Bijl, B.M. ter Haar Romeny, F. Linnebank and G.L. Reijns (1988b) Photograph avoiding complex systems: PACS in Japan 1987, *J. Med. Imaging* 2, 50–55.

de Valk, J.P.J., W.J. Stut Jr., H. Lodder, A.R. Bakker and B.M. ter Haar Romeny (1988c), IMAGIS projects: past, present and future. In: Schneider, R.H., and S.J. Dwyer III (Eds.), Medical Imaging II, *Proc. SPIE* 914, 1136–1140.

Gell, G., G.H. Schneider, M. Wiltgen, M. Becker, G. Seuvert, C. Greinacher and H. Guoyke (1988) PACS Erfahrungen beim Einsatz in der Klinik. In: Schneider, G.H., and E. Vogler (Eds.), Proc. 5. Grazer Radiologische Symposium (Springer, Berlin), pp. 594–600.

Gibson, J.J. (1952) The Perception of the Visual World (Houghton Mifflin, Boston).

Irie, G., Y. Kawakami, Y. Kaneda, K. Miyasaka and T. Kudo (1989) A report on PACS at Hokkaido University. In: Proc. IMAC 89, Int. Conf. on Image Management and Communication, Washington, D.C., pp. 72–76.

Lodder, H., B.M. van Poppel, J.P.J. de Valk, H.B.M. Wilmink, C. Ising and A.R. Bakker (1989) HIS-PACS coupling in practice. In: Schneider, R.H., S.J. Dwyer III and R.G. Jost (Eds.), Medical Imaging III: PACS System Design and Evaluation, *Proc. SPIE* 1093, 301–306.

Lou, S.L., H.K. Huang, N.J. Mankovich, H. Kangarloo, K.S. Park, O.M. Ratib, A. Wong, M. Komori, D. Valentino and Z.L. Barbaric (1989) A CT/MR/US picture archiving and communication system. In: Schneider, R.H., S.J. Dwyer III and R.G. Jost (Eds.), Medical Imaging III: PACS System Design and Evaluation, *Proc. SPIE* 1093, 31–36.

Mattheus, R., M. Ostaux, F. Verhelle and J. van Snick (1990) Four years of PACS development at the University Hospital of Brussels (VUB), EuroPACS 1990, Trieste, Italy.

Medical Informatics (1988) Medical Informatics: an international journal of information processing in health care, special issue on PACS. *Medical Informatics* 13, No. 4.

Mun, S.K., H. Benson, S. Horii, L.P. Elliott, S.H.B. Lo, B. Levine, R. Braudes, G. Plumlee, B. Garra, D. Schellinger and B. Majors (1989) Completion of a hospital-wide comprehensive image management and communication system. In: Schneider, R.H., S.J. Dwyer III and R.G. Jost (Eds.), Medical Imaging III: PACS System Design and Evaluation, *Proc. SPIE* 1093, 204–213.

Ottes, F.P., J.P.J. de Valk, F.H. Barneveld Binkhuysen, H.M.J.A. Kroon and G.W. Seeley (1989) Evaluation of diagnostic image quality using the FEASIBLE software package. In: Proc. CAR '89 (Springer, Berlin), pp. 521–525.

Ottes, F.P., A.R. Bakker, J.M.L. Kouwenberg and B.M. ter Haar Romeny (1990) First phase of the Dutch PACS project (1986–1989): research outcomes and clinical evaluation results. In: Proc. SCAR '90, Symposium for Computer Assisted Radiology, Anaheim, Cal., June 13–16.

Pizer, S.M., and B.M. ter Haar Romeny (1991) Fundamental properties of medical image perception, *J. Digital Imaging* 4, 1–20.

Robb, R.A. (1990) A software system for interactive and quantitative analysis of biomedical images. In: Höhne, K.H., H. Fuchs and S.M. Pizer (Eds.), 3D Imaging in Medicine, *NATO ASI Series F* 60, 333–361.

Roos, P., and M.A. Viergever (1989) Registration and reversible compression of angiographic image sequences. In: Schneider, R.H., S.J. Dwyer III and R.G. Jost (Eds.), Medical Imaging IV, *Proc. SPIE* 1092, 383–391.

Schuttenbeld, H.H.W., and B.M. ter Haar Romeny (1987) Design of a user-interface for a PACS viewing station. In: Schneider, R.H., and S.J. Dwyer III (Eds.), Medical Imaging, *Proc. SPIE* 767, 844–849.

Stut Jr., W.J.J., A.R. Bakker, M.R. van Steen and L.P.J. Groenewegen (1989a) A semantic modelling method to guide simulation-based system development. In: Murray-Smith, D., et al. (Eds.), Proceedings of the third European Simulation Congress, September 1989, Edinburgh, pp. 101–106.

Stut Jr., W.J.J., J.P.J. de Valk, A.R. Bakker and B.M. ter Haar Romeny (1989b) First experiences with the modelling and simulation package MIRACLES applied to a PACS in a clinical environment, *Comput. Methods Programs Biomed.* 28, 63–70.

ter Haar Romeny, B.M. (1989) Implementation aspects of image management, archiving and communication systems. In: Mun, S.K., M. Greberman, W.R. Hendee and R. Shannon (Eds.), Proc. First International Conference on Image Management and Communication Systems in Patient Care: Implementation and Impact, IMAC '89, Washington, June 4–9, IEEE Computer Society, pp. 200–207.

ter Haar Romeny, B.M., and L. Florack (1991) A multiscale geometric model of human vision.

In: Hendee, B., and P.N.T. Wells (Eds.), Perception of Visual Information (Springer, Berlin), in press.

ter Haar Romeny, B.M., J. Meywaard, A. ten Hertog, C.N. de Graaf, P.P. van Rijk and J.P.J. de Valk (1986) Radiological information flow between departments and out-clinics in the Utrecht University Hospital in the Netherlands. In: Schneider, R.H., and S.J. Dwyer III (Eds.), Medicine XIV/PACS IV, *Proc. SPIE* 626, 698 – 702.

ter Haar Romeny, B.M., J.A. Raymakers, P.F.G.M. van Waes, J.C. Helder, C.N. de Graaf, P.P. van Rijk, H. Schuttenbeld, K.J. Zuiderveld, J. Tiemann and B. Scharnberg (1987) The Dutch PACS project: philosophy, design of a digital reading room and first observations in the Utrecht University Hospital in the Netherlands. In: Schneider, R.H., and S.J. Dwyer III (Eds.), Medical Imaging, *Proc. SPIE* 767, 787 – 792.

ter Haar Romeny, B.M., A. Achterberg, F.H. Barneveld Binkhuysen, J.H. Andriessen, K.J. Zuiderveld, J.A. Raymakers, J.J. Stut Jr., B. Scharnberg and J.P.J. de Valk (1988) Procedures to study the impact of PACS on the logistics within a diagnostic imaging department. In: Schneider, R.H., and S.J. Dwyer III (Eds.), Medical Imaging II, *Proc. SPIE* 914, 1159 – 1168.

ter Haar Romeny, B.M., J.M.M. van der Wielen, A.J. Achterberg, F.H. Barneveld Binkhuysen, K.J. Zuiderveld, J.H.T.H. Andriessen and A.R. Bakker (1989) PACS efficiency: a detailed quantitative study of the distribution process of films in a clinical environment in the Utrecht University Hospital. In: Schneider, R.H., S.J. Dwyer III and R.G. Jost (Eds.), Medical Imaging III: PACS System Design and Evaluation, *Proc. SPIE* 1093, 259 – 271.

ter Haar Romeny, B.M., M.A. Viergever, P.F.G.M. van Waes, F.W. Zonneveld, C.N. de Graaf, J.B.M. Wilmink, J.M.L. Kouwenberg and L. Neeleman (1990) Integration of clinical routine digital imaging and advanced image processing through PACS. In: Dwyer III, S.J., and R.G. Jost (Eds.), Medical Imaging IV: PACS System Design and Evaluation, *Proc. SPIE* 1234, 859 – 868.

van Gennip, E.M.S.J., F.P. Ottes, B.M. van Poppel and J.H.T.H. Andriessen (1990) Why do cost-benefit studies of PACS disagree? In: Dwyer III, S.J., and R.G. Jost (Eds.), Medical Imaging IV: PACS System Design and Evaluation, *Proc. SPIE* 1234, 894 – 904.

van Poppel, B.M, A.R. Bakker and J.B.M. Wilmink (1990) A package for cost and critical analysis of picture archiving and communication indicating its true yield (CAPACITY), *Med. Inform.* 15, 67 – 75.

Wilmink, J.B.M., B.M. ter Haar Romeny, F.H. Barneveld Binkhuysen, A.J. Achterberg, K.J. Zuiderveld, P.T. Calkoen and J.M.L. Kouwenberg (1990) PACS in the Utrecht University Hospital: final conclusions of the clinical evaluation. In: Dwyer III, S.J., and R.G. Jost (Eds.), Medical Imaging IV: PACS System Design and Evaluation, *Proc. SPIE* 1234, 915 – 924.

Winter, L.H.L., B.M. ter Haar Romeny, F.H. Barneveld Binkhuysen, F.P. Ottes, H.A.O. Warnars, W.B. Becking, E.J. Haanraadts and G.J. Krabbe (1989) Diagnostic evaluation of a PAC subsystem using phantom chest Röntgenograms: an observer performance study. In: Schneider, R.H., S.J. Dwyer III and R.G. Jost (Eds.), Medical Imaging III: PACS System Design and Evaluation, *Proc. SPIE* 1093, 418 – 422.

Integrated Diagnostic Imaging
Editor: J.P.J. De Valk
© *Elsevier Science Publishers B.V., 1992*

Chapter 14

PACS: in the present lies the past, in now what will be?

A view from the Nijmegen PACS project

Leon J.Th.O. van Erning, Sjef H.J. Ruijs and Wim Guijt

1. Introduction and definitions

Within this chapter the view of the department of diagnostic radiology of the St.Radboud University Hospital Nijmegen (UHN) on developments in the field of integrated medical imaging will be presented. The development of a picture archiving and communication system (PACS) is only one topic in a whole series of projects that relate to integrated diagnostic imaging, i.e., the development of a really complete patient folder. Of course these developments do not originate solely from radiology departments themselves as they reflect the developing technological possibilities within the hospital as well as the worldwide environment. Anno 1992 PACS is just one aspect of the changing infrastructure of the medical environment. Actually we see a trend in the debate about the benefits and improvements for medical care of a PACS towards a more and more expanding field of related topics, i.e., impact on quality of care, legal aspects, influence on the organization, etc. It is to be questioned if all effects can be foreseen. Changes are for the larger part determined by historical, cultural and social developments. Therefore we will start at the beginning of various developments and consider their history.

1.1. The St.Radboud University Hospital Nijmegen

Nijmegen is one of the oldest cities in the Netherlands. The University of Nijmegen was founded in 1923 and the School of Medicine in 1951. The UHN, St.Radboud, opened its gates in 1956. It has grown into one of the largest Dutch university hospitals (940 beds). It is a centre of reference for the southeastern part of the country (over three million inhabitants). It has a large reputation in research and treatment of cancer, e.g., it was one of the first centres in Europe to start bone marrow transplantation. Research to assess the early diagnosis of breast cancer and its treatment has earned international reputation. Currently advanced image processing applications for mammography are being developed to improve pathology detection within the screening program. Connected to the radiology department is the national reference centre for the breast cancer screening. UHN is also a centre for research into and treatment of disorders of the human musculo-skeletal system. The replacement of joints by orthopaedic implants is strongly developed. Dual energy quantitative computed tomography (DEQCT) is applied to improve simulations of bone-(re)modelling. Digitized X-ray film to quantify hip prosthesis migration is applied clinically. A joint project of radiology and orthopaedics considers the set-up of a specific database for these images within a PACS. A joint project of rheumatology and diagnostic radiology concerns the application of DEQCT and dedicated image postprocessing to quantify effects of treatment and fracture risk in relation to osteoporosis.

In cooperation with the University of Nijmegen, the hospital provides teaching programs for over 2000 students, medical specialists and nurses. The hospital handles about 469 000 patients per year of which 27 000 are inpatients (average ten days). The Radboud Hospital information system (RAHIS) is an in-house development. The central service department of radiology has 32 diagnostic rooms with conventional X-ray, computed tomography (CT), digital subtraction angiography (DSA), ultrasound (US) and nuclear magnetic resonance (NMR). The department is a national centre for in-vivo NMR spectroscopy at 2 T. In cooperation with biophysical chemistry, in-vitro as well as in-vivo animal research is performed with up to 600 MHz systems. Radiology has five research lines: evaluation of applied methods, development of new methods, breast cancer, radiation protection and NMR imaging and spectroscopy. To integrate the clinical and research environment a PACS-net of 1000 m connects six diagnostic modalities, two digitization stations and a range of workstations. PACS developments started in 1985 (Bouman et al., 1988; van Erning et al., 1988; Knots et al., 1990) and will be discussed further in Section 4.

1.2. Definitions

Within the scope of this chapter the following definitions will be used.

1.2.1. Hospital information system (HIS)
Hospital information system (HIS), containing all automated procedures in-

volved with the primary process. There exists a large variety of systems all covered by the same indication: HIS. Here the central kernel with patient data needed by all departments is referred to, i.e., general patient data not specific to a department like name, date of birth, etc.

1.2.2. Radiology information system (RIS)

A local system supplying the radiology department with extensive features, like: special departmental scheduling facilities, local management information, radiation dose registration, etc. A RIS should relate to a HIS on a client – server basis.

1.2.3. PACS

A composition of three (separate) systems: a picture, an archive and a communication system. Note that the digital generation of images (e.g., with computed radiology (CR)) on basis of photostimulable plate technology is in our view not specific to PACS although it will change the ratio of analog to digital images significantly and as a consequence influence PACS developments. The strongest incentive for a PACS will be the cost effectiveness when it replaces the current way of working.

For the picture system specific requirements of the medical application of image display and pre- and/or post-processing hold. For a part they differ from other areas of image handling. The major advantages of a digital picture system are:

- the flexibility to manipulate images (a number of post-processing techniques only considers the given set of images, e.g., multi-planar reconstruction (MPR), etc. However, it might be more profitable to consider the raw measurement data first!);
- the enhanced quality (if requirements of spatial resolution (pixels) and contrast resolution (bit planes) are satisfied);
- enhanced speed of access to images;
- reduction of perception errors if image processing supports image reading;
- accuracy to connect diagnostic reports with corresponding images.

For the archive system it is clear that:

- images can always be found, i.e., no image losses;
- images can be sent to various locations at the same time;
- future requirements will also address the archiving of raw measurement data instead of reconstructed images only;
- costs reduction can be expected as image database management techniques can be integrated with RIS (departmental) and/or HIS.

The communication system is no longer the main bottleneck. It becomes more and more clear that communication is a PACS item that is also of crucial importance to the whole field of information technology. For a long time optical-fibre transmission has been too expensive to implement high-speed networks onto every desktop. As the cost-crossover point has been reached now between copper and fibre, even basic telephone services may be realized with fibre. It is clear that these networking facilities become feasible also for image transmission networks. The actual interfacing of various modalities and systems remains a bottleneck, however. Although many efforts to standardize image (ACR-NEMA, 1988) and communication formats (SPI, 1987) are in progress, still a lot of incompatible situations exist within medical research as well as routine environments.

1.2.4. Multimedia systems

Multimedia systems are systems in which audiovisual and computer technologies are integrated (Shandle, 1990; Umeda et al., 1991). From the user's point of view they are able to handle data of various origins (text, graphics, still and full-motion video images and audio signals) in a similar way. These radically different data sets can be integrated in multimedia documents. Multimedia data sets can be accessed from the same user platform in an interactive way. Current personal computer (PC) developments go in the direction of multimedia systems utilizing the capabilities of actual compact disc (CD) technologies like: CD read-only memory (CD ROM), CD interactive (CDI) or CD ROM extended architecture (CD ROM XA).

1.2.5. Integrated diagnostic systems (IDS)

With the advent of computer technology into the field of medicine two specific categories of systems have been developed: (a) the administrative systems for a larger part consisting of the actual HIS and (b) the advanced medical technological systems that are computer controlled. The interaction between user and computer has evolved from a 'programmer' level to a very 'user friendly' level. For a part this is not because the 'more user friendliness' was not recognized earlier but simply because technology was not developed far enough. In Section 3 the future outlook will consider multimedia developments that cover the integrated 'file' (document) concept, like a patient-related data set. From this concept evolves the integration of PACS into HIS providing an integrated patient database, i.e., IDS.

1.2.6. Diagnostic radiology

An area of medicine in which it is tried to visualize the objects about which a specific medical question is put forward. From this visualization it is tried to confirm a diagnosis or to exclude a specific doubt. As this chapter tries to put

PACS developments in a contemporary context it is worthwhile to consider briefly the history of medical imaging.

In 1896 Wilhelm Conrad Röntgen published his discovery of the X-rays. Although Röntgen did not see a medical application at first sight, the americans recognized the medical as well as the industrial importance of his discovery. In the beginning one was unaware of the damage X-rays can cause. But up to now sufficient security measures in the form of radiation protection guidelines and limits have been set up. The further implementation of radiology for medical imaging was stimulated by both World War I and II. Pieces of shrapnel could be localized and X-ray images played a very important role in the surgical treatment. Around the 1930s, radiology became more and more an integrated part in the clinic. It appeared important to get insight into the three-dimensional structures inside the human body by creating two-dimensional images. Clinicians and radiologists had to imagine the three-dimensional structures from a two-dimensional picture. One had to link the knowledge of the 'normal' image to the actual opinions about anatomy while at the same time gathering knowledge about abnormalities and congenital variances. The recognition of structures (perception and interpretation) and the resolving power (resolution) are important therefore. A revolution was the invention of CT in the 1970s by Hounsfield, while the concept of Radon dates from 1917 (Radon, 1917)! It became possible then to create images of transversal slices. These developments very soon found a broad interest within the clinic. However, it was still a two-dimensional technique. The new view on the 'in-vivo' anatomy made it necessary to teach radiologists the items of topological anatomy from which the relations between various objects can be seen. Additionally the difference between 'analog' and 'digital' was recognized. Here digital refers to an image on basis of a (non-film) detector and appropriate processing computer. The digital image consists of pixels that can be displayed on a video monitor in a great variety of ways. However, most commonly images were hardcopied to enable diagnosis from film reading. Note that the concept of a satellite or stand-alone console exists already at the introduction of CT. Looking at the various brochures presently describing PACS consoles one wonders why the clinical applications in this area developed so scarcely. Actually still a number of functions (filtering, etc.) are almost never used in routine diagnostics.

CR or digital radiology systems using reusable photostimulable phosphor screens are the latest X-ray developments. They may simply digitize a number of conventional procedures if it is possible to realize the required spatial resolutions. Contrast resolution (dynamic range of 40000 : 1) can be much better than with film. Like in CT this might compensate for the poorer resolution (pixel size $0.1 - 0.2$ mm) in some cases.

Nuclear medicine (NM) developed from the use of counting techniques for

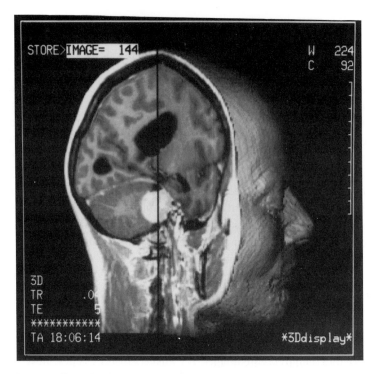

Fig. 1. Various two-dimensional displays of a three-dimensional MRI data set. The real extra information can only become available in interactively manipulating the three-dimensional data set.

detecting ionizing radiation (Webb, 1988). The imaging of radiopharmaceuticals was a logical extension. However, after the first clinical NM scan of the thyroid it still took 16 years before the image formation method was able to produce an 'image' whose contrast could be adjusted a posteriori. Already in 1983 an all-digital NM department was described (Parker et al., 1983).

US applications, based on the pulse-echo principle (RADAR), became possible after the development of fast electronic pulse technology during World War II. Medical use emerged in the 1950s. Meanwhile the technique had been proven to be generally applicable. Although its geometrical resolution is clearly poorer than those of CT or MRI (magnetic resonance imaging), US has the advantage of frame rates up to 50 per second. Also smaller investments for equipment and room requirements are involved. The possible danger of X-rays limited the diffusion of applications over the hospital. As US is not using ionizing radiation, however, its application is less restricted to a specific specialty or department. A number of US scanners are used as a 'stethoscope', i.e., images are only made for inspection or measurement without image storage.

NMR imaging, the last item, enables arbitrary slice selection, i.e., transversal, coronal, sagittal or any oblique direction. It does not require ionizing radiation and provides a safe imaging modality besides US. The creation of three-dimensional images forms a new challenge to the anatomical-medical way of thinking. The medium film is no longer the optimal way to capture the image nor to display it. New techniques have to provide optimal use of three-dimensional information. Computer-controlled devices are placed in between the patient and the resulting image. This enables a vast number of methods (even physiological information may be added) to be applied before the radiologist is to think of the possible answer that relates to the clinician's question. NMR images may be seen as the basis for a new kind of 'three-dimensional anatomy in-vivo', which renders opening of the body superfluous. Figure 1 illustrates the limitations of the two-dimensional display of a three-dimensional data set.

2. PACS 1980–1990

In short one could state: 'PACS has created a number of expectations that were not fulfilled in time'. Some critical notes from the literature may support this (Drew, 1984; Arenson, 1988; Cannavo, 1988; Fischer, 1988; Hendee, 1988; Hodapp, 1988; Ogle, 1988). Maybe the most crucial point in this respect is the difference between the clinical and the research environment. Within the clinical environment a number of standardized procedures are applied that have been developed over a very long time. Most of the people that apply them have not had a technical education. As a consequence for medical technology it appears that the application itself is not of importance but only its clinical relevance. User-friendliness is within limits of minor importance as long as something can be gained with it clinically (remember the aspects of CT imaging). The context in which new technical possibilities develop is of major importance. In the Netherlands windmill technology was used for a long time. Even after the introduction of small steam engines the installation of windmills proceeded until the second half of the nineteenth century. The reasons for this were: windmill operation is small-scaled, transportation costs are low and often the miller could combine his job with some trading or a pub. And thinking of all predictions of the 'less paper' office one should realize that the development of paper industry was not only a consequence of mechanising the industry but also of the development of the newspaper concept, the increasing literacy rate and in general the more important role of written text. It is important to realise the strong correlation between technological and other developments within society. Although computers came into the medical school the insight of most clinicians in the functionality of these systems is only marginal. Within a research environment there is an interdisciplinary cooperation between technologically interested physicians and medically interested physicists and engineers. This enables the use of technological tools by both parties as the primary goal is the development of new techniques for routine use instead of only one successful application. Up to now there are a number of PACS sites worldwide. These systems range from small to large depending on the number of modalities connected, or the number of workstations applied for primary diagnosis. None of these systems has a fully integrated environment, however. It is expected that the integrating step will be made during the next decade.

3. PACS 1990–2000

PACS developments depend on the evolution of related fields of technology in- and outside the medical area. Incentives for a PACS from the clinic are formed by the changing imaging procedures and resulting extra, often quantitative, data. These procedures range from digitized video measurements up to optimized parameter calculations based on synthetic images. A digital infrastructure supports these new possibilities. Note that image requirements differ very much between diagnostic and referring purposes. The following developments in medical imaging will among others contribute to the need of a PACS.

All medical imaging techniques are expected to be digitized in the future. For X-ray applications the CR systems may bring the transition phase. Most three-dimensional imaging applications may be expected from US and MRI. Large three-dimensional data sets from CT are only ethically acceptable if there is an urgent clinical need. Although not yet available at a scale as large as CT, MRI has developed to be the primary modality for neurological and specific soft tissue applications (Goddard, 1991). The developments of MR angiography (MRA) (Axel, 1984) and fast MRI (Cohen and Weisskoff, 1991) are very promising as a substitution of angiography as well as to generate real-time images of movement phenomena (e.g., cardiac disorders and joint movements). Here film is no longer the display mode of first choice. With the development of high-end echographic systems (resolution up to 1 mm) and increased speed (up to 50 frames per second), US has got a very important status. Three-dimensional applications become available in echo-cardiography for an improvement of the determination of three-dimensional morphology (Hottier and Collet Billon, 1990). Three-dimensional US may improve the (exact) measurement of anatomical parameters like distances, areas and volumes. Besides data-acquisition also postprocessing techniques, like MPR and solid three-dimensional rendering, will develop further. Crucial to any rendering technique is an efficient segmentation technique in order to separate different components of an object. Segmentation techniques often vary among applications (e.g., vertebral body (Bisseling et al., 1989), spleen (Karssemeijer et al., 1988), etc.). The actual bottleneck in applying the above-mentioned techniques more easily is the integrated communication (the capital C in PACS) between data-acquisition modalities, general purpose workstations and an archive.

As mentioned before, PACS is not the only developing system within a hospital. And it is certainly not a system that is likely to be the most cost reducing in the near future. Especially the support of a better quality of care is almost impossible to express in terms of cost reduction. That is why PACS introduction will to a great extent depend on technological developments, on general medical requirements and the policy of the hospitals. The available infrastructure in many fields and the short- and long-term goals of the hospital management will steer the introduction. However, PACS developments depend mainly on PACS-related technology itself, i.e., technology of image display and processing, database management systems as well as archiving hardware and communication technology. These directly related fields are characterized by possibilities and needs from the general area of electronic data processing and electronic data communication, by medical requirements and the corresponding choices that will be made within limited budgets. Worldwide costs of health care are discussed. To what part of the gross national product is the level of health care cost to be raised? Differences between diagnostic and therapeutic possibilities are becoming more and more pronounced. Sometimes it is questioned if it is worthwhile to introduce more advanced diagnostic instruments that enable enhanced diagnosis of pathologies for which no therapy exists yet. As developments of US and NMR proceed further, interventional radiological procedures may be performed more often within the department of the medical specialty involved. The application of US has already shown to be useful in a number of cases. Within UHN only six of the total of 36 US units are within radiology. Most units are for inspection or measurement. The observed result is noted in an alpha-numeric value and there is no need for image storage. It is feasible that the new modality NMR will also be used as an instantaneous observation or measurement unit (e.g., NMR spectroscopy) as soon as less costly dedicated systems become available. For various applications there is no need to generate enormous amounts of (three-dimensional) images, which also have to be archived. As NMR proves to be a very rapidly developing 'user-friendly' medical imaging and diagnostic tool, the diffusion of this technique over the hospital also becomes feasible. From a number of cardiology departments it is known that they have their own MRI unit 'in mind'. So a general tendency might develop that a centralized imaging department is not what develops on the long run, making the need for an integrated communication system even stronger. Before 2000, however, in our opinion such a radical change is not to be expected. The past decade showed that infrastructures are not changing as rapidly as technology becomes available to support new ways of working. In this respect the parallel to the predictions of a paperless office is of particular interest. A vicious circle might originate when the developments are gradually because the investments are high and as a consequence diffusion into health care will be slow. Then the slow introduction hinders the fast evaluation that might show PACS to be profitable and efficient. If one extrapolates the experiences from small pilot systems, a number of arguments in favour of PACS indicate that it is worthwhile to set up a complete system, i.e., hospital-wide. The costs estimations show, however, very large differences as different departments put different constraints into sometimes comparable models. Actually research is done to investigate possibilities to develop more reliable medical technology assessment models to predict with more certainty the cost effectiveness of this kind of technology. A factor that is likely to be of importance is the ratio of the technology costs and the materials budget related to the number of hospital beds.

Depending on the developments of data-acquisition modalities the requirements to display, process, communicate and archive images will vary. Therefore main items in PACS are workstations (ranging from simple to extended) (Arenson et al., 1990), network components, archive components and software to be implemented on PACS hardware as well as the clinical environment (RIS and HIS). Note that it is not to be expected that PACS will remain limited to radiology. There are a number of image producing departments (endoscopy, pathological anatomy, radiotherapy) that may use a PACS as well. Workstations are being developed for a large range of applications, e.g., image processing is applied in industrial as well as medical areas. In image and signal processing great changes have to be expected. Manufacturers announce to be able to build neural computers of up to 1152 'neurons' and with a learning processing unit that can handle 2.3 billion operations per second. The USA Defense Advanced Research Project Agency (DARPA) is going to spend $33 million through 1992 to see if neural networks can help solve signal (image) processing problems.

When looking at the future one has to realize that the integration of alphanumerical and image data is not unique to radiology and/or any clinical environment. Integration is proceeding gradually in the form of the multimedia concept. Maybe it will turn out that 1991 will be remembered as the real start-off of a multimedia market. Although a number of prerequisites, like digital signal processing (DSP) coprocessor architectures, control architectures for video, means of distributing multimedia documents, still have to be realized, it is clear that applications become available in every field. Possibilities emerge to run these applications under Windows on PCs that become available at more and more desktops. This makes the hospital-wide distribution of display stations more feasible. Calculations for the UHN indicate that over 1500 lightboxes have to be replaced with image display stations for a hospital-wide PACS. Actually, HIS terminals are already being exchanged for PCs and the next step might be the addition of image display hardware if required or exchange for a multimedia system. Having 600 HIS terminals this would already cover 30% of the image output facilities by simple workstations. An example of a minimal configuration to support image display is an 80286 processor with video graphics array (VGA), 2 Mbytes of system memory and a 360 Mbytes hard disk. Of course multimedia applications do not fully cover all aspects of the high image quality needed for primary diagnosis. On the other hand it is clear that also on the general workstation market huge changes and developments are coming up. For US and endoscopic applications sustained data rates to disk of about 150 Kbytes or 1.2 Mbits/s might turn out to be sufficient.

During the next years the equipment installed in hospitals during the 1980s and still in the early 1990s will not be able to transmit and receive signals at the speed of the actual networks capabilities. While fibre distributed data interconnect (FDDI) interfaces already are being surpassed by newer developments, e.g., fibre distributed video/voice data interface (FDVDI) (Weber, 1989), a large number of the actually installed data-acquisition modalities and workstations are not even able to cope with the actual networking requirements. Most of them are not multitasking yet and are turn-key systems, i.e., shutdown after the last procedure and no longer are accessible from the network. As soon as data-acquisition modalities become more and more controlled by workstations and multimedia applications become available at a larger scale, the reversed situation will occur. Then the newer network technologies will be necessary. The synergy between integrated services digital network (ISDN) and multimedia begins with the coherence between the 1.2 Mbits/s CD ROM data rate and ISDNs 1.5 Mbits/s primary interface. At this point also the compression aspect comes in. Although a number of papers indicated that a lossy compression factor of 20 might be acceptable for certain applications in medical imaging, it still takes too much time to compress and decompress images to be archived. For multimedia applications hardwired DSPs become available that apply the Consultative Committee International Telegraph and Telephone (CCITT)'s Joint Photographic Experts Group (JPEG) algorithm for colour image compression at both still and moving (MPEG) image (cine) applications. Note that although this image quality may not be sufficient for primary diagnosis, it will be sufficient for all referring image display. As was seen in the development of advanced PACS workstations and also for multimedia platforms, the software development is still (far) behind the requirements to be fulfilled. It will not be sufficient to adapt existing programs to new environments because these newer platforms will only be used efficiently if the software takes full advantage of their capabilities. Multimedia applications are a new impulse to the long-awaited paperless office, because they will include compound documents − text and bit-mapped images − at the least. In parallel to PACS one has to state that image management is not the correct problem description in future outlooks. Document management will be the integrated concept, where a document is defined as a collection of information. In the same way a clinician is referring to the material of his patients. The complete patient folder contains a collection of information like anamnesis, blood sample results, reports and images which are not-stand-alone. Then the parallel with the document comes back in that it is constantly updated, not just stored and retrieved. So requirements for the future will go into the direction of a PACS fully integrated into the HIS where the HIS creates the ability to browse through and query the document database.

Another factor that will influence future PACS developments are the results of cost analysis investigations. As long as cost − benefit analyses vary so much between various institutions (van Gennip et al., 1991) it will remain unclear for a larger group to what extend these outcomes can be trusted and the risk to invest in PACS can be taken. Until now it is unclear that in order to determine the amount and type of equipment the same key rules might hold for different hospitals within the same and within different countries. The organization of different hospitals differs so much not only due to the often historical way in which the organization grew but also because health care is differently organized in various countries. This implies that political and social aspects are involved. They will not be changed just by having the technology available to change the infrastructure. If the effectiveness of a system can be proven, a strong incentive to push the developments is available. The problem can be compared to the actual problems in electronic banking. Introduction proceeds only gradually as long as the infrastructure is lacking and one can not fully demonstrate its effectiveness. And not fully demonstrating the effectiveness implies that investments into the infrastructure will be poor thus leading to delay of the demonstration of the effectiveness.

4. PACS, here and now in Nijmegen

Actually the PACS at the department of diagnostic radiology of the UHN integrates a clinical and a research environment. Six clinical modalities are on-line with the PACS MicroVax-II host. They are connected for the following reasons.

- A CT scanner to enable transfer of images and measurement tables from DEQCT for advanced image processing (texture analysis) and input into an alpha-numeric database system (PC);
- two DSA units are connected to transfer images from experimental as well as clinical studies to a postprocessing system which also takes care of archiving series of images;
- a DSA unit to create conference sets of images to add to the film reading and compare MRA with conventional angiography;
- a remote CT scanner at the department of neuroradiology to enable remote reading at the CT's satellite console of centrally generated MR images and enable multi-modality viewing in the future;
- a NMR unit to transfer images for further analysis (parameter optimization, synthetic imaging) and post-processing of spectroscopic data.

The network is connected to a PACS winchester buffer of 1 Gbytes and an optical disc archive of 2×2.4 Gbytes. Patient folders may be viewed on a diagnostic reporting console (DRC-20) having two 1024×1024 screens and a mouse driven user interface. In fig. 2 a diagram is given of this PACS con-

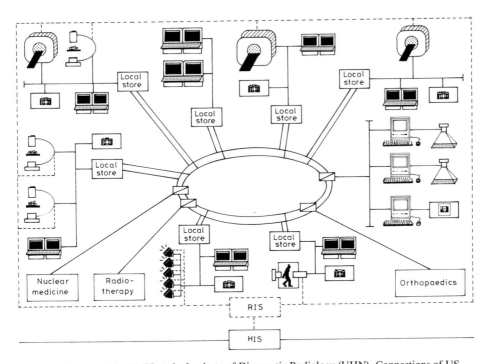

Fig. 2. Diagram of the PACS at the Institute of Diagnostic Radiology (UHN). Connections of US, fluoroscopy, RIS and HIS are in preparation.

figuration as it is realized for the larger part and is expected to be finalized within the next five years. The integration of a second generation console DRC-102 is planned for 1992. Of course this is a projection based on actual expectations. As indicated in Section 3, a number of developments may come-up in the near future. What will become a product depends on the market, however. A RIS will connect the various modalities to the central kernel of the HIS to enable unique patient identification. Additionally actual room occupancy, film usage and radiation dose can be captured automatically. Connections to the departments of nuclear medicine, radiotherapy and orthopaedics are being prepared as there exist clinical needs to have a mutual image exchange: NM because the reading of images from the skeleton in suspicion of metastasis is optimized if NM whole body scans can be compared directly; radiotherapy because treatment planning is done for a number of cases on CT images; and orthopaedics because a joint research project aims at the set-up of a database with digitized images of hip prostheses within the PACS archive. This archive contains four sets of images that are centrally archived and originate from specific patient groups, i.e., osteoporosis, inner ear reconstruction, hip prostheses and mammography. Images in the ACR-NEMA format are read from the central archive by procedures originating from the PACS manufacturer as well as the department itself.

To conclude this chapter it should be stressed that in our opinion PACS can only grow when it is driven from clinical questions. Cost – benefit analysis of various medical technologies have indicated that a technique will be integrated in clinical routine whenever there is a need for it 'no matter' the costs involved. So starting from existing clinical questions PACS may lead to a framework within which research and clinical routine may be combined. The different aspects that refer to the picture, archive and communication system should be considered. For most projects in which a larger patient group is involved, communication of measured data to a standardized, dedicated, often PC-based, analyzing environment is necessary and in general not available. An example that considers the picture system is a receiver operating characteristics (ROC) study considering film and CRT (cathode ray tube) screen reading performed at UHN. The clinical question is: 'Is it possible to reduce the number of carcinomas that are missed within the screening by using image processing techniques?' At first it is important to determine whether it is possible to read mammograms from a CRT screen. If so, processing of the digitized images may be evaluated. Therefore, observer performance tests were conducted based on 240 mammograms to study the visibility of malignancies in digital mammography. The detectability of tumours and of microcalcifications were studied separately. Two sets of images were used, one set consisting of 150 mammograms for tumour detection and one set containing 120 mammograms for microcalcifica-

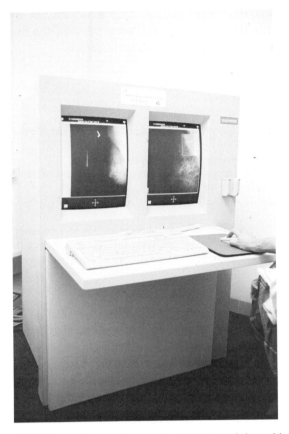

Fig. 3. The Siemens PACS diagnostic reporting console (DRC-20) as it is used in the clinical conferences and ROC study of digitized mammography (see displayed images).

tions. The images were digitized at a resolution of 2048 × 2048 pixels using a 12 bit (4096 × 4096) CCD-camera. Conventional film mammograms were read on a lightbox whereas digital mammograms were read on the PACS console DRC-20 (fig. 3). Two experienced radiologists independently read both sets, and ranked their judgments about the presence or absence of tumours or microcalcifications on a confidence-rating scale. Evaluating the ROC results, no statistical differences were found between judgments based on conventional and digitized mammograms. It should be noted that this study indicates the importance of a thorough consideration of the technical aspects of the digitization procedure. In a number of papers it is reported how insufficient resolution in space and contrast may deteriorate reading performance of digital images.

The way in which PACS will further develop within the next years strongly depends on the extent to which PACS brings improvements of and additions to the current situation. As the history of CT indicated: the emerging of really new information is the most powerful incentive, i.e., the image aspects that represent information that was not available before.

References

ACR-NEMA Publication 300-1988 (1988) Digital Imaging and Communication (NEMA, Washington D.C.)

Arenson, R.L. (1988) Opportunity ahead, *Radiology,* 169, 267.

Arenson, R.L., D.P. Chakraborty, S.B. Seshadri and H.L. Kundel (1990) The digital imaging workstation, *Radiology* 176, 303 – 315.

Axel, L. (1984) Blood flow effects in magnetic resonance imaging, *Am. J. Roentgenol.* 143, 1157 – 1166.

Bisseling, J.T., L.J.Th.O. van Erning, Th.E. Schouten and J.A.M. Lemmens (1989) Automatic CT measurement in lumbar vertebrae. In: Baumann, J.U., and R.E. Herron (Eds.), Proc. Fifth International Meeting Biostereometrics '88 (SPIE, Washington), pp. 146 – 154.

Bouman, H.D., M.J.J. Knots, L.J.Th.O. van Erning and S. Brinkkemper (1988) PACS in practice: the status of the PACS project at the St.Radboud University Hospital in Nijmegen, The Netherlands, Part B: A digital image archive: information analysis and development, *Med. Inform.* 13, 265 – 278.

Cannavo, M.J. (1988) Fitting PACS technology into the hospital of tomorrow, *Diagn. Imaging* 11, 188 – 190.

Cohen, M.S., and R.M. Weisskoff (1991) Ultra-fast imaging, *Magn. Reson. Imaging* 9, 1 – 37.

Drew, P.G. (1984) Many obstacles must be overcome before PACS fulfil their promise, *Diagn. Imaging* 11, 99 – 104.

Fischer, H.W. (1988) Danger ahead?, *Radiology* 169, 267.

Goddard, P.R. (1991) MR imaging overtakes CT in clinical oncology, *Diagn. Imaging Int.* 5, 32 – 38.

Hendee, W.R. (1988) Transforming medical imaging from a craft into a science, *Diagn. Imaging* 11, 97 – 103.

Hodapp, T.E. (1988) Imaging industry's growth boom should hit its peak in 1989, *Diagn. Imaging* 12, 58 – 73.

Hottier, F, and A. Collet Billon (1990) 3D echography: status and perspective. In: Höhne, K.H., H. Fuchs and S.M. Pizer (Eds.), 3D Imaging in Medicine, *NATO ASI Series F* 60, 21 – 41 (Springer, Berlin).

Karssemeijer, N., L.J.Th.O. van Erning and E.G.J. Eijkman (1988) Recognition of organs in CT-image sequences: a model guided approach, *Comput. Biomed. Res.* 21, 434 – 448.

Knots, M.J.J., L.J.Th.O. van Erning, J. Scaf, W. Guijt and J.H.J. Ruijs (1990) PACS in practice: on-line communication in daily routine, *Med. Inform.* 15, 11 – 14.

Ogle, P.L. (1988) All-digital department: don't bet on it just yet, *Diagn. Imaging* 12, 5.

Parker, J.A., H.D. Royal, R.F. Uren, D. Front, J.G. Bliss, M. Rabuzzi, D. Jansons and G.M. Kolodny (1983) An all-digital nuclear medicine department, *Radiology* 147, 237 – 240.

Radon, J. (1917) Über die bestimmung von Funktionen durch ihre Integralwerte entlang gewisser Mannigfaltigkeiten, *Ber. Verh. Saechs. Akad. Wiss. Leipzig Math. Phys. Kl.* 69, 262 – 277.

Shandle, J. (1990) Who will dominate the desktop in the '90s?, *Electronics* 2, 48 – 55.

Standard Product Interconnect (SPI) (1987) Siemens UB Med, Erlangen and Philips CHF Müller Hamburg, Federal Republic of Germany (in-house publication).

Umeda, T., K. Ihamura and K. Inamoto (1991) Multi-media PACS integrated with RIS/HIS employing magneto-optical disks. In: Jost, R.G. (Ed.), Medical Imaging V: PACS Design and Evaluation, *Proc. SPIE* 1446, 199 – 210

van Erning, L.J.Th.O., M.A.O. Thijssen, N. Karssemeijer and W. Guijt (1988) PACS in practice: the status of the PACS project at the St.Radboud University Hospital in Nijmegen, The Netherlands, Part A: Introduction and the picture system, *Med. Inform.* 13, 255 – 264.

van Gennip, E.M.S.J., B.M. van Poppel, A.R. Bakker, F.P. Ottes (1991) Comparison of worldwide opinions on the costs and benefits of PACS. In: Jost, R.G. (Ed.), Medical Imaging V: PACS Design and Evaluation, *Proc. SPIE* 1446, 442 – 450.

Webb, S. (1988) In the beginning. In: Webb, S. (Ed.), The Physics of Medical Imaging (Adam Hilger, Bristol and Philadelphia), pp. 7 – 19.

Weber, S. (1989) Looking ahead to FDVDI, *Electronics* 11, 99 – 100.

Integrated Diagnostic Imaging
Editor: J.P.J. De Valk
© *Elsevier Science Publishers B.V., 1992*

Chapter 15

Evolution of PACS concepts

Osman Ratib

1. Introduction

The concept of management and archival of medical images in digital form appeared and slowly matured during the 1980s. A rapidly growing number of concrete implementations of these systems will certainly flourish during the 1990s. Such systems are a logical consequence of the development of digital imaging modalities in medicine. Initially limited to some nuclear medicine studies, the number of digital images has grown exponentially since the early 1970s with the appearance of the computed tomography scanners and later with the introduction of magnetic resonance imaging technique. In parallel to these new imaging technologies, conventional X-ray imaging techniques were progressively converted to digital form. Digital capture of X-ray images from image intensifiers led to significant progress in digital subtraction angiography and to a substantial improvement in the diagnostic performance of such investigation technique. Recent development of photostimulated luminescence digital radiography allows now-a-day to capture X-ray images digitally without film. All these new digital imaging techniques produce a tremendous amount of digital images and data that required special technical developments for their management and storage. Such systems are usually referred to as image management and communication systems (IMACS) or picture archiving and communication systems (PACS).

2. PACS 1980 – 1990

2.1. Early PACS projects

In November 1981, Dr. Samuel J. Dwyer III from the University of Kansas presented a novel seminar on PACS for medical imaging to the Biomedical Engineering Division and the Department of Radiology, University of Iowa. Soon after, Dr. H.K. Huang together with Dr. Edmund Anthony Franken Jr., Chairman of the Department of Radiology, started to plan a PACS project for the Radiology Department. In 1982, Dr. Huang moved to the University of California in Los Angeles where he became in charge of a newly created image processing laboratory in the Department of Radiological Sciences. He then rapidly moved into an ambitious PACS project to try on the concept of a digital radiology department in a real clinical environment.

Several groups in the United States and in Japan followed these early developments and moved on very early towards centralized digital archives connected to different imaging sources where images can be stored and retrieved for review on display workstations. Among all the projects we would like to mention a few who played a leading role in the development of clinical PACS in the early 1980s.

- *The University of California in Los Angeles (UCLA)* was a pioneer in the field with a first clinical PACS in the department of pediatric radiology. Under the leadership of Professor H.K. Huang, this group contributed to the development of PACS concepts and technology in a large extent. They demonstrated the feasibility of an open-architecture PACS with the acquisition and storage of images from different modalities obtained with equipment from different vendors. Their work in the field of system integration, image compression, high-resolution workstations and recently in high-speed networks is widely acknowledged and has been the subject of a very large number of publications (Huang et al., 1988).
- *The University of Arizona*, where several research projects focused on the evaluation and modelling of the requirements for PACS networks, database and structure. They contributed in defining some innovative approaches for the architecture of distributed databases (LiuSheng et al., 1990) for medical images and the evaluation of such systems through computer modeling tools.
- *The University of Kansas* has done extensive work in the clinical implementation and development of PACS. They particularly focused their efforts in the development and integration of different network systems for PACS and teleradiology. They also carried out several clinical studies for the evaluation of the acceptability of high-resolution workstation in clinical practice (Dwyer III et al., 1990).
- *The University of Pennsylvania* was involved in digital image management systems since 1982. Their initial work on digital subtraction angiography systems was subsequently extended by a significant effort in the field of

high-speed optic networks (Arenson, 1984). They also developed useful methodology to design and evaluate PACS (Arenson et al., 1989).

- *Washington University in St. Louis* has contributed to the field of PACS development in collaboration with the Mallinckrot Institute of Radiology. Among other PACS developments one could mention their work in experimenting with ISDN networks on a PACS testbed (Blaine et al., 1990).

- *Georgetown University in Washington* is known for its work in the field of PACS and particularly for implementing a wide-scale, fully digital neuroradiology service based on AT&T CommView system. They also contributed to several studies on the requirements and specifications of a total digital radiology department. Part of this research was supported by grants from the department of defense and helped establishing the requirements for fully digital PACS for the armed forces (Mun et al., 1989).

- *Tokyo University Hospital* is among the leading institutions in Japan to develop and implement PACS and digital image management systems. They elected to develop a multivendor PACS with the first clinical implementation of the MIPS-87 standard (Kimura, 1989).

- *Kyoto University Hospital.* The PACS project named KIDS (Kyoto University Hospital image database and communication system) was initiated in spring 1985. In 1988, a second-generation system was introduced to integrate several major digital imaging modalities such as DSA (digital subtraction angiography), CR (computed radiography), CT and MRI with a new 100 Mbit/s network and high-speed image workstations. The KIDS is also used for teaching purposes where images can be directly visualized on large screens in the lecture hall of the medical school (Minato et al., 1990).

- *Hokkaido University Hospital.* A PACS project was already discussed at the Hokkaido University in Sapporo as early as 1980. In 1985, they received a budget from the government for research co-operation with industry. A joint development with NEC (Nippon Electric Company) was undertaken with a significant investment from the industry. Because most of the equipment is still under development and several component are not commercially available, the Hokkaido University decided to rent this equipment instead of buying it. Since June 1989 a clinical PACS (called HUPACS) is fully operational and is also integrated with the HIS (hospital information system) (Irie, 1990). The imaging equipment include three CT scanners, one MRI, three FCR computed radiography systems and two film laser scanners (Irie et al., 1990).

- *Utrecht University Hospital and the BAZIS group, the Netherlands* played the role of pioneer in Europe with the development of the IMAGIS project (image information system). In this project, carried out with the support of Philips, they put a noticeable effort in the integration and coupling of a

PACS with a radiology information system (RIS). They designed and developed methods for modelling and simulation and performance evaluation of PACS components. They also designed tools for technology assessment and cost – benefit analysis (Ottes et al., 1989).

– *University Hospital of Brussels (VUB)*. In 1987, the Vrije Universiteit Brussels (VUB) created the 'Pluridisciplinary Research Institute for Medical Imaging Sciences' (PRIMIS) for the study of the applications of digital imaging techniques. One of the PRIMIS project was a PACS project at the University Hospital. This system was designed on an open and distributed architecture based on a distributed sub-network topology (Mattheus and Osteaux, 1990).

– *University consortium of Nantes, Rennes and Villejuif*. In 1989, the University of Rennes initiated a project for a distributed PACS architecture (Sirene project). At the University Hospital of Nantes, a PACS was implemented for nuclear medicine (DIMI project) and in Villejuif a PACS is in building in the Gustave Roussy Institute (Simbad project). Recently, these three institutions created a consortium (NRV consortium) for PACS development and collaborative research (Vermont et al., 1990).

2.2. Meetings related to PACS development

Although the concept of archiving medical images in digital form and distributing them to remote workstations for review was conceived in the late 1970s, it is not until the assembly of the first International Conference and Workshop on PACS for Medical Applications in Newport Beach, California, in January 1982 that this idea received sufficient attention by the radiological community (Duerinckx, 1982). This meeting for the first time brought together researchers in both the academic and private sectors. The word 'PACS' was then unofficially adopted as the acronym for picture archiving and communication systems. Since then, an annual meeting sponsored by the International Society for Optical Engineering (SPIE) was held under the title of 'Applications of Optical Instrumentation in Medicine and PACS for Medical Applications' (Dwyer III, 1983). The last meeting, held in 1986, is also known under its abbreviated name 'Medicine XIV and PACS IV' and was replaced the following year by the new title of 'Medical Imaging' (Schneider and Dwyer III, 1984, 1985, 1986). In their introductory notes of the first Medical Imaging meeting in 1987, Roger Schneider and Samuel Dwyer, chairman and editors of the series, reported that the change in name reflected the general feeling that medical imaging had matured to the point that it must be considered in its entirely – from detector physics to database management and display – to optimize its clinical utility (Schneider and Dwyer III, 1987). From 1987 to 1990 this meeting was held every year in Newport Beach and was considered by all the experts in the field as the reference meeting for PACS development and related research.

In November 1987, for the first time, the Radiological Society of North America (RSNA) had a special focus session on PACS during its 73rd Annual Assembly in Chicago. Since that year, there has been an increasing number of sessions dedicated to PACS in the following RSNA meetings.

During this period, the first Japanese PACS (JPACS) meeting was held in Tokyo in July 1984, and the meeting has convened annually since then. In 1984, a European PACS society (EuroPACS) was founded in Europe with the aim to 'promote the exchange of information and research in the development and use of digital systems for acquisition, storage, transport, processing, display and reproduction of medical pictures'. One of the major activities of this society is to organize an annual meeting on PACS in Europe. Every year the meeting is held in a different country and there is an increasing number of communications presented every year, including ones from the United States and Japan.

2.3. Technical challenges of PACS

Several papers published on PACS in the early years predicted that it would only take three to five years before PACS and filmless radiology departments become a clinical reality. History showed that these predictions were overoptimistic and that it took more than ten years for PACS technology to mature and to become available for the 1990s. A serious underestimation of the technical difficulties was responsible for this phenomenon. Although most technical problems seemed easy to solve, it is the cumulative effect of putting together all the components of a PACS to achieve the goal of a fully digital radiology department that was underestimated. In addition to all the technical challenges, the problem of system integration was responsible for many additional difficulties. Besides, the high cost of PACS development was also responsible for the limited number of successful projects. In addition to the cost of the equipment itself, the manpower and resources necessary for PACS implementation turned out to be a substantial additional cost of the development.

2.3.1. Digital image acquisition

One of the first objectives of a PACS is to collect radiological images in digital form for archival and communication (Huang, 1987). Although there is an increasing number of radiological images that are acquired directly in digital form (CT, MRI, nuclear medicine, etc.), most manufacturers would not provide an easy way to access the images in their original digital form. It is only in the late 1980s that some industry standards emerged to allow images to be transferred from the acquisition devices to PACS environments. Most PACS projects had to deal with serious difficulties in extracting the images from the acquisition devices. Customized interfaces had to be developed for the different devices to connect PACS equipment. These developments could only be undertaken with a contribution from the manufacturers. These developments are usually very costly, because individual technical solutions are always more expensive than more generic ones that can be reused in different configurations. For the same reasons it is more difficult to integrate imaging equipment from different manufacturers and some PACS projects were often limited to equipment from a single manufacturer. Such a solution is generally not acceptable in large academic hospitals where state-of-the-art imaging equipment is required and can only be obtained by selecting the best equipment from different manufacturers.

Another difficulty encountered with the development of PACS is the acquisition of conventional X-ray images traditionally acquired on films. Two major solutions were adopted: high-resolution laser scanners and photostimulated luminescence digital radiography (PLDR). Laser scanners only provide a partial solution to the problem since they require images to be obtained on films first and then to be scanned digitally. In addition to the technical problem of loss of image quality, this solution also requires extra manpower for handling the digitization process. PLDR is undoubtedly a more adequate solution.

The PLDR imaging techniques use the properties of certain kinds of phosphors called photostimulable luminescence (PSL). With proper addition of energy, the electrons in the phosphor which usually stay in the valence band move up to the trap band and stay there. With the addition of another energy, the migrated electrons in the trap band will fall back to the valence band. At this time the phosphorus luminescence phenomenon occurs. Therefore, if X-rays are used as the first energy, a plate containing a uniform layer of PSL phosphor crystals will be able to retain a part of the absorbed X-ray energy in the trap band in the form of electrons. The distribution of these electrons forms a latent image just as that in a film-screen receptor. The latent image can be read by a second energy source such as a laser beam. After the latent image is erased with an intensive light source, this phosphor layer can be used over and over again.

The PSL phenomenon was discovered in the middle of the nineteenth century, but it has been almost ignored because of the lack of industrial applications. In 1975, PSL phosphor was proposed to be used as an image receptor. In 1982, the first radiographic imaging device using the PSL phosphor was built in Japan. The phosphorus crystal used was $BaFX : Eu$ ($X = Cl$, Br, I). Stimulation of the latent image in the plate by a laser beam gives emission of luminescence radiation corresponding to the absorbed X-ray energy.

One of the first commercial PLDR systems, also called Fuji computed radiography (FCR) system, was manufactured by Fuji Photo Film Co., Ltd., Tokyo, Japan. The PSL phosphor plate, called an imaging plate in the FCR system, is housed inside a cassette just like a film-screen system. After the imaging plate is exposed to X-rays and a latent image is formed in the plate (similar to a film-screen detector), it is processed through the FCR for extracting the radiographic image. There are four major components in the FCR: the image reader, the image processor, image storage devices and the image recorder.

Although the output of this system is digital, the first commercial systems only provided analog images printed on conventional films. The reason for this restriction was to maintain film consumption similar to the conventional X-ray equipment. Early PACS projects encountered some difficulties in interfacing these devices with a PACS network. Even after several main manufactures have provided commercial PLDR systems, only a limited number of installed equipment were digitally interfaced to PACS. Often special interfaces had to be developed to transfer the digital data. The first institution to develop such a system was UCLA (Ho et al., 1987), where a FCR system was connected to a PACS network.

2.3.2. Storage devices

The storage of radiological images in digital format is a non-trivial problem due to the very large volume of data that these images contain. Projectional X-ray images require very high resolution to be clinically acceptable. Such images must be acquired and stored in image matrices of more than 2000×2000 pixels, with a dynamic range of $8-12$ bits per pixel. This represents between $4-8$ Mbytes per image. Digital imaging modalities such as computed tomography or magnetic resonance imaging generate images with smaller matrices (typically 256×256 or 512×512 with a dynamic range of $12-16$ bits per pixel), but the difficulty there comes from the very large number of images generated at each patient examination. One examination can generate between twenty and sometimes more than one hundred images. This corresponds to storage requirements between 10 and 50 Mbytes per study. The rapid development of very high capacity optical disks that can also be handled in large numbers inside optical disk libraries called 'jukeboxes' offer a practical solution to the storage problem. The major problem of optical disk storage is the fairly slow throughput of these disks. Reading and writing data on optical disk is significantly slower than on all other disks. Besides accessing images from large number of optical disks may require frequent swapping of the disks in the jukeboxes which is a slow mechanical operation. In order to overcome this speed problem, the design of optical disk archives for PACS requires large-capacity magnetic disk caching to maintain a rapid access to most recent and most frequently accessed images. Only a well-adjusted combination of

magnetic disk and optical disk storage space will allow adequate performance
of the archival and retrieval tasks of the PACS.

Despite the rapid development of high-capacity optical disk storage devices
with constant increase in storage capacity and decrease in cost, proper archive
of images will also require data compression. For radiological images, existing
lossless or reversible methods achieve compression ratios with an upper bound
near 3 : 1. More typically the ratio is in the range of 1.5 to 2.0. Irreversible
methods can achieve higher compression ratios at the expenses of image fideli-
ty. Irreversible image compression can provide significantly higher reduction in
data volume ranging from 5- to 20-fold. However, to be acceptable, a compression algorithm requires clinical validation tests. Such tests must be carried out
on a large number of images and should involve a large number of clinicians
to ensure that the diagnostic accuracy is not jeopardized by image compression.
The technique consists of comparing receiver operating characteristic (ROC)
curves of compressed and uncompressed images for different imaging
modalities and for different diagnostic signs (Harrington, 1990). Such studies
are expensive and time consuming but are mandatory before the application of
any compression algorithm. Clinical validation is not the only difficulty encountered with image compression; most compression algorithms require long
computation time particularly on large images. Hardware implementation of
the compression algorithm necessary to provide the appropriate speed of compression and decompression of images in a PACS environment. The UCLA
group designed a compression algorithm based on full-frame cosine transformation and they have implemented it in hardware (Ho et al., 1988). Subsequent clinical validations showed that this compression algorithm could provide
compression factors up to 20 : 1 for conventional chest X-rays and up to 5 : 1
for tomographic images without significant loss of clinically relevant information. With the hardware implementation these compressions are performed
within a few seconds even for very large images.

2.3.3. Workstation design and performance

The display workstation is an essential part of PACS mainly because it is the
most visible part to the radiologists. It should primarily allow the radiologist
to handle digital images on a monitor in the same way as he does in daily practice when manipulating radiographs on a lightbox. In addition to simply viewing images, the workstation is expected to bring some additional functionalities
that were not available in a film-based system. Among the major added features
one can mention image processing and enhancement tools, dynamic displays,
image analysis and quantification tools, and access to image-related data such
as report and clinical record. The greatest challenge, however, is to provide the
basic functionalities of image display in a way that is at least as convenient as

the lightbox. Radiologists are used to review very large number of images on alternators, where images can be brought up very rapidly and several images can be displayed side by side for comparison. This convenient and very rapid access to the images is often the most difficult task to achieve on a viewing station. Due to hardware limitations it is often difficult to access very large images and display them as quickly as is possible on the alternator lightbox. Large amount of RAM memory, special high-speed parallel disks, and fast display devices are needed to allow such a performance. Besides, for image comparison, the workstation should be equipped with several high-resolution monitors. This kind of hardware is still very expensive and can only be implemented in a limited number in a PACS.

Most studies showed that in a PACS several types of workstations are necessary. For primary diagnosis the radiologist needs a workstation that provides the best possible performance with the highest resolution. For review and clinical conferences the requirements are less stringent and do not require the same high performance. Finally, a third type of workstations can be envisioned for image processing and analysis. This third category should provide more specific tools for image analysis of certain type of images and provide the best possible user interface to allow easy access to these tools by non-computer-oriented users.

2.3.4. Network design

In large-scale PACS, the network performance is a crucial element of the whole system. Early systems often relied on fast point-to-point communication interfaces. With the development of a larger number of acquisition and display nodes, the point-to-point communication channels can no longer be used and a distributed network is then required. Most projects adopted the most widely available industry standard, namely the IEEE 802.3 Ethernet standard. However, several authors reported that the Ethernet performance is insufficient for a departmental or hospital-wide PACS. High-speed optical fiber networks were then designed with a transfer rate of an order of magnitude faster than Ethernet. Several systems designed by the manufacturers were closed networks in the sense that only the components from the same manufacturer can be connected to the network. Recent development of the FDDI technology seems to emerge as a standard for optical local network based on the IEEE 802.5 token-ring standard. It is intended for the connection of high-performance mainframes, workstations and peripheral equipment and to provide a backbone connection for lower-speed local-area networks. FDDI operates at a speed of 100 Mbits/s and should allow an effective transfer rate of image data for up to 80 Mbits/s (Stewart, 1990).

Beyond the departmental or hospital PACS, there is an increasing need for image transfer between institutes through wide-area networks (WAN) and metropolitan-area networks (MAN). Among the most promising systems is the integrated services digital network (ISDN). This public network is intended to simultaneously provide end-to-end digital communication of voice and all types of packet-switched and circuit-switched data.

2.4. Emergence of industry standards

From early on, most groups doing PACS-related work have encountered the problem of acquiring images and image-related data from different manufacturer's equipment. This problem was debated among the radiology community through the American College of Radiology (ACR). The manufacturers also began to realize that there was little to be gained by keeping image format proprietary. In early 1983, the ACR/NEMA Digital Imaging and Communication Standards Committee was founded. The original objective of the committee was to develop an interface so that images and related information could be exchanged between a piece of medical imaging equipment and whatever was on the other side of the interface (Horii et al., 1990). In defining this as the objective, the committee restricted its range of activity. The resulting standard would not be a full PACS standard, nor a database standard, nor a network standard. However, the ability to bring digital image information out of a piece of equipment over standard hardware using a standard format was felt to be a goal worthy of such concentrated research. Within two years, a standard evolved that was felt to meet all the requirements set forth by the committee. It was distributed at the Radiological Society of North America meeting in 1985 and published as a NEMA standard (ACR-NEMA, 1988) in the same year. The first revision of the standard (revision 2.0) was approved and published in 1988.

In 1984, the Japan Industries Association for Radiation Apparatus (JIRA) created a committee to establish a medical image transfer standard for medical image processing system (MIPS), to be used as a standard for transfer of both image data and demographic data for medical imaging hardware. Soon afterwards, the ACR/NEMA published its own standard. The current version, namely the MIPS-87, is basically similar to the ACR/NEMA version 1.0 minimum requirement, with some minor modifications, mainly with regard to the handling of text data. The MIPS standard had undergone major revisions and an update version was issued early 1990 (MIPS 89).

Two other committees were also founded in Japan: the committee for Personal Health Data (PHD) and the Image Save And Carry (ISAC) Committee. Dr. S. Ikeda from the National Cancer Institute of Japan proposed in 1982 that every citizen should have his medical record on digital media. Dr. Ikeda and his colleagues had proceeded in the development and evaluation of PHD system between 1982 and 1987 under the support of the Japanese Ministry of International Trade and Industry (MITI) and the Japanese Ministry of Welfare. The work done by this committee has been followed by ISAC committee for the image data handling aspect. The ISAC committee organized four working groups (WGs) for the development of the standard: WG-1 for disk format, WG-2 for image data file, WG-3 for software development and WG-4 for technology assessment. The WG-2 already stated that image data file format on MO disk in ISAC standard should have the same format as the MIPS standard. WG-3 and WG-4 began their activity in 1990.

3. PACS 1990 – 2000

It is through the contributions of the early researchers dedicated to this field that the PACS concept has matured. PACS research is beginning to bear fruit as we now see a few working PACS modules in clinical operation.

In a recent meeting on PACS that was held in Evian in October 1990, several encouraging observations could be made from the contributions presented at this meeting leading to believe that the technology of PACS is available for the 1990s. During the meeting, Professor H.K. Huang from UCLA observed in his opening keynotes that the clinical implementation of PACS can be carried out through three typical ways:

(1) PACS implementation can be carried out by a multidisciplinary team within a department or a hospital for PACS development and integration;

(2) PACS can be designed by a team of experts who write the specifications

Type	Advantages		Disadvantage	
(1)	–	Built to specs	–	Difficult to assemble a team
	–	State of the art	–	One of a kind system
	–	Continuous upgrade	–	Service and maintenance cost
	–	Indep. from manufacturer		
(2)	–	Specifications are written for certain clinical environment	–	Specifications tend to be over-ambitious
	–	Implementation is delegated to manufacturers	–	Underestimate technical and operational difficulties
			–	Manufacturers lack clinical experience
			–	Expensive
(3)	–	Lower cost	–	Too generic
	–	Easier maintenance	–	No state of the art

and leave the implementation and development to be carried out by the manufacturers;

(3) PACS can be purchase as a 'turn-key' system fully designed, developed and implemented by manufacturers.

Most PACS developments reported are of one of these three types, or in some cases a combination of those. There is however, some advantages and disadvantages to each type.

Most interesting in the evolution of PACS concept between 1980 and 1990 is the trend towards distributed and open architectures. The early PACS designs were geared towards a centralized system where images and data are stored in a central archive node and then distributed upon request to peripheral workstations. With the development of network facilities and intercomputer communication systems it became possible to design distributed archives where images and data can be stored at different node of a network and still be accessible in any other part of that network. The choice between the centralized and distributed architecture will depend on the type of PACS and the flow of images that need to be supported (fig. 1). The advantages and disadvantage of centralized versus distributed systems are the following:

Centralized architecture:

Advantages	Disadvantages
– Shareable resources	– Limited performance (network load)
– Easier management of all images in a centralized directory	– Variable and inconsistent response time depending on the workload
– Maintenance of a single system	– If the central host computer is down all workstations are inoperable

Distributed architecture:

Advantages	Disadvantages
– Higher performance through distributed tasks	– Network performance limitations
– Allows easy development of modular software applications	– Difficult support and maintenance in inhomogeneous environments
– Part of the system can remain operational when some other are down	– Requires special development of data traffic management and interprocess communications

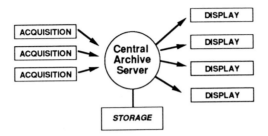

Centralized Architecture

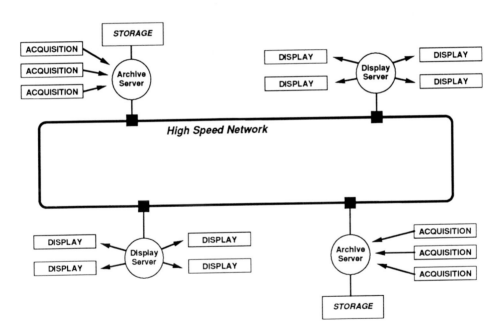

Distributed Architecture

Fig. 1. Schematic illustration of different PACS architectures. The figure above displays a centralized approach with central archive of all image data that are then distributed to different display stations. The figure below shows a distributed network of multiple archive and display servers.

The other sign of evolution in PACS design is the move towards an open architecture with multivendor equipment based on industry standards for interconnection of imaging devices and other PACS components. This trend is made possible by a similar evolution among the manufacturers who tend to support established standards and to be less protective about the integration of their equipment with other equipments. The emergence of these standards from a joint effort between the academic community and the manufacturers (such as ACR/NEMA standard) together with standards of the computer industry (such as UNIX, Ethernet protocols, FDDI, etc.) have played a major role in this evolution.

4. PACS at the University Hospital of Geneva

The University Hospital of Geneva initiated a hospital-wide PACS project that officially started the third quarter of 1989. The aim of this project is to develop an integrated image management system for radiological as well as non-radiological medical images. The main characteristic of this PACS is that it is directly part of a large-scale hospital information system. Since 1975, the medical informatics division of the hospital has developed one of the widest hospital information systems in Switzerland, called the Diogene system (Scherrer et al., 1990). The evolution of the Diogene HIS from a centralized system to a distributed architecture promoted the concept of the integration of the PACS directly as a part of the HIS. In this architecture, the images are viewed as another type of information to be handled by the HIS. This leads to a new concept of ward information system (WIS) where physicians and nurses could review and update their patient's medical record directly in digital form. The Geneva PACS is based on an open architecture with heterogeneous systems and multi-vendor equipment. It is built around a set of widely available industry standards, namely: UNIX as the main operating system of all computers, TCP-IP as network protocol currently implemented on Ethernet networks but soon supported transparently by high-speed networks, as well and an SQL-based distributed database (INGRES) that handles both the PACS and the HIS. The PACS is based on a distributed architecture of large number of servers. Two main types of servers are designed: the archive servers connected to the sources of images and equipped with large storage capacity using optical disk libraries (jukeboxes), and display servers distributed over the hospital for temporary storage of images of current patients (fig. 1).

4.1. PACS architecture

4.1.1. The archive servers
Several archive servers allow for the acquisition and storage of image from different imaging modalities. Each of these servers is designed with a hierarchical cache system that consists of sufficient RAM memory space (32 – 128 Mbytes), large capacity magnetic storage disks (2 – 4 Gbytes) and very large optical disk jukeboxes (approximately 1 Terabytes). This cache system allows a better performance and more rapid access to recent images that are kept in RAM and magnetic storage space.

A special file transfer management software is developed for the distribution of the images to predefined display servers where images can be accessed by the users. Images can thereby be distributed to several display servers simultaneously to be available at different locations in the hospital such as the radiology reading room and the medical ward, for example. Images from previous examinations are extracted from the image database and sent through the same path either together with the current images or in advance prior to the requested examination.

4.1.2. The display servers
Display servers are equipped with magnetic or opto-magnetic disks for temporary storage of images. One server supports a cluster of several display workstations. The user of a given workstation can only access the images available on the corresponding display server. If the user requires an image that is not available on the local display server, provided he has the proper privilege to access these images, a special request can be posted from the workstation to the archive server through a query to the PACS database. The corresponding images are transferred from the archive to the display server in batch mode according to priority schemes and depending on the network load. The user is notified when the requested images are available on his local server. A queueing system allows to control the network load at all time and avoid excessive traffic due to large number of simultaneous requests that may be submitted to the archive servers.

4.1.3. The imaging workstations
Different types of workstations are required for different usage in a hospital-wide PACS. High-performance workstations equipped with multiple high-resolution displays are needed for review and primary diagnosis by the radiologists. Multipurpose workstations for accessing images and other clinical information are to be designed to support all the functionalities of the HIS.

Finally, there is an increasing demand for more quantitative analysis workstations, for image processing and computer-assisted image interpretation.

In order to provide a more uniform user interface on a variety of different
workstations, a common platform was developed for image display and
manipulation and can be ported on different workstations. A software package
called OSIRIS was designed based on X-11 windowing system and OSF/Motif
extension (Ligier et al., 1990). Such a platform is intended to be portable to any
computer running UNIX and equipped with a graphic display system running
X-11. This software is developed in the object oriented language C+ + to be
easily expandable and easily adaptable to different needs and requirements. The
OSIRIS user interface is described in more details later in this chapter.

4.2. Specific developments

4.2.1. Image file format

A standard image storage format was developed based on the ACR/NEMA
standard of image communication (ACR-NEMA, 1988). This file format,
called the PAPYRUS format, allows to store sets of images as a sequence of standard ACR/NEMA messages in an 'encapsulated' file format (Ratib et al.,
1990). A 'folder' structure allows to keep a directory of related images in a
single file or in different files. All images obtained from different modalities
are converted to the PAPYRUS format prior to archiving.

The PAPYRUS file format is a tagged file format based on the ACR/NEMA
specifications for data communication until a final agreement about the
ACR/NEMA file format is reached. The fields in the headers are of variable
length and are always preceded by a label and the length of the field in bytes.
The file resembles an ACR/NEMA message and could be directly read as such
(Ratib et al., 1990). The only difference is that in order to allow for multiple
images to be stored in a single file or in separate files, an additional group of
data called the 'folder information' was added. This additional group contains
the number of images actually in the file and a set of pointers to the location
of these images. The first version of the PAPYRUS format has been extensively
modified after its evaluation by a technical working group of the European
teleradiology project ('TELEMED' project). After several technical meetings,
the different partners of TELEMED came to an agreement that required a few
functionality to be added to the original proposal. Among the modifications
two features supported by the SPI (standard product interconnect for compatibility of digital imaging) were discussed: the unique image identification
code and the image folder concept that contains references to image data sets.
Related images can be distributed in separate files or directly in the folder file.

Each image of a given radiological procedure and its associated information

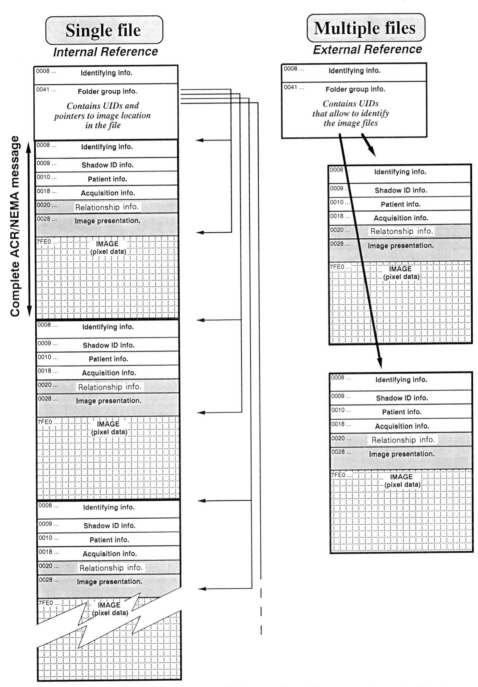

Fig. 2. Description of the PAPYRUS image file format. Sets of images can be stored either in a single file or in multiple files. A folder data set contains the appropriate information for identifying every image of the set.

can be stored in the same file (like in an ACR/NEMA message), and are organized into groups representing the general categories of information. Each group is further subdivided into related data elements. Within each group there are data elements which are mandatory and some which are optional. The mandatory items provide data necessary to display an image and to interpret it. Optional data elements may be included to provide supplemental information.

Images are stored as 'image data sets'. Each image data set contains only one image and corresponds to a complete ACR/NEMA message. As such, each image data set consists of a list of ACR/NEMA groups of elements necessary to form a complete message.

Image sets can be stored in sequence in a single file preceded by a folder structure. A folder is a means of associating sets of related data sets. In the context of the PAPYRUS format, a folder is simply a data set type which incorporates, either by reference or by value, other data sets. As defined here, a folder is not a display metaphor, a query mechanism, a directory structure or a data base structure. It is only a data set that permits the definition of association information about other data sets. Two types of references to sets of images are supported:

– internal references (pointers to data sets in the folder file);
– external references (references to data sets stored in other files).

A schematic representation of these two reference types is shown in fig. 2.

4.2.2. Interactive software for image display

Part of PACS development, a portable software package called OSIRIS for the display and manipulation of images is being developed. This project is based on preliminary exploratory work in this area at UCLA where a prototype of such a software called CALIPSO (Ratib and Huang, 1989) was developed on a Macintosh computer. During the development and evaluation phase of the project, the Macintosh was found to be an excellent training platform for clinicians and residents to familiarize themselves with different image processing and image analysis techniques and to explore their effects on different imaging modalities. During this first phase, a clinical survey showed that none of the users seemed to be confused by the large variety of tools that the program offers. On the contrary, most of the users made suggestions of additional tools that they would like to have. Thus, there is a general demand for more sophisticated analysis tools if they are made available in a user-friendly interface which does not require extensive computer manipulation skills. This confirms our hypothesis that if complex analysis tools are made available in simple systems one can expect a wide acceptability by the radiologists and clinicians. Another important observation is that when physicians are exposed to such analysis tools, their imaginations are stimulated and almost all the users that were interviewed had envisioned specific applications of some of these tools in their daily work.

In the design of the OSIRIS program special care was taken to provide a very consistent approach with the different image processing tools. The way the different tasks are performed are always very similar allowing the user to rapidly become familiar with the operation of all the features of the program. This consistency in the design and operation of a large variety of analysis tools applicable to different imaging modalities is unique and non-existent in currently available commercial imaging systems. Most manufacturers implement image processing and analysis programs that are manufacturer and modality specific. Recent developments of PACS led the manufacturers to provide systems that can handle and display images from different modalities. Very little effort was made, however, to unify the different image analysis techniques in a unique set of standard tools. The OSIRIS software is developed under X-11 and OSF/Motif windowing environment to ensure its portability to any UNIX platform.

Image display in windows
In graphic softwares designed to display medical images it is necessary to define the way images should be displayed and handled in a window. Because medical images often come in sets (sequential images or set of different views or sections) the window must provide a way of handling more than one image at a time. The OSIRIS software supports two modes of presentation of a set of images:
– tiled images;
– stacked images.

The user can switch from one mode to another at anytime.

In the tile mode, the images are displayed side by side in a grid that is optimized to be as square as possible based on the number and the size of images to be displayed. The user can further modify the image distribution. The scroll controls of the window allow the user to move across the set of images. The whole set behaves as a single large image. Therefore, zooming or reducing the images automatically change the magnification factor of the whole set.

In the stack mode, the images are virtually displayed in a stack. The user is then able to 'browse' through the stack up and down using a special control. In a movie mode, the user can also dynamically display the images in sequence. This mode was found to be very helpful not only for viewing dynamic images, but also for browsing into sets of contiguous tomographic images (fig. 3).

Image contrast and intensity adjustments
The most essential tool in medical image manipulation is the adjustment of con-

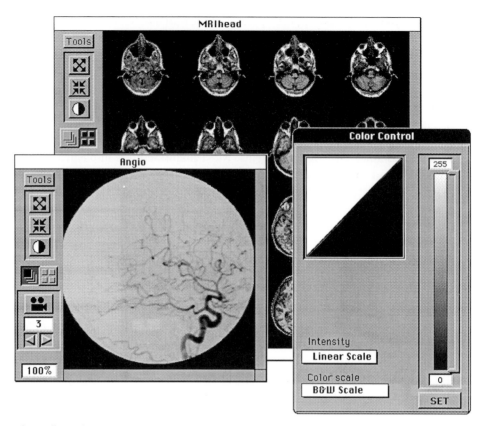

Fig. 3. Illustration of a 'multi-window' user interface for image display and management. This example is obtained from the OSIRIS software and shows the two modes for displaying image sets: the stack mode (for the angiography images up front) and the tile mode (for the MRI images in the back). A switch on the tool palette on the left of each window allows to switch from one mode to another easily. The window on the right shows the intensity and contrast adjustment tool.

trast and intensity (window width and window level). In the OSIRIS software the user is able to adjust the contrast and intensity of an image interactively in real-time. A set of linear and non-linear intensity transformation functions (ITF) are selectable. Finally, the user has the choice to display the images in black and white or in pseudocolour scales. Sets of standard as well as custom color look-up tables (CLUT) are available.

Because the dynamic range of some images may largely exceed the range of intensity levels that can be displayed at one time on a screen, it was important to allow for optimal mapping of the image values into the subset of intensity (or color) values available for display. Typically medical images will have an intrinsic dynamic range of up to 12 or 16 bits deep while most of the common display systems support 8 bit displays that will allow only 256 levels to be displayed at one time. The interactive adjustment is done in real time on the available dynamic range of the display (typically 256 levels) and when done, the image in its full dynamic range is remapped to the screen.

Also, because images displayed in different windows could be used for comparative evaluations, each window is adjustable separately. Due to hardware constraints, it is often not possible to perform this adjustment in each window individually in real time. It is therefore usually accepted that in some configurations the real-time adjustment will affect the whole screen (including all the windows displayed on it) and when done, only the active window (the top most in the stack of windows) is readjusted to match the setting that was selected interactively.

Annotations and image-related information
Medical images are usually accompanied with clinical information and related data. Three types of annotations and data presentations are supported and accessible from the workstation.
(1) For each image window, a secondary window containing the image interpretation report as well as any clinical information related to the images can be displayed.
(2) Annotations can be added to the image when needed in form of short text that can be positioned anywhere in the image. All the annotations are always handled as 'objects' separate from the image itself that can be moved, altered and deleted at will.
(3) In order to allow for longer text to be attached to an annotation, a 'Post-It' window is also accessible. Such a window should act as a pop-up window that is activated by clicking on a selected annotation on the image. When a Post-It is available the corresponding annotation should have a visual clue that allows the user to know that there is more information available.

Processing and analysis tools
Because the OSIRIS software is intended to be used with images from different imaging modalities, two different types of image manipulation tools are designed. One set of generic image processing and analysis tools and a set of specific quantitative analysis tools that can be implemented modularly depending on the needs of the different users. The general image manipulation and processing tools are divided into the following categories:
Image manipulation tools
- zooming and panning,
- contrast and intensity adjustment,
- magnifying glass,

– rotation and flipping,
– reordering images;
Image processing tools
– filters,
– adaptive histogram equalization,
– isocontours,
– image combinations,
– display of global and regional histogram,
– cross section histogram;
Annotation and drawing tools
– annotations,
– arrows and lines;
Standard analysis tools
– coordinates, angles and local density measurement,
– regions of interest (ROI): copy and paste an ROI between images,
– clear or delete a ROI,
– reshape and resize ROIs,
– merge of several ROIs in one single ROI,
– generate a ROI from the intersection of two ROIs,
– shrink and grow of a ROI.

In addition to this list of general purpose tools, specific clinical tools will also be implemented. Usually, such tools are more specific to certain types of images. Among the most commonly used clinical tools one can mention ejection fraction calculation, vascular stenosis evaluation, flow measurement, dynamic tracer washout analysis, etc.

4.3. Current implementation

As mentioned earlier, the Geneva PACS is designed by a development team that is in charge of the development and implementation of the different components of the PACS. A modular development of the hospital-wide PACS will allow to develop clusters of sub-PACSs in different sections of the hospital. The general architecture is based on sets of archive servers, each of them supporting a groups of image sources. Images are then distributed to display servers, each of them supporting one or several workstations.

The current status of the project is schematically shown in fig. 4 and includes the following parts:

(1) A software development laboratory equipped with a variety of workstations for the development of software tool for image management and communication as well as the OSIRIS image manipulation software.

(2) The first PACS module currently implement consist of a cluster regrouping

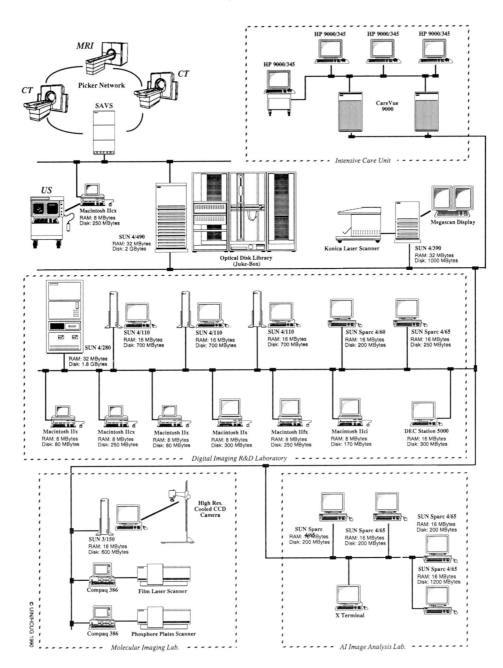

Fig. 4. Schematic diagram of the Geneva PACS imaging network around the first clinical sector (see text for details).

two CT scanners, an MRI scanner and an ultrasound unit. All the images from these imaging units are stored on the same archive server consisting of a SUN 4/490 server and a Cygnet jukebox with ATG optical disk drives for 6.4 Gbyte platters for a total capacity of approximately 1 Tbyte.

(3) A prototype project for implementation of a multimedia workstation in an intensive care unit. This project developed in collaboration with Hewlett Packard will focus on the development of workstations where the data obtained from patient monitoring systems can be reviewed together with the laboratory results, medication, nursing observations and the radiological images. It is a first step toward a completely integrated bedside workstation for a ward information system.

(4) A laboratory for acquisition and analysis of non-radiological images such as autoradiography, electrophoresis and histological images. This laboratory is equipped with a high-resolution laser scanner and a table-top phosphor plate computed radiography system and several workstations for image display and analysis. Clinical images obtained from this laboratory will be incorporated in the PACS database as well.

(5) A special laboratory for development of automatic image analysis software and artificial intelligence tools is also implemented.

4.4. Future planning

The choice of a very modular architecture with clusters of archive and display servers allows for a progressive planning of the PACS implementation on a hospital-wide scale. Different PACS modules will be progressively implemented. After the completion of the first module for cross-sectional images (CT, MRI and US) expected in the middle of 1991, the following modules are planned:
- PACS for intensive care units;
- PACS for molecular biology images;
- PACS for emergency room;
- PACS for nuclear medicine;
- PACS for digital angiography;
- PACS for cardiology.

All these modules will be developed on a similar architecture even if the hardware choices may differ depending on the availability of new and more performing equipment. A distributed database allows the access to all images from the different modules. Prefetch algorithms are being developed to anticipate the needs and regulate the traffic of images between the archive servers and display servers.

Also a pilot project for teleradiology and remote consultation is currently underway as part of the European TELEMED project. This projects includes developments of videoconferences and remote expert consultation systems, establishment of a radiology reference image database and PACS-to-PACS communication systems. The University Hospital of Geneva will be able to test high-speed communication lines (2 Mbit/s) for the transfer of images with other partners of the TELEMED project in Europe (Sweden, Norway, Germany, France, Spain, Italy and Greece). The PAPYRUS image file format proposed by Geneva was adopted as a standard file format for image communication in this project. As an extension of this project it is also planned to use the same technology for transferring images to and from remote clinics affiliated to the Geneva Hospital and located in different parts of the city.

References

ACR-NEMA Publication 300-1988 (1988) Digital Imaging and Communication (NEMA, Washington D.C.).

Arenson, R.L. (1984) Automation of the radiology management function, *Radiology* 153, 65–67.

Arenson, R.L., S.B. Seshadri, H.L. Kundel and D. DeSimone (1989) PACS at Penn. In: Schneider, R.H., S.J. Dwyer III and G. Jost (Eds.), Medical Imaging III: PACS System Design and Evaluation, *Proc. SPIE* 1093, 50–59.

Blaine, G.J, R.C. Ferguson, J.W. Sudt and R.A. Whitman (1990) ISDN: early experiments as a wide-area extension to LAN-based PACS. In: Dwyer III, S.J., and R.G. Jost (Eds.), Medical Imaging IV: PACS System Design and Evaluation, *Proc. SPIE* 1234, 140–147.

Duerinckx, A.J. (Ed.) (1982) Picture Archiving and Communication Systems (PACS) for Medical Applications, First International Conference and Workshop, *Proc. SPIE* 318.

Dwyer III, S.J. (Ed.) (1983) Picture Archiving and Communication Systems (PACS) for Medical Applications, Second International Conference and Workshop, *Proc. SPIE* 418.

Dwyer III, S.J., G.G. Cox, L.T. Cook J.H. McMillan and A.W. Templeton (1990) Experience with high resolution digital gray scale display systems. In: Dwyer III, S.J., and R.G. Jost (Eds.), Medical Imaging IV: PACS System Design and Evaluation, *Proc. SPIE* 1234, 132–138.

Harrington, M.B. (1990) Some methodological questions concerning ROC analysis as a method for assessing image quality in radiology, *J. Digital Imaging* 3, 211–218.

Ho, B.K., C. Morioka, N.J. Mankovich, B. Stewart and H.K. Huang (1987) Image acquisition for the pediatric radiology PACS module. In: Schneider, R.H., and S.J. Dwyer III (Eds.), Medical Imaging, *Proc. SPIE* 767, 554–557.

Ho, B.K., K.K. Chan, Y. Ishimitsu, B. Stewart, S.C. Lo and H.K. Huang (1988) High speed image compression system, prototype and final configuration. In: Schneider, R.H., and S.J. Dwyer III (Eds.), Medical Imaging II, *Proc. SPIE* 914, 786–791.

Horii, S., D. Hill, H. Blume, D. Best, B. Thompson, C. Fuscoe and D. Snavely (1990) An update on american college of radiology-national manufacturers association standards activity, *J. Med. Imaging* 3, 146–151.

Huang, H.K. (1987) Elements of Digital Radiology: A Professional Handbook and Guide (Prentice-Hall, Englewood Cliffs NJ)

Huang, H.K., N. Mankovich, R. Taira, P. Cho, B. Stewart, B. Ho, K. Chau and Y. Ishimitsu

(1988) Picture archiving and communication systems (PACS) for radiological images: state of the art, *CRC Crit. Rev. Diagn. Imaging* 28, 383–428.

Irie, G. (1990) Clinical experience: 16 months of HU-PACS. In: Picture Archiving and Communication System (PACS) in Medicine, Evian, *NATO ASI Series* (Springer, Berlin), pp. 183–188.

Irie, G., K. Miyasaka, K. Miyamoto, T. Kojima, I. Yamamoto and T. Kudo (1990) PACS experience at the University of Hokkaido Medical School. In: Dwyer III, S.J., and R.G. Jost (Eds.), Medical Imaging IV: PACS System Design and Evaluation, *Proc. SPIE* 1234, 26–32.

Kimura, M. (1989) Inter-vendor connection between components of a picture archiving and communication system (PACS) using the MIPS-87 image standard at Tokyo University Hospital, *Med. Rev.* 33, 21–25.

Ligier, Y., M. Funk, O. Ratib, R. Perrier and C. Girard (1990) The OSIRIS user interface for manipulating medical images. In: Picture Archiving and Communication System (PACS) in Medicine, Evian, *NATO ASI Series* (Springer, Berlin).

LiuSheng, O.R., H.M. Chen Garcia, C.P. Wei, T. Ozeki and P. McNulty (1990) Distributed database design and modelling for PACS. In: Dwyer III, S.J., and R.G. Jost (Eds.), Medical Imaging IV: PACS System Design and Evaluation, *Proc. SPIE* 1234, 256–269.

Mattheus, R., and M. Osteaux (1990) PACS and PACS-related research in Belgium. In: Picture Archiving and Communication System (PACS) in Medicine, Evian, *NATO ASI Series* (Springer, Berlin), pp. 251–258.

Minato, K., M. Komori, Y. Nakano, K. Okajima, I. Kimura, T. Takahashi, J. Konishi, M. Abe, Y. Gotoh and K. Sato (1990) Present status of PACS at Kyoto University Hospital: image workstation for clinical education. In: Dwyer III, S.J., and R.G. Jost (Eds.), Medical Imaging IV: PACS System Design and Evaluation, *Proc. SPIE* 1234, 180–186.

Mun, S.K., H. Benson, L. Elliott, F. Goeringer, A. Saarinen and D. Haynor (1989) Total digital department: implementation strategy. In: Schneider, R.H., S.J. Dwyer III and R.G. Jost (Eds.), Medical Imaging III: PACS System Design and Evaluation, *Proc. SPIE* 1093, 133–139.

Ottes, F.P., J.P. de Valk, H. Lodder, W.J. Stut, I.E. van der Horst-Bruinsma, P.L. Hofland, B.M. van Poppel, B.M. ter Haar Romeny and A.R. Bakker (1989) Results of IMAGIS project 1986–1989; facts and fallacies. In: Schneider, R.H., S.J. Dwyer III and R.G. Jost (Eds.), Medical Imaging III: PACS System Design and Evaluation, *Proc. SPIE* 1093, 133–139.

Ratib, O., and H.K. Huang (1989) CALIPSO, an interactive software package for multimodality medical image analysis on a personal computer, *J. Med. Imaging* 3, 205–216.

Ratib, O., R. Appel and J.R. Scherrer (1990) PAPYRUS: a multimodality image file format for PACS and teleradiology, *Radiology*, 177(p), 320.

Scherrer, J.R., R. Baud, D. Hochstrasser and O. Ratib (1990) An integrated hospital information system in Geneva, *M.D. Computing* 7, 81–89.

Schneider, R.H., and S.J. Dwyer III (Eds.) (1984) Application of optical instrumentation in medicine XII, Vol. 454, Society of Photo-Optical Engineers, Bellingham, Washington.

Schneider, R.H., and S.J. Dwyer III (Eds.) (1985) Picture Archiving and Communication Systems (PACS), Third International Conference and Workshop, *Proc. SPIE* 536.

Schneider, R.H., and S.J. Dwyer III (Eds.) (1986) Medical XIV/PACS IV, *Proc. SPIE* 626.

Schneider, R.H., and S.J. Dwyer III (Eds.) (1987) Medical Imaging, *SPIE* 767.

Stewart, B. (1990) Three tiered network architecture for PACS clusters. In: Picture Archiving and Communication System (PACS) in Medicine, Evian, *NATO ASI Series*, (Springer, Berlin), pp. 113–119.

Vermont, J., P. Cinquin and J. Demongeot (1990) PACS and PACS-related research in France, Picture Archiving and Communication System (PACS) in Medicine, Evian, *NATO ASI Series* (Springer, Berlin), pp. 267–272.

PACS in Japan

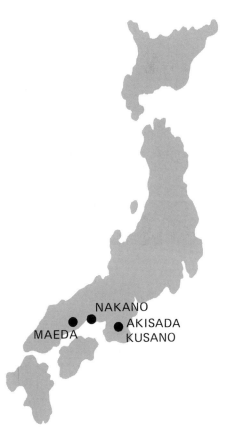

NAKANO

AKISADA

KUSANO

MAEDA

Integrated Diagnostic Imaging
Editor: J.P.J. De Valk
© *Elsevier Science Publishers B.V., 1992*

Chapter 16

The present and future aspects of PACS activities in Japan

Masayoshi Akisada, Michio Kimura and Yukihisa Saida

1. Japanese PACS industry in the present and future

1.1. Introduction

In the end of the eighteenth century, the industrial revolution has led the material civilization caused by power revolution and energy revolution. The technical revolution and renovation born of computer and other technological advancements in the latter half of the twentieth century have established an infrastructure for a superior information society. In 1984, the information industry generated a production worth two trillion yen in Japan (6.4% of GNP). It is predicted that it will reach 14 trillion yen by the year 2000 (20.7% of GNP).

The optics industry in Japan generated a production worth over 80 billion yen in 1980, over 900 billion yen in 1985 and over 2 trillion yen in 1990. Production has increased quite rapidly, and it is predicted that it will reach 12 trillion yen by the year 2000. The industry is comprised of optics components, 22%, optics devices, 42%, and optics communication systems, 36%.

The information industry is already the leading industry of Japan. It is safe to assume that the medical information industry including the PACS (picture archiving and communication system) industry will show the same trend. It is quite possible that PACS wil be easily implemented and accepted in the image age of the twenty-first century when the technologies related to PACS are improved and PACS implementation becomes cost effective.

In 1974, before digital imaging such as X-ray computed tomography was introduced, Dr. T. Iinuma presented a concept of a network system for radiology image processing and management in the medical practice (Iinuma, 1974). He discussed functionality, effectiveness and feasibility of such a systematic management network capable of image filing, image compression, and image transmission in and out of the hospital. At that time, lack of adequate technologies prevented the implementation of the new concept.

Many new desirable technologies are now available and the need for PACS technology has become very clear in Japan. A number of companies, hospitals and radiologists are now actively involved in making PACS a reality addressing the needs of modern radiology.

Many Japanese companies are actively engaged in developing PACS-related products and services. Several organizational efforts were formed to promote PACS and to study the technology and understand the needs of modern radiology practice. The program is aimed at facilitating graceful implementation of the sophisticated and complex technology into the clinical environments. The organizational efforts were driven by the industry and by academic and clinical users.

Three PACS organizations in Japan (1991) are:

(a) Japan PACS (J-PACS) (Chairman: J. Tsujiuchi);
(b) Japan Association of Medical Imaging and Technology (JAMIT)-PACS (Chairman: M. Akisada);
(c) PACS Comittee of the Japan Radiological Society (JRS-PACS) (Chairman: M. Akisada).

In this chapter three views of Japanese PACS as seen from the industries and users sides are presented, i.e.: (1) Japanese PACS Industry in the present and future (M. Akisada), (2) Tokyo University Hospital PACS − (medical image processing system standardization) (MIPS) image standard implementation (M. Kimura), (3) a reporting system in Tsukuba University Hospital (Y. Saida).

Table 1
Present and tentative goals of PACS keytechnologies in Japan.

Item		Present status	Tentative goal
Optical fiber network	Transmit speed	100 Mbitps	400 − 600 Mbitps
	Interface	ACR/NEMA & MIPS	Standard
Diagnostic image work-station	Processing speed (cycle time)	> 100 ns	10 ns
	Data acquisition	< 1 Mbytesps	3 Mbytesps
Optical disk	Data transfer	< 330 Kbytesps	1 Mbytesps
	Memory capacity	< 3 Gbyte	10 Gbyte
	Data compression	$\frac{1}{2}$ (reversible)	$\frac{1}{20}$ (irreversible)
Image digitizer	Digitizing speed	> 30 s	10 s
Laser image printer	Printing speed	> 30 s	10 s

1.2. Forecasting the Japanese PACS industry in the future

It is difficult to make a prediction on PACS status/movement in the twenty-first century because PACS technology contains many technical elements which are developing at a rapid speed and in an ever changing environment.

Table 1 shows the PACS technologies status of present and future which was published in early 1988 (Okabe, 1988). Some tentative goals in this table have already been achieved and commercialized, for example, an optical fiber network with a throughput rate of 600 Mbitsps (Mbit/s) workstation with 3Mbytesps acquisition speed, and 7 GByte optical disk. Progress in technologies has been faster than anticipated.

Along with these advances, almost 100 hospitals in Japan have already introduced digital filing systems for diagnostic images. However, PACS needs an additional merit to blossom in the twenty-first century. And PACS should be continuously assessed in order to match with the current trend. If necessary, its direction for development may be drastically altered regardless of the past.

Furthermore, the following should be emphasized.

1.2.1. Cost – benefit analysis

Hidden by the term 'cost – benefit analysis', many worthy PACS research projects have not ever seen the light of a day. We must consider the reason why many Japanese companies have already introduced computers for their managements, designing and manufacturing fifteen years ago. Computerization itself could not bring 'cost – benefit' situation, but has brought high quality management/designing/manufacturing that have made them to be superior in the world. The same situation may be rightly said to PACS in radiology departments.

1.2.2. Globalization and standardization

Japan will enter a global age in the twenty-first century. Obstacles such as the complexity of the Japanese language which contains three different types of characters (katakana, hirakana, and kanji) and Japan being geographically isolated will be addressed and dealt with in the twenty-first century. Standardizations on many important PACS technologies, for example, LAN, optical disk, diagnostic viewing workstation, interface, digitizer, hard copy, image compression, etc. should be unified. Standards (ACR/NEMA, MIPS and others) must be expanded to accomodate HIS/RIS connectivity, off-line storage media formats*, and true networking in order to play a major role in the future of the imaging environment of the twenty-first century.

---

* For example, IS&C (Image Save and Carry) system for an off-line use (Ohyama, 1989) is promising to solve the problems with on-line PACS of centralized database. The disk and logical formats have been standardized.

1.2.3. PACS individualization

A radiologist has individual needs and preferences in image design. The radiologist preferences often affect their performances as PACS should satisfy their needs. Image display should be attractive and user-friendly to its users.

1.2.4. Simplicity and accessibility of PACS images

The current PACS systems are inflexible and used under limited conditions. Many radiologists who are not accustomed to handle a complex machine/ equipment will certainly stay away from the PACS display units. Image access by PACS should be easy, less complex and more efficient. PACS should be more flexible and accommodating to diverse situations and needs.

J.H. Perry stated that separation of the physician's viewing system, the image archival system, and the image documentation system from the modality would simplify the modality while providing the services more generally and consistently in a situation. An additional possibility is to see PACS workstations as operator's control systems, further simplifying the design of the core modality (Perry, 1989). Radiologists in the twenty-first century should be able to utilize PACS without any hesitation.

2. Tokyo University Hospital PACS – MIPS image standard implementation

2.1. Introduction

The authors have designed and constructed a small image management and communication system (PACS) for X-ray CT scanners, called TRACS (Tokyo University, radiologic image archiving and communication system), at Tokyo University Hospital. In this system, several X-ray CT scanners and an image filing system are connected using the MIPS-87 protocol, an image standard proposed by the Japan Industries' Association for Radiation Apparatus (JIRA) which is basically similar to the ACR/NEMA standard (American College of Radiology/National Electrical Manufacturers Association) minimum requirements. This is the first practical implementation of the MIPS-87 standard, which was proven valid and reasonable. This section comprises an overview of TRACS, description of the implementation of MIPS-87, and discussion of the problems with MIPS-87 which were discovered at the time of implementation.

2.2. TRACS system profile

TRACS currently comprises three X-CT scanners, an image data archive, image display workstations, and a workstation for patient data processing. Image data of three CTs are sent to DATAVIEW. DATAVIEW sends data to TDIS-FILE by interconnection with MIPS-87. TDIS-FILE sends patient data of image examinations to AS3160. An image examination database is constructed at AS3160. AS3160 makes interconnection with HIS and RIS. J3100 is a terminal of AS3160, located at referring departments. AS3160 and J3100s control image displays (fig. 1). The unique character of TRACS is that it puts emphasis on the management of the patient data of image examinations. For this purpose. TRACS employs a 32-bit workstation to control image display, interface with users, and communicates with HIS.

The TRACS configuration is as follows. The three YMS/GE (Yokogawa Medical System, General Electric) X-CT scanners at the hospital and the medical image filling system Toshiba TDIS-FILE (Toshiba diagnostic imaging system (Shigemura et al., 1987) cannot be connected directly, because of insufficient image tranformation features and different image data standards. Therefore, it was necessary to connect the X-CT scanners to a local image station, DATAVIEW (Takarabe et al., 1989) with TDIS-FILE connected to this local image station. MIPS-87 standard (MIPS Committee, 1988) is used for the image standard between these two. The MIPS-87 standard is similar to the ACR/NEMA standard (ACR-NEMA, 1988), with minor modifications concerning Japanese character processing. (One Japanese character needs two bytes.) In every X-CT examination, image data is sent automatically to TDIS-FILE, where it is archived on optical discs (fig. 2).

The 32-bit workstation for patient data processing and user interface is a

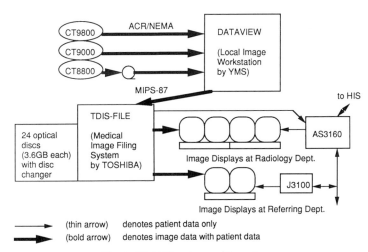

Fig. 1. TRACS system configuration.

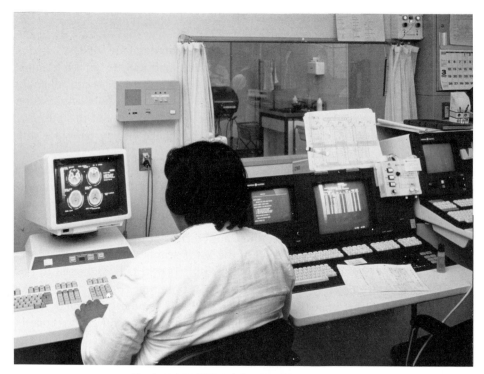

Fig. 2. DATAVIEW (left), GECT9800 (right).

Toshiba AS3160 (model 3160 of series AS3000, which is an OEM of SUN 3/160). With a Japanese language word processor and installed RDBMS (relational data-base management system), this workstation provides examination history, and diagnostic report, on the same window manager of the workstation. Every time image data arrive to TDIS-FILE, patient data of the examination (patient's name, ID, examination data and time, method, etc.) is sent automatically to AS3160. This data and the diagnostic reports form the database of X-CT examinations at the workstation. AS3160 issues commands to TDIS-FILE which images to display, on which CRT, in what window width/level, etc. (fig. 3).

TDIS-FILE has optical discs and magnetic discs. The capacity of the former is larger (3.6 Gbytes per disc), but the access time is much longer than that of the magnetic discs. On the other hand, the capacity of the latter (120 Mbytes, basic configuration, expandable up to 6 Gbytes) is very crucial for image data. If image data which are expected to be viewed (i.e., the new images and also

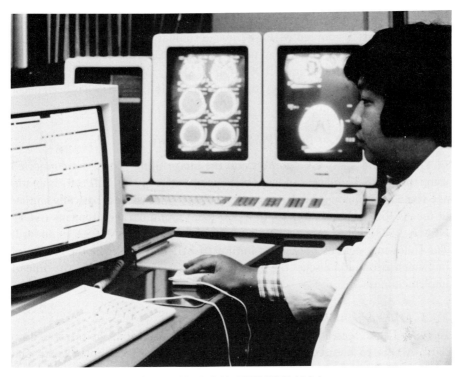

Fig. 3. AS3160 (left), TDIS-FILE (right).

the patient's old images for comparison) were copied from the optical discs to magnetic discs, the user would not complain about the slow access to optical discs. This prefetching can be done according to data on patient submission and examination reservation. This data can be acquired from the HIS.

Compared to other PACS, TRACS has the following specifications:

(a) Imaging modalities included in TRACS are three X-CTs, while CR images are also handled at UCLA (Hegde et al., 1986; Huang et al., 1987; Boechet et al., 1988; Cho et al., 1988; Irie et al., 1989; Mun et al., 1989; Taira et al., 1989).

(b) There is currently no PAC system which has image displays throughout the hospital. TRACS has them at radiology department and one referring department.

(c) Only TRACS handles demographic data of image examinations more precious than mere RIS, which handles diagnostic results, for example, only as a string of characters.

(d) Most PACS are based on single vendor configuration. TRACS includes GE/YMS CTs and Toshiba image filing system.

(e) Connections between imaging apparatus are based on local protocols, while TRACS adopted MIPS-87 image standard (Kimura et al., 1989).

(f) TRACS is among the few systems (IMAGIS (De Valk et al., 1986, 1988; Lodder et al., 1989), new-KIDS (Komori et al., 1987; Minato et al., 1989) and at Hokkaido University) for which interaction with HIS has been deeply in mind.

2.3. Implementation of the MIPS-87 image standard

In TRACS, the X-ray CT scanners and the image filing system are connected using the MIPS-87 image standard (MIPS Committee, 1988). MIPS-87 is an image standard which has been proposed by JIRA, and which is basically similar to the ACR/NEMA version 1.0 (no. 300-1985) minimum requirements (ACR-NEMA, 1988). TRACS is the first system to implement the MIPS-87 standard. The following sections present an outline of MIPS-87, describe the results of implementation, and discuss the problems which were discovered at the time of implementation.

2.3.1. MIPS and ACR/NEMA

In 1984, JIRA created a committee to establish a medical image transfer standard, MIPS, to be used as a standard for transfer of both image data and

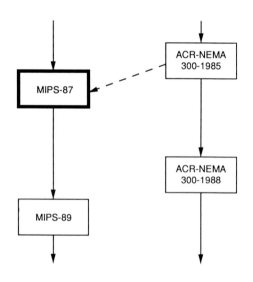

MIPS-87 ≈ ACR-NEMA 300-1985 minimum requirement

Fig. 4. MIPS and ACR/NEMA.

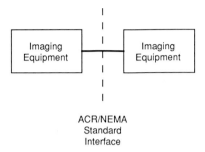

Fig. 5. Location of standard interface, without a network.

demographic data for medical imaging hardware. Soon afterwards in 1984, ACR and NEMA created a committee in the United States to establish an ACR/NEMA standard with the same intent. Eventually, MIPS-87 is basically similar to the ACR/NEMA version 1.0 (no.300-1985) minimum requirements, with some minor modifications mainly with regard to the handling of text data. Both the MIPS and ACR/NEMA standards are currently undergoing revision (fig. 4).

The standards specify the hardware interfaces, a minimum set of software commands, and a consistent set of data formats for communication across an interface between an imaging device and a network interface unit or another im-

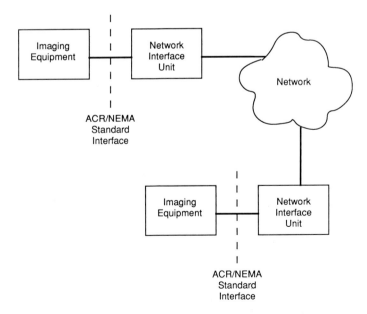

Fig. 6. Location of standard interface, with a network.

aging device. Figure 6 shows a typical PACS network configuration and the location of the standard. Figure 5 shows point-to-point connection without a network. These standards describe only the basic protocols for imaging devices to communicate with other imaging devices. Therefore, simply adopting these standards does not, in itself, result in an effective medical image management and communication system. Many other factors must be taken into consideration in the design of a workable medical imaging system. In the design of these standards, efforts were made to conform to the ISO-OSI (open system interconnection) reference model for networks (ISO, 1983). This reference model has seven layers: physical, data link, network, transport, session, presentation, and application. In the image transfer standards, standards are defined for each of these layers. A 50 pin EIA485 connector is the main specification in the physical layer. Commands for communication (send, receive, echo, etc.) are defined in the presentation layer. However, up to now, no standards have been defined for the top application layer (Spilker, 1989). This is why the following statement is included in the ACR/NEMA standard publications (ACR-NEMA, 1988).

"This publication specifies a minimum set of necessary attributes for an imaging device interface to communicate succesfully with other devices that also meet the specification. The standard is not intended to be an overall PACS or workstation specification, nor an archive or magnetic tape transfer standard, nor a network standard."

2.3.2. Implementation of MIPS-87 in practice

In TRACS, connections for image transfer are point-to-point, as shown in fig. 1. Ideally, the three YMS/GE X-ray CT systems and the TDIS-FILE should be connected directly. However, some older X-ray CT systems (for example, in our case, the CT/T9000 and GECT8800) do not have provisions for image tranfer based on the ACR/NEMA or MIPS standards. This is why the DATAVIEW was employed to connect the three X-ray CT scanners to the TDIS-FILE.

Figure 1 shows the system configuration used to connect the YMS DATAVIEW to the Toshiba TDIS-FILE. Both of these systems are provided with interface board for the MIPS-87 protocol, and the systems are connected with the 50 pin cable specified in the standard.

The maximum data transfer speed is 8 Mbitps. In TRACS, the two systems are separated by a distance of about 50 m. The actual transfer time for a single CT slice (512 × 512) is about seconds. The authors consider this to be an acceptable transfer time, provided that the data transfer is point-to point. Almost half of the transfer is spent in memory access in both systems. Therefore, the use of faster disks, cache memory, or perhaps an efficient buffer should result in significant improvements in transfer time.

Error handling is a major concern when making inter-vendor connections. However, we have seldom observed hang-ups. The sender automatically repeats sending if image transmission is unsuccesful, checking the messages from the other side, under the protocol described at lower layers of the standard. No errors have occurred in sending typical axial scan images. Errors have occurred when sending images containing information which is not supported by the system, as described in the following section.

2.3.3. Problems with the MIPS-87 and ACR/NEMA standards

The authors have discovered a number of problems with MIPS-87 through this practical implementation of the standard.

(a) It is impossible to send the exact scan time (precise to the seconds) of each slice. A 'study time' (group 0008, element 0030) is included in the standard, but 'study' here refers to a series of slices. This item is not used to send the scan of each slice, but the time the examination is started (the time of the first slice). In TRACS, the CT9000, CT8800, and DATAVIEW are connected by GE net. Therefore, the DATAVIEW receives the scan time for examinations performed using these scanners. On the other hand, the CT9800 is connected to the DATAVIEW by an ACR/NEMA connection, and scan time information is lost. In any case, this information is lost by the MIPS-87 connection between the DATAVIEW and the TDIS-FILE. This loss of scan time information is a major problem when interpreting dynamic bolus studies, for example, to differentiate a hemangioma from a hepatocellular carcinoma. However, the image time, acquisition time, and series time are all specified in the updated ACR/NEMA version 2.0 (no. 300-1988) standard. The new version of MIPS should also include these frames.

(b) There is no indication of 'end of study' or 'number of slices in the study', which would allow the receiving system to check that all the slices of a study have been received. Clinicians are aware that an X-ray CT study comprises a series of slices. Image standards, on the other hand, typically apply to single images. In TRACS, where the image data network is point-to-point, the system can simply assume that the start of reception indicates a new study, and long-term silence indicates the end of a study. However, in advanced network architectures, this implicit information may not be valid. In any case, the receiving system must be able to sort the images of a study after reception. Without the information described above, the system cannot determine when to 'close' a study. In the next revision of ACR/NEMA standard, the 'folder' concept is going to be introduced. This folder can fold not only a series of images of an examination like PAPYRUS standard, but also demographic data. This new data structure will be utilized in the data transfer. Among image examination apparatus, however, no current modality of any manufacturer can send a series of images as a folder. At most of the current X-ray CT scanners, the 'end of study' information, which allows file system to close a folder, is originated by a push of 'new patient' button. This button is sometimes left unpushed after the last examination of the day. The author proposes manufacturers to be ready for producing image examination apparatus which can make full use of the new image tranfer standard.

(c) Images containing overlay information cannot be sent. Radiologists often place information on images, such as distance measurements, CT values, etc. This is done using the region of interest (ROI) features of the imaging system. Such image-information images superimposed on original images are called overlay information images. In the ACR/NEMA standard, these images are sent as bitmap data for each of the three primary colors. The MIPS-87 standard, on the other hand, does not have any provisions for overlay information. Overlay information was deleted from the MIPS standard in order to simplify implementation, but such information is important in a clinical setting. The authors do not maintain that ACR/NEMA's approach is ideal but some provisions must be made for overlay information. Some overlay information could be regenerated at the PACS workstation. The measurements placed on an image by the radiological at the scanning site serve as message to the referring physican and other radiologists, and eliminating such information would present difficulties. Moreover, the slice-position guidelines on scout views could not be reproduced. Once again, to simplify implementation, it has been suggested to send two scout view images, one with guidelines and the other without. To permit this, and also for teleradiology conferences (where ROIs are interchanged in real time), the imaging system must be designed with the ability to separate the original image data from overlay information.

2.3.4. Comparison of image communication in various PACS

As noted above, this is the first practical implementation of the MIPS-87 image standard. This is also the first case known to us of inter-vendor interconnection using this kind of standards.

In most PACS implementations, interconnections are made using protocols such as DR11-W, which is a point-to-point protocol for the connection of two DEC computer buses (Huang, 1987). Ethernet is widely used for network interconnections. These type of protocols, however, have definitions only for the lower layers of the OSI model. As a result, medical image interconnections usually incorporate custom hardware and software. Usually, such customization is undertaken under the supervision of the manufacturer of the medical imaging device, because detailed understanding of the imaging device is required. This is one reason that there are so few inter-vendor interconnections in PACSs.

By adopting the MIPS-87 standard, the authors have eliminated the need for any custom hardware other than the MIPS-87 interface boards, manufactured by each vendor, Yokogawa and Toshiba installed in the DATAVIEW and the TDIS-FILE. This is the primary reason for defining standards, and this implementation has demonstrated the usefulness of such standards. In a later implementation, in the PACS at Hokkaido University (which also includes YMS/GE X-ray CT systems), Yokogawa Medical Systems has employed an identical system configuration. The same MIPS-87 interface boards were installed to make interconnection to an NEC NEPACS.

2.3.5. Proposals for a better standard

As noted before, the authors regarded the speed of image transfer as acceptable. It is only acceptable provided that the image transfer is by point-to-point configuration, which may be found in local data transfer of a large network communication. MIPS and ACR/NEMA are not the standards of protocols for a large PACS, as noted in the standard publications. They cannot be used in a large network because of the limitation of lower layer definitions of themselves. 8 Mbyteps data transfer by a 50 pin cable, as their lowest physical layer define, is not fast enough for large network configuration (fig. 7). Moreover, they have no definition for network addressing. Their higher layer definitions, on the other hand, is nice for examination image/demographic data transfers. Therefore, the authors propose an improved standard definition

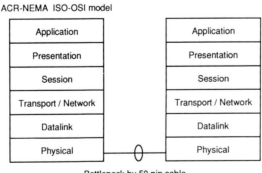

Fig. 7. ISO-OSI model of the standard, and its bottleneck.

which has alternative lower layers with the same higher layer. Ethernet, TCP/IP, and FDDI are examples of network protocols, which are faster than the protocols defined in the current standards.

Demographic data (patient data) should be utilized fully at PACS (Lodder et al., 1989). Their data origins differ. Patient name, ID, etc., should come from RIS and HIS, but in most cases, they are re-typed at the apparatus console. Examination time, methods, etc., are supplied by modalities and can be sent to other system using the image standards. Contents of diagnostic reports are from radiologists. So, man – machine interface of the system should be sophisticated enough for radiologists to promote integration of these data. Patient case histories, etc., should come from HIS. In any case, PACS – RIS – HIS coupling is indispensable for integrated use of PACS. Both MIPS and ACR/NEMA committees are making efforts to include PACS – RIS – HIS integration protocols. In the same time, modalities should be ready for receiving and sending these kinds of data from/to RIS or HIS.

2.4. Final remarks

A number of problems with the MIPS-87 standard were discovered in the implementation at TRACS. The authors hope that PACS with this kind of standards will be implemented at other sites. It is through such practical implementation that standards will be improved. In addition, the authors hope that manufacturers will begin to produce medical imaging devices which conform to these standards, and continue to be involved in the development of requirements for medical imaging systems.

3. Reporting system in Tsukuba University Hospital

The number of diagnostic radiologists in Japan is not as large as in many western countries and unfortunately the radiological reporting system in Japan

Table 2

Outpatients charts	177 000
Inpatients charts	57 000
X-ray films	1 673 000
Cine-angio reels	17 000
Endoscopy cases	52 000
EEG cases	21 000
Functional studies	165 000

From Akisada (1989).

is not sufficiently developed, although the number of members of the professional Japanese radiologists organization has recently steeply increased (Akisada, 1988). It indicates that in some Japanese institutions, all radiological examinations are not always interpreted and there are some examinations having no change to be interpreted by radiologists. With recognition of this fact, we reached to our basic principle that no radiological images are allowed to be distributed without proper interpretation. Reporting issues should preceed every other PACS problem in Japan (Saida et al., 1991).

The radiology department of Tsukuba University performs almost all diagnostic examinations with exception of cardiac, pediatric, and gynecologic contrast studies, where all the medical records have been gathered in one library of 1186 m². During 11 years from November 1976 to October 1987, the deposits were as shown in table 2.

There are several important concepts regarding to develop a reporting system along with PACS in Tsukuba University Hospital. The main issue in our system is how to assure perfect matching between each radiological examination and its report. To give an ID to each examination (examination ID) is a way of solution to this problem. After diffusion of instrumental attachments to read bar code transformed from the examination ID throughout the hospital, both report making and report reference become smoother and more reliable. An isolated terminal may access to the system with using this examination ID and it means that theoretically the integration of HIS and PACS is realized without actual construction of a fiberoptic network.

To avoid troublesome and time-consuming manipulation of key board on our medical work station (MWS) for radiologists reporting system should be supported by a transcriber work station (TWS), which through a dictation system can give more comfortable circumstances for reporting. TWS should be constructed based on the widely used and easy handling computer terminals in order to keep optimal man – machine interface.

It is emphasized that a double check system in report making is mandatory. A double check system needs longer times to release the reports in comparison to a simple reporting system. However, for maintaining the standard quality of diagnostic performance and for providing proper training and education system to students and young doctors (Selzer et al., 1981), a double check system should be prepared in PACS.

The last requirement is to establish a well-organized diagnostic system to realize the immediate reference of previous medical images from the viewpoints of both clinical and researching aspects. To reduce the excessive efforts of radiologists to input the diagnostic code number to each examination, and to avoid a more power depending system, it is desired to develop a self-operating diagnostic file system which is able to extract key medical terms automatically from the reporting sentences.

4. Conclusion

The number of radiologists is relatively small in comparison with internists or surgeons in Japan. In some instances, especially in smaller facilities, the radiology is conducted by self-styled 'Fachradiologe'. However, since the number of younger radiologists, with more exposure to computer technologies are increasing rapidly, more radiological diagnoses are being performed by radiologists.

While we are facing many problems in managing film-based radiology service, Japan is experiencing a period of rapid introduction of PACS technology into the university hospitals for the following reasons.

(a) Once positive results of PACS projects are obtained from the aforementioned university hospitals, the Japanese government will fund similar projects at other hospitals within a few years.

(b) The demand for quality control of images and radiology service from users is very strong and the use of PACS is expected to help to meet such demands.

(c) Japan has a strong and suitable technological and industrial bases to develop and implement PACS technology.

References

ACR-NEMA Publication 300-1988 (1988) Digital Imaging and Communication (NEMA, Washington D.C.).

Akisada, M. (1988) Present status of PACS activities in Japan, *Med. Inform.* 13, 289–293.

Akisada, M. (1989) Present status and perspective of PACS activities in Japan, Proc. IMAC 89, 25–31.

Boechet, M.I., et al. (1988) Clinical experience with a PACS module in pediatric radiology; clinical viewpoint and system viewpoint (consecutive two papers). In: Schneider, R.H., and S.J. Dwyer III (Eds.), Medical Imaging II, *Proc. SPIE* 914, 1036–1056.

Cho, P.S., et al. (1988) Clinical experience with a digital remote viewing system in coronary care unit. In: Schneider, R.H., and S.J. Dwyer III (Eds.), Medical Imaging II, *Proc. SPIE* 914, 1057–1064.

de Valk J.P.J., et al. (1986) PACS reviewed: possible and coming soon? Proc. MEDINFO-86, 990–995.

de Valk J.P.J., et al. (1988) IMAGIS projects: past, present and future. In: Schneider, R.H., and S.J. Dwyer III (Eds.), Medical Imaging II, *Proc. SPIE* 914, 1136–1140.

Hegde, S.S., et al. (1986) AT&T PACS architectures. In: Schneider, R.H., and S.J. Dwyer III (Eds.), Medicine XIV/PACS IV, *Proc. SPIE* 626, 618–625.

Huang, H.K. (1987) Elements of Digital Radiology: a Professional Handbook and Guide (Prentice-Hall, Englewood Cliffs NJ).

Huang, H.K., et al. (1987) PACS at the University of California, Los Angeles. In: Schneider, R.H., and S.J. Dwyer III (Eds.), Medical Imaging, *Proc. SPIE* 767, 547–584.

Iinuma, T. (1974) Image processing in clinical medicine - considerations of a system, *Bull Tokyo*

Women Med. 44, 152 (in Japanese).

Irie, G., et al. (1989) A report on PACS at work in Hokkaido University, Proc. 6th JAMIT-PACS symposium, *Med. Imag. Technol.* 7, 227 – 228.

International Organization for Standardization (ISO) (1983) Information processing systems – Open Systems Interconnection – Basic reference model, ISO 7498 – 1983.

Kimura, M., et al. (1989) Tokyo University Hospital PAC System: TRACS – importance of non-image data management and integration to hospital information system, Proc. MEDINFO-89, 385 – 388.

Komori, M., et al. (1987) Pilot PACS with on-line communication between an image workstation and CT scanners in a clinical environment. In: Schneider, R.H., and S.J. Dwyer III (Eds.), Medical Imaging, *Proc. SPIE* 767, 744 – 751.

Lodder, H., et al. (1989) HIS-PACS coupling in practive. In: Schneider, R.H., S.J. Dwyer III and R.G. Jost (Eds.), Medical Imaging III: PACS System Design and Evaluation, *Proc. SPIE* 1093, 301 – 306.

Minato, K., et al. (1989) PACS prototype at Kyoto University Hospital, Proc. MEDINFO-89, 389 – 392.

MIPS Committee (1988) MIPS-87 image standard, JIRA (Japan Industries Association of Radiation Apparatus) Publications (in Japanese).

Mun, S.K., et al. (1989) Completion of a hospital-wide comprehensive image management and communication system. In: Schneider, R.H., S.J. Dwyer III and R.G. Jost (Eds.), Medical Imaging III: PACS System Design and Evaluation, *Proc. SPIE* 1093, 204 – 213.

Ohyama, N. (1989) Transportable Image Recording Media, a proposal of ISAC (Image Save and Carry) System, Proc.1st IMAC, June 4 – 8. Washington DC (IEEE Comp. Soc. Press) pp. 250 – 255.

Okabe, T. (1988) PACS Chapter 8, Recent development of diagnostic imaging modalities (in Japanese) (Asakura Publ. Tokyo) pp. 240 – 269.

Perry, J.H. (1989) Imaging in the Twenty-First Century: The impact of the networking on image system design, Abstracts of Plenary Symposium on Images of the 21st Century. 11 Annual Int'l Conf. Nov. 9 – 12. Seattle, p.15.

Saida, Y., et al. (1991) PACS and the reporting system. Present status of PACS in the University of Tsukuba, *Comput. Methods Programs Biomed.* 36, 89 – 92.

Selzer, S.E., S.J. Hessel, P.G. Herman et al. (1981) Resident film interpretations and staff review, *Am. J. Roentgenol.* 137, 129 – 133.

Shigemura, N., et al. (1987) Development of a medical image filing system. Proc. 4th JAMIT-PACS symposium.

Spilker, C. (1989) The ACR-NEMA digital imaging and communictions standard: a nontechnical description, *J. Digital Imaging* 2, 127 – 131.

Taira, R.K., et al. (1989) Performance evaluation of a clinical PACS module. In: Schneider, R.H., S.J. Dwyer III and R.G. Jost (Eds.), Medical Imaging III: PACS System Design and Evaluation, *Proc. SPIE* 1093, 406 – 417.

Takarabe, K., et al. (1989) DATAVIEW: network image station. Proc. 6th JAMIT-PACS symposium, *Med. Imag. Technol.* 7, 215 – 216.

Integrated Diagnostic Imaging
Editor: J.P.J. De Valk
© *Elsevier Science Publishers B.V., 1992*

Chapter 17

Picture archiving and communication system at the Kitasato University East Hospital: promises and problems

Shoichi Kusano and Yoshitaka Okada

1. Introduction and definitions

A major change in radiology, i.e., from analog to digital imaging, was triggered by the development of computed tomography (CT) by Hounsfield (1973), a change that has had an enormous clinical influence. At approximately the same time, direct computer diagnosis (Hall et al., 1971) in which an image was converted into a digital one was begun. However, it is clear that the appearance of CT accelerated the subsequent development of ultrasonography (US), digital subtraction angiography (DSA) (Kruger et al., 1979), magnetic resonance imaging (MRI), emission computed tomography (ECT) and computed radiography (CR) (Sonoda et al., 1983). The concept of the picture archiving and communication system (PACS) (Templeton et al., 1984) came about when central processing units (CPU) became greater in number and capacity in imaging in medicine applications.

The fundamental components of PACS are a database of digital images, workstations (WS) for imaging diagnosis and a network. The number of imaging modalities in the network and the number and frequency of use of WS define the scale of PACS, while the integration of information through the system, radiology information systems (RIS) and hospital information systems (HIS) enhance the efficiency of communication through PACS. This chapter describes the past, present and future of PACS on the basis of our experience with the system in Kitasato University East Hospital between 1986 and 1990.

2. Background of PACS introduction

Central management of radiological images was performed for the first time at a Japanese university hospital in Kitasato University Hospital in 1971 (Hashimoto et al., 1972). Since then, radiological images have been filed in an individual film jacket with an ID number for each patient. On the other hand, the number of X-ray films used has increased, together with a subsequent increase in imaging diagnostic examininations, to exceed 450 000 X-ray films annually by about 1980. The number of images stored has thus increased rapidly. Therefore, one of the big problems in the Department of Radiology of Kitasato University Hospital in the 1980s was obtaining storage space for images. The disadvantage of this analog storage system is that a great deal of manpower and space is required for storage and management. Therefore, images will have to be thrown away eventually.

When Kitasato University East Hospital was planned as a second educational hospital in 1985, there were three important problems to be solved in the Department of Radiology: the development of a long-term management system for images; the establishment of methods for quick and easy creation of radiology reports and referencing of past reports, and for integrating information with that from other divisions, e.g., pathology or surgery; and the clinical application of a digital image database.

Unlike the time when Kitasato University Hospital was established, US, CT, and DSA had been developed and introduced, CR had been developed, enabling replacement of plain X-ray examinations by the film and screen (F/S) system with CR, and image processing speed of CR had progressed to a level approximately equivalent to film developing time of the F/S system when Kitasato University East Hospital was planned. Therefore, in the planning stage, the management of analog images could be largely changed to the management of digital images by introducing CR. However, when the hospital was opened in April, 1986, no apparatus for on-line management of digital images had yet been developed. Therefore as many as possible digital imaging modalities were employed, and the following studies were performed in cooperation with Toshiba Co. in order to solve the above-mentioned problems:

(1) development of RIS by personal computer (PC);
(2) construction of a network between RIS and HIS and integration of diagnostic information among divisions;
(3) development of a system for on-line construction of an image database;
(4) compression of images for efficient management; and
(5) development of a system for the clinical application of an image database.

3. PACS in the present

Figure 1 shows the radiology information management system in Kitasato

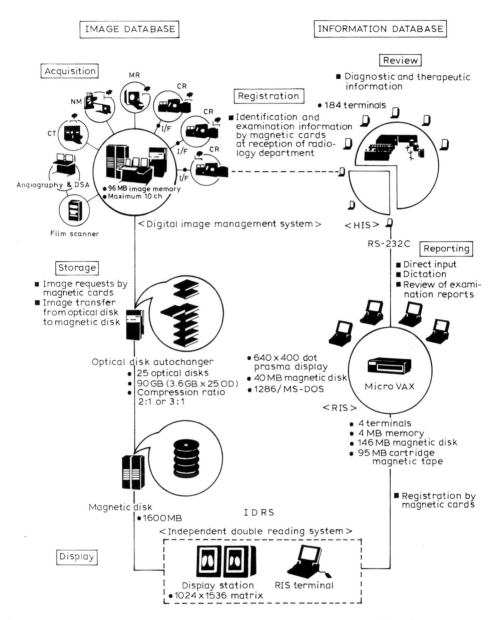

Fig. 1. Schematic illustration of the image acquisition management and the double reading system.

University East Hospital. The system is currently composed of a RIS, digital image management system (DIMS), a HIS and an independent double reading system (IDRS).

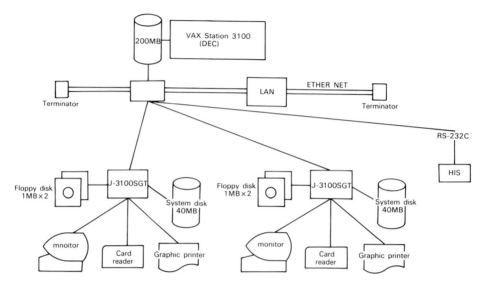

Fig. 2. Configuration of the reporting console.

4. Kitasato University East Hospital

Kitasato University East Hospital, which is composed of three centers (digestive organ diseases, psychoneurotic diseases and chronic intractable diseases), has 500 beds and treats approximately 850 outpatients per day. The Radiology Department operates three CR units, three special radiography units (one equipped with CR), one polytomography, one CT scanner, one MRI unit, one angiography unit (with DSA), one gamma camera, and five portable radiography units. On average about 18 000 radiographs are taken per month, resulting in 3800 examination reports.

5. Radiologic report management system

5.1. Radiology information system (RIS)

In the Kitasato University Hospital, it was difficult to retrieve database information on a real-time basis using a system in which general-purpose CPU was used for registration and retrieval of radiological reports (Sakurai et al., 1975). Furthermore, input information was restricted to the patient's basic information, information on the examination requested, and diagnostic code, and the efficiency of the system was low. To solve these problems, a database of radiological reports was constructed using a PC terminal as WS with LAN, and a RIS which would allow reference to past reports when making a diagnosis was developed. The system and our experience in the early stage have been reported (Murata et al., 1989). To enhance performance, the PC was changed from a Toshiba Pasopia 1600 microcomputer to a Toshiba workstation laptop J3100 and the CPU from a Toshiba Total-Ran/PB file server (130 Mbyte) to a DEC VAX system 3100 (400 Mbyte) (fig. 2). This new hardware was better able to respond to increases in the volume of diagnostic information and number of examinations caused by the increasing number of patients. The number of WSs was also increased from 4 to 5 units, vastly improving the system. There are two methods of input: direct input by a radiologist from the RIS terminal J3100 and a dictation system, by which data are tentatively recorded into a magnetic tape and are input from the terminal by a typist.

5.2. A communication between RIS and HIS

RIS information , which includes the patient's basic information, information on the examination performed, and the diagnostic code and keywords for reference, is transmitted to the HIS via an RS-232C interface, and requested report can be reviewed by any physician, at any time, from any of the 184 HIS terminals (Hitachi 2020 personal workstation). The host computer of the HIS is a Hitachi M 600 H which has a 23 Gbyte database. More than 800 users operate the system, resulting in 160 000 transactions a day with a maximum of 22 780 transactions per hour.

5.3. Integration of diagnostic information

Efficient confirmation of past radiologic reports is essential for the radiologist. While past reports can be read on the HIS terminal at present, not every examination room has a terminal. Even if there is a terminal, repeated development of the information needed may be required. Therefore, for CT, nuclear medicine, MRI and angiography examinations, previous radiology and pathology reports and past diagnoses are output in the evening on the day preceding examination. Then this summary file is beneficial for easy reference and image reading. By a method similar to the aforementioned one, one month after the radiologist has entered his report, the information is output from the HIS database and a copy is given to the radiologist who made the diagnosis. This enables the radiologist to review the results of his report without undue effort, making it easier to maintain a high work standard.

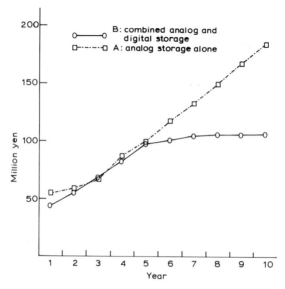

Fig. 3. The prospect of cost by means of analog and digital storages in the Kitasano University East Hospital. (A) The storage of analog images alone. (B) The combined storage of both analog and digital images. Inactive images, which are defined as being films not used for the past five years sequentially, reach 50% of all patients who visit the hospital. These 5-year-old inactive films are abandoned while all digital images and key films of analog images are continued to be stored on optical disk (OD) for reference because a few percent of the inactive patients possibly visit the hospital later. The cost for indivisual editing of retrieved images in the OD and the image worksta-tion for examination, investigation or teaching is included.

6. Image information management system

6.1. Image modality

Two special radiography units and conventional angiography are performed with the F/S system. All information from other units is digital in origin, about 88% of all radiological examinations are based on digital images. Among these examinations, the percentage of plain X-ray examinations is the highest, 66%, most of which (more than 95%) are taken by CR. The images selected as key films from images taken with the F/S system are digitized using a film digitizer and stored on optical disc (OD).

6.2. Image database

The recording medium for storage of images is an OD of 3.6 Gbyte. CR and CT images are stored by on-line transmission and MRI images are stored off-line. Nuclear medicine data are stored in a magnetic tape, but will be stored on-line in the future. Since 25 ODs can be built in an OD autochanger, information can be retrieved from image database totalling 90 Gbyte.

6.3. Image workstation (WS)

There are two CRT with a matrix of 1024×1536, and at most 24 images can be displayed on one CRT. There is one CRT for letter use. Image processing includes gradation processing, frequency processing, gray scale reversal, magnification and subtraction.

6.4. Characteristics of storage of images in OD

Images have been stored in 200 ODs during the past $4\frac{1}{2}$ years; CR and CT images and F/S images are stored on-line and by film digitizer, respectively. The difference between analog storage and on-line OD storage is that the cost of the former continues to increase linearly, while the cost of the latter has been gradually decreasing. Manpower and storage requirements are reduced with the latter system, although the initial expenditure is high. We compared the two systems in our hospital which is located on expensive urban land. One system used storage of actual analog images, the other one on-line storage on OD with the irreversible compression rate of 1 : 10. Digital storage was found to be lower in cost than analog storage after six years (fig. 3.).

7. PACS (image integration)

7.1. Independent double reading system (IDRS)

When radiographic procedures are performed with portable X-rays units, a referring physician wants to receive the films as soon as possible. Such images have been sent without reading by a radiologist to the referring physician because there was no system for emergency reading. Since radiological reports of the examinations that lack a reading by a radiologist are not included in the RIS database, the quality of the database is eventually decreased. To solve this problem, we developed a system (IDRS) which allows output of data stored in digital image form in the image WS from the image database following sending images to the referring physician, reading on the CRT by a radiologist, and communication between the radiologist and the physician by sending the report from the RIS to HIS (Kusano et al., 1991).

7.2. Hardware

The hardware consists of a magnetic card that starts the system, image WS, RIS

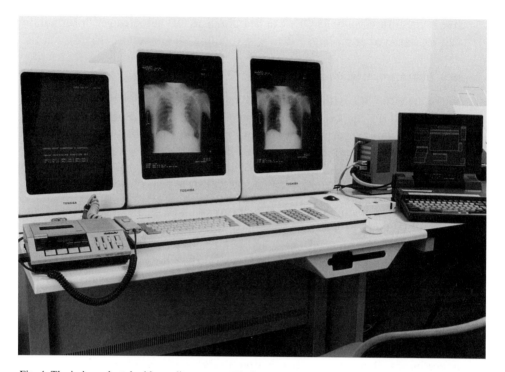

Fig. 4. The independent double reading system. The image display is seen at the left, while the RIS terminal is on the right.

terminal and a 'mouse' that operates the system (fig. 4). The system is placed in the reading room as well, and radiologists are able to read the images.

7.3. Software

The software, named CRT image-review support system (CRISS), is constructed of two major functions, preliminary work and reading as shown in fig. 5. Since reading takes place in a darkroom, reports are prepared by dictaphone. The data are then input by a typist, transported from the RIS to HIS, and viewed on the HIS terminal.

About 15 portable X-ray examination reports are read daily with this system at present. The rate of reading of plain X-ray examination reports by the radiologists increased markedly by the system. Because operation of the WS by the 'mouse' has been made easier than conventional keyboard operation, it can be handled easily, without special knowledge. This system is also less troublesome than the film jacket viewing system when comparing images. One problem is the limited recording capacity of a magnetic disk, 1600 Mbyte, another is that the system can only be used in the evening because the magnetic disk is used for archiving of CR and CT images in the daytime. Since the recording capacity of the OD autochanger is 90 Gbyte, the number of patients whose reports can be read is restricted when many examinations are performed on a particular patient in a short time. These problems, however, will be resolved soon because the irreversible compression at ratio of 1 : 10 for CR images begin in September, 1990.

8. PACS ten years from now

An ideal PACS is considered to be similar to the one described in a report by the Kansas University research group (Templeton et al., 1984). It is, however, difficult to obtain the ideal system immediately. Study of PACS has progressed by concentrating on partial aspects of the system rather than the total system at many institutes (Huang et al., 1990). Ten years from now, a major problem is how partial PACS will be integrated. This is because the more expanded the system becomes, the larger its social impact will be.

For radiologists, it is of major importance how well we use PACS to improve the quality of radiological examinations. The target of future study may be oriented to the clinical application of digital image database with PACS to suit clinical needs. For this purpose, systematic editing of individual image data will be required. Since our IDRS is limited to CR images, it may be regarded as be-

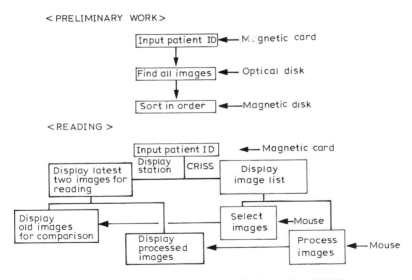

Fig. 5. Flow chart of the software in the display station (CRISS).

ing a modality PACS. We are now developing a system that allows editing of CT images and key film images of angiography necessary for interventional radiologic clinic for the outpatients. These are output from the images database by a method similar to that in IDRS and observed with the image WS.

Because storage space for analog images is limited, we are discussing abandoning this system in favor of digital management. In this case as well, individual editing of retrieved images is required, as in IDRS. We are discussing the development of a system in which digital images on the OD are re-edited on the disk individually by OD autochanger. They can be displayed and observed on the CRT when needed for examination, investigation or teaching, and hard copies can be output.

In conclusion, we spent most of the past five years constructing the digital image database essential for implementation of PACS. From our study on PACS and image archiving during that period, the target of the next five years of study will be oriented to the development of a system which enables the clinical application of the digital image database as needed in the clinical setting. How these systems will be integrated during the next ten years is a matter of utmost concern and interest. The development of such a system seems to depend on new technology enabling to cope with problems such as standardization of whole images, CRT performance as well as WS, communication speed, financial problems, and so on.

Acknowledgements

The authors wish to thank professor Sadayuki Miura (manager of Kitasato University East Hospital) and employees of Toshiba Inc. and Toshiba Medical Inc. for their help in developing the system.

References

Hall, D.J., G.S. Lodwick, R.P. Kruger, S.J. Dwyer and J.R. Townes (1971) Direct computer diagnosis of rheumatic heart disease, *Radiology* 101, 497–509.

Hashimoto, S., T. Matsubayashi, A. Shirai, A. Ogihara and Y. Yamada (1972) Radiology information system, *Image Technol. Inform. Display 4,* 43–50 (in Japanese).

Hounsfield, G.N. (1973) Computerized transverse axial scanning (tomography), Part I: Description of system, *Br. J. Radiol.* 46, 1016–1022.

Huang, H.K., H. Kangarloo, P.S. Cho, R. Taira, B.K. Ho and K.K. Chan (1990) Planning a total digital radiology department, *Am. J. Roentgenol.* 154, 635–639.

Kruger, R.A., C.A. Mistrella, T.L. Houk, S.T. Riederes, C.G. Shaw, M.M. Goodsitt, A.B. Crummy, W. Zwiebel, J.C. Lancaster, G.G. Rowe and D. Flemming (1979) Computerized fluoroscopy in real time for nonivasive visualization of the cardiovascular system, *Invest. Radiol.* 130, 49 – 57.

Kusano, S., Y. Okada, T. Endow, M. Kanai and H. Murayama (1991) Independent double reading system; Application of digital image management database, *Comput. Methods Programs Biomed.* 36, 113 – 117.

Murata, K., S. Kusano, M. Izutsu, N, Higuchi and H. Murayama (1989) Development and evaluation of a radiologic reporting system for use with a personal computer, *Med. Inform.* 14, 71 – 83.

Sakurai, K., T. Matsubayashi and S. Hashimoto (1975) Computer application in storage and retrieval of X-ray diagnostic information, *Nippon Acta Radiologica* 35, 430 – 438 (in Japanese, abstract in English).

Sonoda, M., M. Takano, J. Miyahara and H. Kato (1983) Computed radiography utilizing scanning laser stimulated luminescence, *Radiology* 148, 833 – 838.

Templeton, A.W., S.J. Dwyer III, J.A. Johnson, W.H. Anderson, K.S. Hensley, S.J. Rosenthal, K.R. Lee, D.F. Preston, S. Batnitzky and H.I. Price (1984) An on-line digital image management system, *Radiology* 152, 321 – 325.

Integrated Diagnostic Imaging
Editor: J.P.J. De Valk
© *Elsevier Science Publishers B.V., 1992*

Chapter 18

A practical system for patient care using PACS with emphasis on the evaluation of a CRT-based diagnostic system

Tomoho Maeda, Hitoshi Nishimoto, Masuyoshi Yachida, Shuichi Ohara, Masatoshi Nishioka, Yasuhiko Tohyama and Yasuhiro Kitazoe

1. Introduction

The concept of a picture archiving and communication system (PACS) has been introduced for the primary purpose of medical image management (Lehr, 1983). Alongside, one can think of a second purpose, i.e., to develop a new method of image analysis through image processing and subsequent display of the results, taking advantage of the digital character of the images and the application of a computer for image control (Blume et al., 1986; Taira et al., 1987; Honii et al., 1989; Lo, 1989).

Thereafter, the concept made a further evolution, owing to the employment of an CRT (cathode ray tube) display, for reading three-dimensional images (Rusinek et al., 1989; Levin et al., 1989; Ehricke, 1990) and dynamic images (Fujita et al., 1987; Lam et al., 1990; Maeda et al., 1990). In this way, medical images are now analyzed and read with three-dimensional and/or dynamic functions, giving an added-value to the image by the introduction of image processing technology. This could be considered as one of the effects produced by CRT diagnosis.

The author attempts to construct a PACS which would be more practical, more economical and clinically more valuable, from the stand point of a clinical doctor.

2. The CRT display device

In the PACS mechanism, the medical doctor has a direct relation with the CRT display, of which the performance is critical to the establishment of filmless radiology. Therefore, we hereby present a basic and clinical evaluation of the CRT display and, thereafter, explain the CRT diagnosis procedure which will offer added-value to the digital images.

2.1. Basic evaluation

2.1.1. CRT display device for image diagnosis

Figure 1 shows the scheme of the CRT diagnostic systems which are installed in the Radiology Department of Kochi Medical School Hospital. The 20 inches CRT display of the main device displays an image matrix of 1024×1536 portrait type. In the Toshiba system, images are displayed at a rate of 40 frames/s interlaced with a scarcely recognizable flicker.

Figure 2 shows the result of a precision study of this CRT by the employment of the SMPTE (Society for Motion Pictures and Television Engineers) pattern of a super high resolution image generator OPIX (made by Quantum Data).

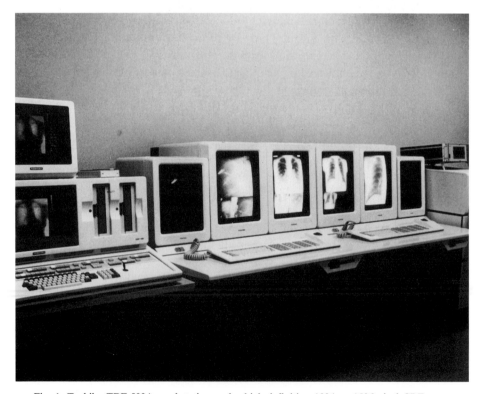

Fig. 1. Toshiba TDF-500A workstation and a high-definition 1024 × 1536 pixel CRT.

A sufficient resolution could be confirmed with 1024 × 1024 pixels. With a 65.4 kHz horizontal line frequency and an 80 Hz field frequency, the CRT proved to be a high-quality display device.

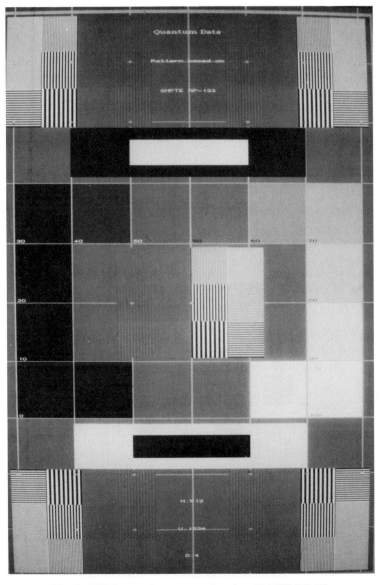

Fig. 2. CRT image of test pattern based on SMPTE RP-133.

2.1.2. An optimum display condition for CRT images: influence of room light

The brightness of the CRT is as low as 1/10 of that of a lightbox. Therefore, in the case of reading chest X-ray images which bear a large gray-level difference in one image, we need to make a prior evaluation of the room light influence on the CRT. Figure 3 shows the relationship between the CRT video signal level (%) and the relative brightness.

Under normal room light, the CRT does not produce the full contrast which it has under dim light, due to the reflection on the CRT, and such a delicate image recognition as that of a dark portion of a chest X-ray image might not be possible. In conclusion, the consultation room which requires normal room light would not be suitable for sophisticated image reading with detailed image processing.

Therefore, when a detailed disease status needs to be displayed by a combination of gray-scale manipulation and spatial frequency modulation, a suitable viewing environment, i.e., a dim light reading which is usually found in the radiology department, needs to be used (fig. 4).

2.1.3. Image processing on the CRT

We evaluated the influence of image processing on an X-ray image using a 15 mm acrylic resin Burger phantom.

(1) *Recognition performance in relation to a gray-scale processing.* By gray-

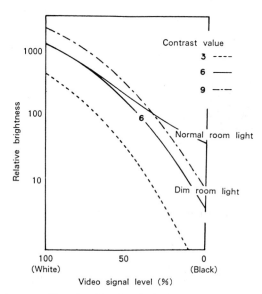

Fig. 3. Comparison between video signal level and relative brightness of CRT using SMPTE test pattern.

scale manipulation the recognition performance is increased on the CRT image compared with the original X-ray image, and by comparing the two images, one at a 200 μm and another at a 100 μm sampling pitch, the slight difference can be recognized (fig. 5).

(2) *Recognition performance improvement by black and white inversion.* A change of brightness by a change of the hole-depth in 7 mm diameter holes in a Burger phantom was measured using a brightness meter (MINOLTA LS -100). Figure 6 shows the negative and positive image result, which sug-

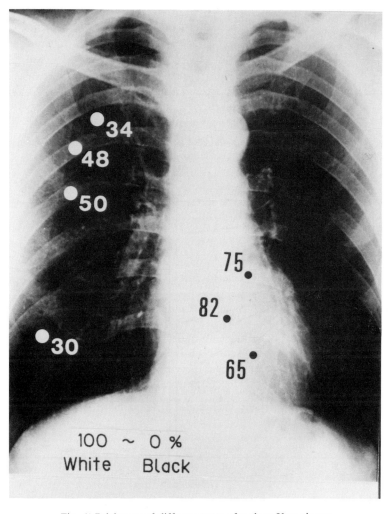

Fig. 4. Brightness of different parts of a chest X-ray image.

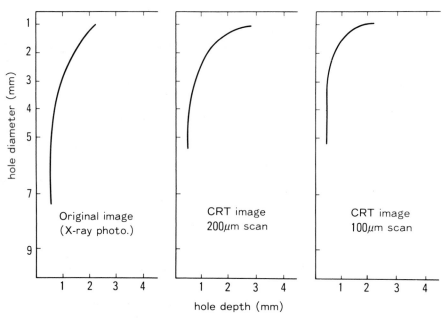

Fig. 5. Comparison between X-ray image and CRT image taken as 200 μm and 100 μm in sampling pitch size.

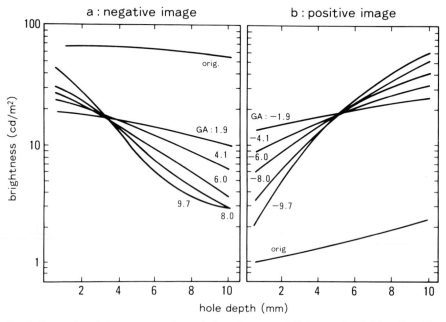

Fig. 6. Comparison between gray-scale gradation of gamma shift in negative (left) and positive (right) image.

gests that the less the hole-depth is, the easier the recognition is for the positive image.

(3) *Spatial resolution by the line chart.* Adding spatial frequency processings on top of the gray-scale processing, a slight improvement of the spatial resolution was witnessed.

In summary, there is a high number of studies on sampling pitch size and image quality. These studies seem to tell that a sampling pitch size of $100 - 200$ μm and a 1024×1024 matrix CRT are the optimum, which coincides with the conclusion of our study. There is a report which says that for mammography (Chan et al., 1990) and skeletal radiography (Merphey, 1989), a $40 - 50$ μm sampling pitch seems to be required and, therefore, that for mammography the conventional film image is still superior to the digital image.

2.2. Clinical evaluation

Plain X-ray images were digitized by a laser digitizer at a sampling pitch of 100 μm and 200 μm. Thereafter, image processing such as gray-scale manipulation and spatial frequency enhancement were performed to each of the 100 μm and 200 μm sampling pitch images. Then a comparison of the two images (100 μm, 200 μm) was made concerning a disease status in the chest image and a diagnosis in the knee joint image.

2.2.1. Influence of the sampling pitch size upon the image quality

Five cases of a chest tomography image showing a lung tumor shadow and five cases of a plain X-ray image showing pulmonary fibrosis were used.

For CRT images to which gray-scale manipulation was applied over the ROI (region of interest), there was no discrimination between the 100 μm and 200 μm sampling pitch sizes (table 1).

Table 1
Discrimination between 200 μm and 100 μm using five confidence levels.

	Pulmonary carcinoma		Pulmonary fibrosis	
Confidence level	200 μm	100 μm	200 μm	100 μm
5	2%	0	1	0
4	38	37	22	25
3	48	51	24	24
2	12	12	3	1
1	0	0	0	0
Average	3.30	3.42	3.42	3.48

However, when a spatial frequency processing was added on top of the gray-scale manipulation, using a reduced masking area and a larger enhancement, the difference of the two was conspicuous and a trivial noise was discovered on the 200 μm image (fig. 7).

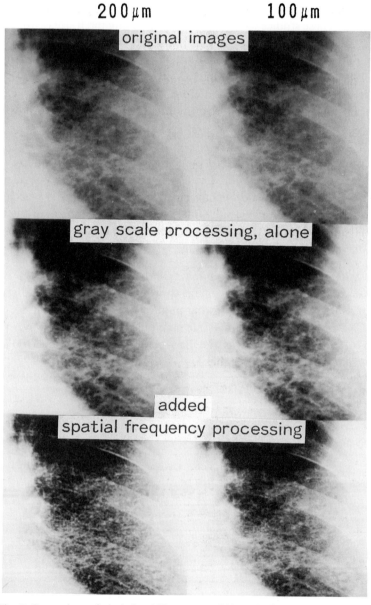

Fig. 7. Comparison of pixel size, 100 μm versus 200 μm (pulmonary fibrosis).

This illustrates the importance of the sampling pitch size at a magnification operation.

2.2.2. Obtaining a disease status with the chest X-ray image

The plain X-ray image and/or tomographic X-ray image were digitized using a He – Ne laser type film digitizer at a 200 μm sampling pitch and 10 bits gray level.

Then gray-scale manipulation and a spatial frequency processing were applied before viewing on the CRT for a comparison with the original image concerning the level of disease status recognition.

2.2.2.1. Tumor shadow.

Images with the following known diagnosis were used: sharpness/unsharpness of the tumor boundary, notch, spiculae, evenness/unevenness of the shadow inside the tumor as well as a cavity in the mass shadow, pleural indentation, compression image, air bronchogram and lymphangiosis.

Concerning many diagnostic findings, the CRT image and the (original) X-ray image showed almost equivalent display ability while the CRT image was superior in approximately 25% of the cases.

Above all, spiculae along a boundary of the mass shadow were better expressed in the CRT images and, in several cases, a change of a constricted bronchus in the tumor was also better recognized in the CRT images (fig. 8).

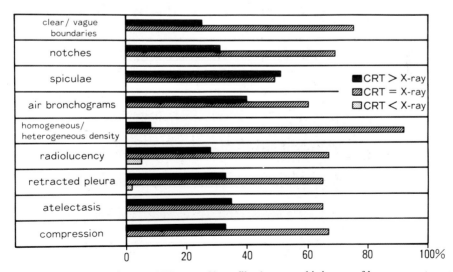

Fig. 8. Comparison of images, CRT versus X-ray film (tomographic images of lung cancer: tumor shadow).

2.2.2.2. Infiltration shadow. Diagnosis of air bronchograms, air alveolograms, unsharpness of the boundary and lesion fusion trends were used.

The originating diseases were 16 cases of pneumonia and 4 cases of pulmonary edema. Among these cases, air bronchograms and air alveolograms are better presented in CRT images employing gray-scale manipulation while a boundary unsharpness is sometimes better expressed in the X-ray image (fig. 9).

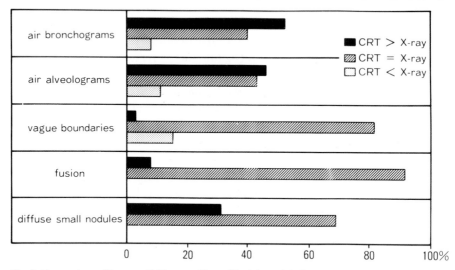

Fig. 9. Comparison of images, CRT versus X-ray film (chest plain images of inflammatory disease).

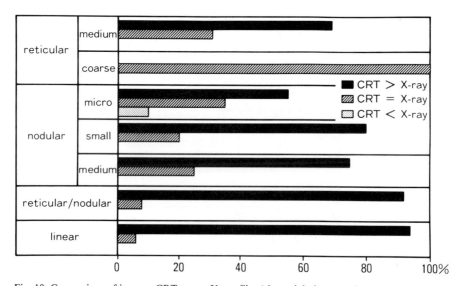

Fig. 10. Comparison of images, CRT versus X-ray film (chest plain images of pulmonary fibrosis).

2.2.2.3. Linear/reticular shadow. As to linear/reticular shadows which express interstitial changes, features can be more easily recognized through a proper gray-scale manipulation accompanied by spatial frequency processing.

Moreover, medium thick linear or reticular shadows are more easily recognized than large nodular shadows.

However, in some cases of micronodular shadows, better recognition was found for the X-ray film (fig. 10).

2.2.3. Knee joint X-ray image recognition
Twenty-two cases of knee joint images were read by five radiologists with three to nine years experience, using the three types of images described below. The plain X-ray film (original), a hard copy image printed after image processing and a CRT image displayed on the CRT were read applying image processing.

2.2.3.1. Visualized degree of bone trabeculae. Images were classified into three categories, i.e., (a) well visualized, (b) moderately visualized and (c) poorly visualized. For each case, the observers classified images into category (a) or (b) or (c). The result is shown in table 2. For original images, the percentage of 'well and moderately' is 53% and 44%, respectively, while with the CRT, the percentages are 81% and 16%. The result shows that with the CRT, there was a better recognition.

With images printed after image processing, their evaluation showed an inclination toward 'moderately and poorly' perhaps because of the frozen image processing, leaving a substantial difference with the other two images.

It also can be said that with the X-ray image, relevant exposure conditions decide the level of an easy recognition, while with the CRT, the displayed images can be changed to better recognizable ones as a result of the most suitable image processing.

Table 2
Comparison of three types of images, visualized degree of bone trabeculae in lateral radiograph of knee joint.

Visualized degree	Sorts of image		
	Plain X-ray image (%)	Post processed hard copy (%)	Gradation processing CRTs (%)
(a) well	53	9	81
(b) moderately	44	44	16
(c) poor	3	47	3

2.2.3.2. Recognition of periosteal reaction and detection of an arterial shadow in the soft tissue. ROC (receiver operating characteristic) analysis was performed in order to perform an objective evaluation of these three types of images, using images showing a periosteal reaction and an arterial shadow in the soft tissue (fig. 11). The periosteal reaction which consists of information in a relatively high-frequency area was best recognized on the CRT while the CRT is inferior in the detection of an arterial shadow in the soft tissue which is an information in a relatively low-frequency area. In this low-frequency area, DSA (digital subtraction angiography) is an advantageous method of diagnosis.

However, the bone X-ray image is meant for the recognition of a bone tissue change and, therefore, it can be duly said that the CRT image reading with the application of the relevant image processing is superior for obtaining a correct diagnosis of the bone.

Summarizing the above-mentioned, on a high-resolution CRT, we can obtain a satisfactory diagnosis more easily than on the X-ray film, if several suitable conditions for image reading are fulfilled. Such conditions are: an image reading environment in dim room light, and application of the image processing method which is the most suitable for the purpose.

3. A CRT diagnostic system which will support the diagnosis with value-added images

The human being is dynamic by its nature and the best way of image reading would therefore be dynamic image reading. However, the conventional viewing method (using the film-screen system) is a static image viewing of a fixed infor-

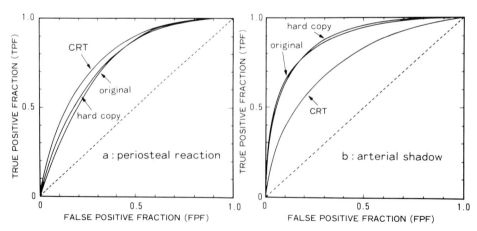

Fig. 11. ROC curves of periosteal reaction and arterial shadow in lateral view of knee joint.

mation volume. By digital imaging, however, using the CRT display as a viewing media, it became possible to view in real-time the result of image processing as well as to view three-dimensional images and dynamic images.

As to dynamic image viewing, high-speed recording and display are necessary. The current continuous X-ray exposure method and X-ray cine-filming methods, however, cannot be easily integrated into daily diagnosis.

In a PACS which handles digital information, it is currently difficult, because of technical and economical aspects, to support high-speed recording of a huge volume of image information. Therefore, we conceived a system in which dynamic images (e.g. movements of various joints of the body, the digestive organs, the heart and the lung etc.) are acquired through the I.I. (image intensifier) and of which the output will be A/D converted. The A/D converted output is stored on an optical disk at 30 frames/s for subsequent viewing on the CRT monitor. The system also enables an objective evaluation of the dynamic object through the employment of computerized measurements (fig. 12).

We called this system 'Hybrid PACS' which supports the management and diagnosis of dynamic images using both analogue and digital images (Maeda et al., 1990). The Hybrid PACS enables a dynamic image evaluation as an added-value.

If you perform 90 seconds of dynamic image filming with this Hybrid PACS, the radiation to the patient is approximately 6% of 90 seconds of X-ray cine-filming and equivalent to 6 general X-ray exposures. This could be considered as another aspect of the added-value. In consequence, the radiation can be dramatically reduced resulting in the same amount of information.

Currently, the system is mainly applied to cases of the orthopaedics area for

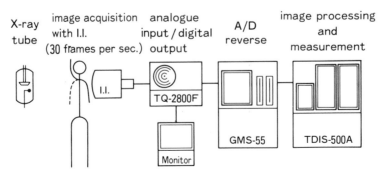

Fig. 12. System configuration of Hybrid-PACS.

an evaluation of 'early diagnosis of irregularities of joint movements by application of dynamic images'.

In comparison with a conventional diagnosis which uses static images, the new method of diagnosis by dynamic images carries a drastically increased information volume, enabling a conspicuous display of precise movements of the joint as well as a relation between the joint movement and related pain.

4. Basic concept of PACS in Kochi Medical School

In Kochi Medical School, a large-scale PACS is conceived for the possible application of medical images to education, research and medicare. Relevant research and development is in progress.

The image production volume of the radiology department is approximately 5.5 Gbytes daily (table 3).

Figure 13 shows the outline configuration of the Kochi Medical School experimental PACS where the Toshiba TDIS F-500 and GE-YMS CRT display unit are the major components.

The Toshiba TDIS F-500 is mainly used as a filing system for X-ray images obtained via imaging plate technology. It can also digitize and file a conventional X-ray image using a film digitizer attachment. With the Toshiba system, images produced on computed radiology (CR) are transmitted to the included optical disk (OD) after data compression. Thereafter, the images stored on the optical disk will be transmitted to a magnetic disk of the TDIS-file for a prompt retrieval by the console No. 1. Images stored in these image files will be transcribed into a file memory as frozen images, after image processing. Thereafter, images will be displayed under control of a lap-top personal computer contained in physicians view stations which are located in the outpatient

Table 3
Daily image volume in Kochi Medical School Hospital.

	Bits/image	No. of exposures	Bits
X-ray image	$2048 \times 2048 \times 12$	900	4.5×10^{10}
CT	$512 \times 512 \times 12$	800	2.5×10^{9}
RI static	$256 \times 256 \times 8$	10	0.3×10^{8}
dynamic	$64 \times 64 \times 8$	50	2.5×10^{6}
DF	$1024 \times 1024 \times 10$	600	0.6×10^{10}
MRI	$512 \times 512 \times 10$	500	1.6×10^{9}
Total	–	2860	5.5×10^{10}

Outpatient 650/day; numbers of beds 600.

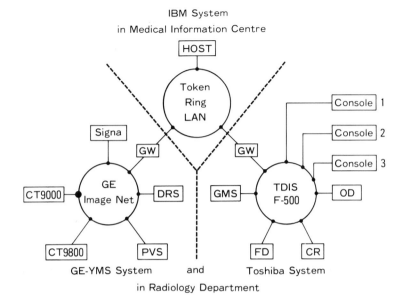

Fig. 13. Scheme of experimental study connecting GE-YMS System, Toshiba System and IBM System.

wards of the internal medicine (console No. 2) and orthopaedics (console No. 3).

With the GE system, images produced on the CT 9800 and 9000 are transmitted via GE image net to a diagnostic CRT (DRS) on which level and window processing can be done. Thereafter, the images will be transmitted to the physician review station (PRS) located in the outpatient ward of internal medicine for a practical clinical application.

Each operation mode maintains its own image database with which a primary image reading and subsequent erasure are performed. A benefit for the outpatient care is that an outpatient was formerly requested to visit the hospital twice, the first visit for an examination and the second visit for hearing the result. Now, the patient needs to visit the hospital only once and a treatment plan can be decided quickly.

Figure 14 shows a near future plan, where a workstation is being conceived which would integrate various operation modes by its functions of integrated image diagnosis, compilation of various images and producing value-added images. These images are transferred via a gateway to the database of the Medical Information Center as a compressed image or a frozen image for a later delivery to each outpatient department and ward where normal room light is usually used. Currently, the system is still under clinical evaluation. The development

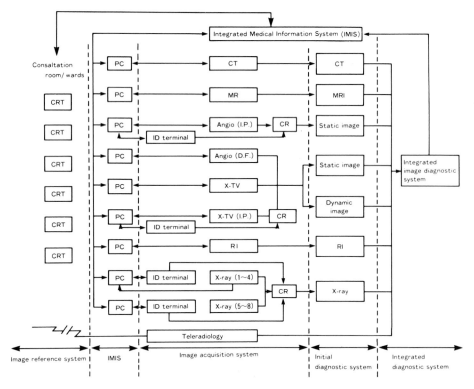

Fig. 14. Configuration of PACS in Department of Radiology with subsidiary connection to medical information centre, Kochi Medical School Hospital.

of the datalink is, however, finished, which will transmit images of these two systems into the IBM database (using DASD: direct access system device magnetic disc) located in the Medical Information Center through a gateway. These transmitted images are already frozen and complicated image processing is not necessary. These images can be promptly and easily retrieved and displayed on the IBM PS/55 terminals in the consultation room in the ward.

In the meantime, we have been evaluating teleradiology (Weber et al., 1973; Seeley et al., 1989; Batnitzky et al., 1990). The result of the evaluation tells that, by teleradiology, the spatial resolution of images may decrease but that the gray-scale resolution is scarcely affected. Considering these observations, teleradiology limited detailed diagnosis of chest X-ray images and bone X-ray images while a proper diagnosis of CT and MRI could be made without significantly affecting the image quality.

In an experimental study we are performing an image transmission between Kochi Medical School Hospital and 2 other hospitals located 40 km from Kochi

Medical School. Utilizing teleradiology, we recently experienced in three cases that a prompt operation was performed for a neurosurgery case which required an emergency treatment and in three other cases that timely and proper treatment were performed to patients of lung cancer who required a prompt radiation therapy and after treatment results show a favorable progress.

This teleradiology is included in 'Kochi Medical School PACS' (fig. 14), a development which is still in progress.

In recent years it appeared difficult to introduce computer equipment without economical effects. Above all, PACS still requires further research on its implementation even though PACS contributes much to medicine (Mun et al., 1988).

In this article, we explained our ideas, limiting the discussion to the CRT which has direct relations with medical doctors. It turned out that a construction of PACS as a value-added system is also important at a cost as low as possible. Various PACS (Saarinen et al., 1989; Arenson et al., 1990) which would meet the size and operation of various hospital categories are studied based on models. These models always need to go through a clinical evaluation (validation).

References

Arenson, R.L., et al. (1990) The digital imaging workstation, *Radiology* 176, 303 – 315.

Batnizky, S., et al. (1990) Teleradiology: an assessment, *Radiology* 177, 11 – 17.

Blume, H., et al. (1986) A versatile image processor for digital diagnostic imaging and its application in computed radiography. In: Schneider, R.H., and S.J. Dwyer II (Eds.), Medicine XIV/PACS IV, *Proc. SPIE.* 626, 314 – 324.

Chan, H.-P., et al. (1990) Improvement in radiologists' detection of clustered microcalcifications on mammograms: the potential of computer-aided diagnosis, *Invest. Radiol.* 25, 1102 – 1110.

Ehricke, H.-H. (1990) Problems and approached for tissue segmentation in 3D-MR imaging. In: *Proc. SPIE* 1233, 128 – 137.

Fujita, H., et al. (1987) Basic imaging properties of a large image intensifier/TV digital chest radiographic system, *Invest. Radiol.* 22, 328 – 335.

Honii, S.C., et al. (1989) Environmental designs for reading from imaging work stations: ergonomic and architectural features, *J. Digital Imag.* 2, 156 – 162.

Lam, K.L., et al. (1990) Dynamic digital subtraction evaluation of regional pulmonary ventilation with nonradioactive Xenon, *Invest. Radiol.* 25, 728 – 735.

Lehr, J.L. (1983) Impact of manual & computer assisted PACS for automated PACS. In: Dwyer III, S.J. (Ed.), Picture Archiving and Communication Systems (PACS) for Medical Applications, Second International Conference and Workshop, *Proc. SPIE* 418, 6 – 13.

Levin, D.N., et al. (1989) Surface of the brain: three-dimensional MR images created with volume rendering, *Radiology* 171, 277 – 280.

Lo, S.B. (1989) Development of pictorial directory workstation for rapid image presentation. In: Schneider, R.H., S.J. Dwyer III and R.G. Jost (Eds.), Medical Imaging III, *Proc. SPIE* 1091, (26).

Maeda, T., et al. (1990) Development of new method image diagnosis through Hybrid PACS — with a special concern to a dynamic image. In: Dwyer III, S.J., and R.G. Jost (Eds.), Medical Imaging IV: PACS System Design and Evaluation, *Proc. SPIE* 1234, 294–301.

Merphey, M.D. (1989) Digital skeletal radiography: spatial resolution requirements for detection of subperiosteal resorption, *Am. J. Roentgenol.* 152, 541–546.

Mun, S.K., et al. (1988) Cost analysis for the developing digital imaging network. In: Schneider, R.H., and S.J. Dwyer III (Eds.), Medical Imaging, *Proc. SPIE* 767.

Rusinek, H., et al. (1989) Three dimensional rendering of medical images: surface and volume approach. In: Schneider, R.H., S.J. Dwyer III and R.G. Jost (Eds.), Medical Imaging III, *Proc. SPIE* 1091 (26).

Saarinen, A.O., et al. (1989) Modeling of the economics of PACS: What is important? In: Schneider, R.H., S.J. Dwyer III and R.G. Jost (Eds.), Medical Imaging III: PACS System Design and Evaluation, *Proc. SPIE* 1093.

Seeley, G.W., et al. (1989) Evaluation of the De Pont teleradiology system. In: Schneider, R.H., S.J. Dwyer III and R.G. Jost (Eds.), Medical Imaging III: PACS System Design and Evaluation, *Proc. SPIE*, 1093, 106–108.

Taira, R.K., et al. (1987) Operational characteristics of paediatric radiology image display stations. In: Schneider, R.H., and S.J. Dwyer III (Eds.), Medical Imaging, *Proc. SPIE.* 767, 713–716.

Weber, M.M., et al. (1973) Telecommunication of image in the practice of diagnostic radiology, *Radiology* 109, 71–74.

Integrated Diagnostic Imaging
Editor: J.P.J. De Valk
© *Elsevier Science Publishers B.V., 1992*

Chapter 19

Present status of PACS in Kyoto University Hospital: trials carried out to put the system into clinical use

Yoshihisa Nakano, Masaru Komori, Kotaro Minato, Ishu Kimura, Kaoru Okajima, Junji Konishi and Kazuhiro Satoh

1. Introduction

Many trials have been performed to put the picture archiving and communication system (PACS) into clinical use (Mun et al., 1988; De Valk et al., 1988; Huang et al., 1990a). A survey in July, 1989, indicated that there are approximately 50 systems installed in Japan and about 30 installed or to be delivered in the United States and Europe (Huang et al., 1990b). However, PACS concept, although generally regarded as important, has not been well accepted in the radiology community.

PACS project named KIDS (Kyoto University Hospital image database and communicating system) began in spring, 1985. This project was set up to study the feasibility of integrating all digital imaging modalities currently in use at the hospital. On-line data acquisition, long-term archiving, the function of the image workstations, communication between devices and man – machine interface have been tested (Komori et al., 1987; Minato et al., 1988, 1989). In this chapter, we describe the present status of our PACS and the tests carried out to put the system into clinical use.

2. The first experimental system: old KIDS

The first goal was to link an X-ray scanner (GE CT/T 8800) and a magnetic resonance imaging (MRI) scanner (GE Signa) provided a central archiving system. The image workstation has three 20-inch black-and-white cathode-ray tube (CRT) screens with a resolution of 1024×1024 pixels. The optical disk library was a jukebox-style system consisting of 32 12-inch optical disks, each with a capacity of 2.6 Gbyte. A laser film printer was linked using a 10 Mbits/s

(Mbps) token ring optical fiber network. A general purpose interface bus (GPIB, IEEE 488 standard bus) was used between the scanners and the network interface unit. The system was completed in April, 1988.

Trials of primary diagnosis on CRT screens have met with little success. Radiologists agreed on the images of the CRT, but preferred conventional means; unfamiliarity with the system, the slow response of the imaging operation and the limited number of the CRT screens were among the reasons. After three years working with KIDS, we concluded that in order to study the feasibility of PACS even in a limited clinical environment, all clinical images would need to be on the CRT screen; i.e., all digital filmless imaging should be achieved.

3. System description of the current system: the new KIDS

The new KIDS has been implemented since mid-summer 1988 (fig. 1). The purpose of the project is to expand the old KIDS and to integrate several major digital imaging modalities. Digital subtraction angiography (Hitachi DFA-3) and computed radiography (Fuji CR101) are connected to the system in addition to already existing X-ray computed tomography (CT) and MRI. A film digitizer is also connected to the system. The new image workstation and the new 100 Mbps fiber optic local area network constitute two major technical improvements.

The storage device of the image database module increased to two 83.2 Gbyte

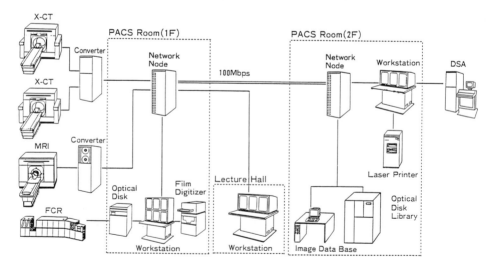

Fig. 1. Block diagram of the new KIDS.

optical disc libraries (ODLs). The image database is managed by a minicomputer (micro-VAXII). Messages such as a retrieval request from workstation to the minicomputer are transferred by low-speed RS-232C. Data on the optical disks are managed by the relational database system (RDB, DECs Rdb/VAX) in the minicomputer. The keys of the RDB are: patient ID, date of examination, type of modalities and volume name of platters. Retrieval can be carried out with any combination of these keys.

Figure 2 is a block diagram of the workstation. A 64 Mbyte RAM is used to increase the image handling speed. A 2 Mbyte image memory (1024 × 1024 pixels, 16 bit) is available for each CRT. The 1.2 Gbyte magnetic hard disk system is used for intermediate storage. The workstation can display 96 (256 × 256) images from screen to screen, setting images from different files side by side and making close-ups. It is controlled by a mouse and has various image processing capabilities such as intensity windowing, histogram equalization, three-dimensional displays and editing and retrieving.

The fiber optic local area network system (LAN) for PACS has been newly developed. The physical architecture of the 100 Mbps token ring is logically divided into eight high-speed (10 Mbps) lines and 121 low-speed telephone lines. The physical layer protocol for the high-speed lines is RS-422 with RS-232C control line. HDLC (high level data link control) protocol has been adopted for the datalink layer. Functionally, the LAN looks like a distributed PBX (private branch exchange) of the same speedlines. V. 25-bis is used for the high-speed network control for line switching. The logical architecture of the LAN, which has eight 'leased' lines for picture transmission and line switching, is suitable for connection among several imaging modalities, workstations and an optical disk library.

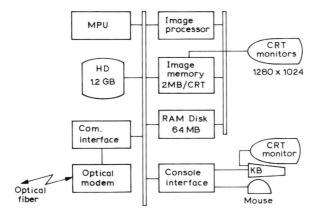

Fig. 2. Block diagram of the image workstation.

4. Current status of the system

Figure 1 is a diagram of the system. Optical disk libraries, a workstation with three CRT screens, and a control node (loop control station: LCS) for the network are installed in the database room. A laser film printer is attached to the workstation with six CRT screens and a remote network node (input – output station: IOS) are located in the reading room. A whole body X-ray scanner is connected to the IOS. A CR unit is linked to the workstation through an independent optical disk system. A film digitizer and another laser film printer are connected to the workstation.

Data acquisition from two CT scanners is continually operated. Data from other modalities are partially transferred. Conventional X-ray films from other hospitals are digitized by a film scanner. Since image data of the previous CT and MR stored on the magnetic tapes has been transferred to the optical disk library, the optical disk library has contained body CT image data for the last ten years and MRI data for the last five years. Table 1 shows the image data in the database.

Compared to conventional film and magnetic tape archiving systems, the advantages of using the on-line optical disk library are easy accessibility, automatic registration, space-saving and a complete resolution of the problem of lost films.

Table 1
Statistics of the image data stored in ODL[a].

	Body CT	Head CT	MR	CR	DSA
Number of					
patients	7.303	5.064	6.660	169	16
examinations	17.787	11.189	8.764	191	17
images	260.754	123.045	491.360	576	2.050
Amount of data (Gbyte)	53.4	25.2	64.4	3.2	2.9
Images per patients	36	24	74	3	181
Data per patients (Mbyte)	7.3	5.0	9.7	19	91
Images per examination	15	11	56	3	171
Data per examination (Mbyte)	3.0	2.3	7.3	5.6	86
Stored images in PACS	98%	25%	100%	< 1%	7%

[a] ODL: optical disk library; PACS: picture archiving and communication system; CT: computed tomography; MR: magnetic resonance imaging; CR: comupted radiography; DSA: digital subtraction angiography.

5. Problems in primary diagnosis using the image workstation

We have attempted primary diagnosis using the PACS image workstation. In comparison to the current film system, the ODL corresponds to the film library, the magnetic disk to film jackets of scheduled patients, and the RAM disk memory to the film viewing box or the alternator. Problems we encountered include the increased requirements for data storage, the speed of data transmission, and in particular its presentation. Out trial showed that the speed of the image presentation is critical for primary diagnosis in the PACS image workstation.

Current image workstations are able to show image data of less than 64 Mbyte instantaneously. However, when seeing image data of more than 64 Mbyte, such as DSA, the average data amount of which is 81 Mbyte, it is necessary to wait another 90 s for the other part of the image data to be loaded. During primary diagnosis, these images that are to be read should be transferred to the image memory for simultaneous viewing.

Figure 3 shows the amount of image data per patient. Sixty-four Mbyte image memory is not sufficient for patients who have already undergone many examinations, for whom digitized film images, or DSA images, already exist.

The decrease in the cost of DRAMS within a few years may solve this problem. However, recent developments in the quality of the digital modality image has resulted in an increased demand to PACS. For example, recent X-ray CT is 512×512 12 bit, and DSA is 1024×1024 10 bit, respectively. The image data will probably have to be decreased in order to control the image data.

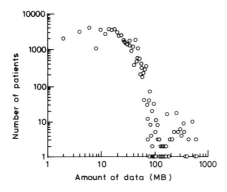

Fig. 3. Data amount of one patient.

6. PACS reporting system

Once images are reviewed, the radiologist can select key images for examination. Eliminating redundant information is important for PACS in terms of storage, display and communication. However, key images alone may be difficult for understanding the condition of the patient. We combined the personal computer with the PACS image workstation to link the key images with the report, the most effective way of image data compression.

Figure 4 is the block diagram of the reporting system. The report is filled out using a personal computer (NEC 9801) which is connected to the image workstation. Figure 5 shows the procedure of transfer of the report to the image workstation.

Prior to reading, images of the previous examinations are transferred from ODL to the image workstation. During the reading, the key images from the new and previous examinations are selected. Key images from the conventional films are also selected and digitized during the reading, and an image summary of key images of the patient is made. Reports are filled out and stored in the

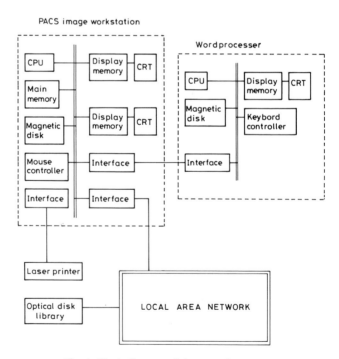

Fig. 4. Block diagram of the reporting system.

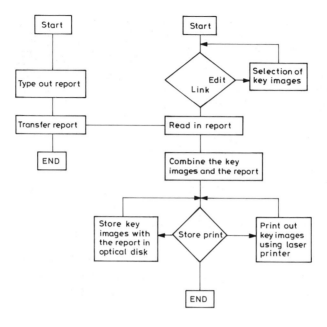

Fig. 5. Procedure of the reporting system.

personal computer. Then the report is transferred to the workstation to combine the key images with the report (fig. 6).

During the last eleven months, 20% of the CT reports were compiled in the personal computer by a word processor. However, only 3% of all cases were reports with image summaries, as the procedure is tedious and time-consuming. This procedure corresponds to $\frac{1}{10} - \frac{1}{100}$ data compression and helps both radiologist and the referring physician to obtain a general view of the image history of the patient.

At present, the procedure of compiling an image summary with the report is too time-consuming. We are now working on software which can create key images with the report with the lowest user-overhead. If information such as ID of the patient, date of examination and slice number of the key image is in the report, it will be possible to make key images with the report automatically, by transferring the information to the PACS image workstation.

The advantage of the PACS reporting system is that the system creates an image database for both teaching and research activity. By using the commercially available database software in a personal computer, key image can be found easily by searching the key words in reports, word by word.

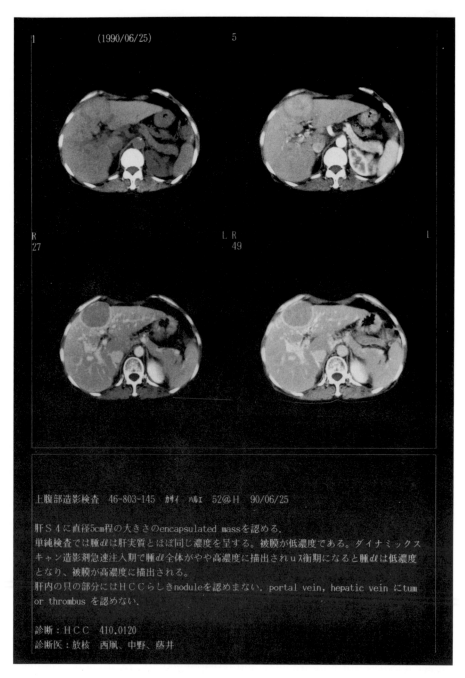

Fig. 6. Key images with the report printed out by the laser printer.

7. Current plan of the system

Demand to the department of radiology is to increase the number of CT and MR examinations because the waiting time for the examination is too long. In order to increase the number of the study, installation of the new scanner and people who operate the scanner, i.e., radiologist, technologist, nurse, etc. are necessary. Although the recent technical development decrease the cost of the scanner, the radiologist and trained technicians are not easily available. We are planning the new workstation where one radiologist or trained technician can control the two or three scanners. On-line real-time transfer of the image data from the scanner to the image workstation, image hard copy by the laserprinter and performance of the primary diagnosis will be necessary in the new PACS image workstation.

8. Conclusion

KIDS has all the basic components of a hospitalwide PACS and has been used for five years in clinical environments. Since the long-term archives of the image data and the increase in the number of image modalities cause the system to be overloaded, efforts should be made to reduce the image. Our current approach is to reduce image data by creating the image summary with the report using the PACS image workstation. Although the results obtained with the current system are limited, our approach is the most effective way of image data compression and it may enable us to expand KIDS to include all images in the hospital.

References

De Valk, J.P.J., F.P. Ottes, W.J.J. Stut et al. (1988) Background of the demonstrated IMAGIS activities and future expectations, *Med. Inform.* 13, 327–329.

Huang, H.K., H. Kangarloo, P.S. Cho et al. (1990a) Planning a total digital radiology department, *Am. J. Roentgenol.* 154, 635–639.

Huang, H.K., P.S. Cho, R.K. Taira, B.K. Ho and K.K. Chan (1990b) Picture archiving and communication systems in Japan: 3 years later, *Am. J. Roentgenol.* 154, 415–417.

Komori, M., K. Minato, Y. Nakano et al. (1987) Pilot PACS with on-line communication between an image workstation and CT scanners in a clinical environment. In: Schneider, R.H., and S.J. Dwyer III (Eds.), Medical Imaging, *Proc. SPIE* 767, 744–751.

Minato, K., M. Komori, Y. Nakano et al. (1988) Experience with a small scale all digital CT and MRI clinical service unit: present status of Kyoto University Hospital image database and communication system. In: Schneider, R.H., and S.J. Dwyer III (Eds.), Medical Imaging II, *Proc. SPIE* 914, 1356–1361.

Minato, K., M. Komori, Y. Nakano et al. (1989) PACS development at Kyoto University Hospital: toward integration of digital imaging modalities. In: Schneider, R.H., S.J. Dwyer III and R.G. Jost (Eds.), Medical Imaging III: PACS System Design and Evaluation, *Proc. SPIE* 1093, 20–23.

Mun, S.K., H.R. Benson, B. Lo et al. (1988) Development and technology assessment of a comprehensive image management and communication network, *Med. Inform.* 13, 349–359.

Subject index